Tin and Malignant Cell Growth

Editor
J. J. Zuckerman
Deceased
Professor
Department of Chemistry
University of Oklahoma
Norman, Oklahoma

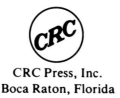

CRC Press, Inc.
Boca Raton, Florida

Library of Congress Cataloging-in-Publication Data

Tin and malignant cell growth/editor, J.J. Zuckerman.
    p. cm.
  Bibliography: p.
  Includes index.
  ISBN 0-8493-4714-9
  1. Organotin compounds--Testing.   2. Cancer--Chemotherapy-
-Evaluation.   3. Organotin compounds--Physiological effect.
I. Zuckerman, Jerry J.
RC271.O73T55 1988
616.99'407--dc19

This book represents information obtained from authentic and highly regarded sources. Reprinted material is quoted with permission, and sources are indicated. A wide variety of references are listed. Every reasonable effort has been made to give reliable data and information, but the author and the publisher cannot assume responsibility for the validity of all materials or for the consequences of their use.

All rights reserved. This book, or any parts thereof, may not be reproduced in any form without written consent from the publisher.

Direct all inquiries to CRC Press, Inc., 2000 Corporate Blvd., N.W., Boca Raton, Florida, 33431.

© 1988 by CRC Press, Inc.

International Standard Book Number 0-8493-4714-9

Library of Congress Card Number 87-36741
Printed in the United States

THE EDITOR

Dr. Jerold J. Zuckerman, George Lynn Cross Research Professor of Chemistry at the University of Oklahoma, died while on sabbatical leave at the University of Hawaii on December 4, 1987.

Professor Zuckerman was born in South Philadelphia on Leap Year Day in 1936. In 1957, he received a bachelor of science degree from the University of Pennsylvania, and in 1960 he obtained his first doctorate at Harvard University. Later, in 1962, Dr. Zuckerman completed a second Ph.D. at the University of Cambridge. During this time, he spent his summers in the research laboratories of Smith, Kline & French, Inc., (Philadelphia, PA, 1956), Houdry Process Corporation (Marcus Hook, PA, 1957) and at the M.I.T. Lincoln Laboratories (Lexington, MA, 1958). He held scholarships and fellowships from the Philadelphia Board of Education, the University of Pennsylvania, the U.S. Public Health Service, and the National Science Foundation.

In the same year that he received his second Ph.D., Professor Zuckerman began his academic career at Cornell University. In 1968, he accepted the position as Director of Research at State University of New York (SUNY) at Albany. While at SUNY, he presided over the Board of Trustees of the Brunswick Common School District for Rensselaer County, New York.

In 1973, he was a Senior Fellow of the Alexander von Humboldt Foundation and Visiting Professor at the Technical University of Berlin, Germany. In 1976, Dr. Zuckerman was awarded an Sc.D. degree from the University of Cambridge and also accepted the chair position at the University of Oklahoma at which he served until 1980. He was Professeur Associe at the Universite d'Aix-Marseille III in 1979 and 1982, and was awarded a doctorate *honoris causa* from that institution in 1982. He was elected a Fellow of the American Association of the Advancement of Science in 1981 and was made George Lynn Cross Research Professor at the University of Oklahoma in 1984.

Professor Zuckerman authored more than 200 scientific articles, numerous reviews, and was regional editor of *Inorganic and Nuclear Chemistry Letters*. He also co-edited the multi-volume *Determination of Organic Structures by Physical Methods,* and prepared with F. C. Nachod the English translation of R. Steudel's *The Chemistry of the Non-Metals.* In 1976, he completed the article "Molecular Structure" for the 15th edition of *Encyclopedia Britannica,* and co-authored with I. Haiduc of the Babes-Bolyai University, Cluj-Napoca, Romania, the textbook *Basic Organometallic Chemistry* (William de Gruyter, 1985). At the time of his death, Dr. Zuckerman was in the midst of editing the 18-volume *Inorganic Reactions and Methods*, which surely would have been his greatest editorial accomplishment.

He organized the 1970 Organosilicon-Award Symposium at SUNY-Albany and a Symposium on Organotin Compounds at the New York City Centennial ACS Meeting, Chaired the Mossbauer Effect Methodology Symposium at the 1973 American Physical Society Meeting, the National Research Council Panel on Mossbauer Spectroscopy, the Committee on Nominations and Symposia Planning of the ACS Division of Inorganic Chemistry, and was the Division's 1976 Program Chairman. He organized the Karcher Symposia on Energy and the Chemical Sciences, on the Structural Aspects of Homogeneous, Heterogeneous and Biological Catalysis and on the Origin and Chemistry of Petroleum in 1977 to 1979 at the University of Oklahoma, and co-edited with S. D. Christian, G. L. Guggenberger, and G. Atkinson the resulting books. He co-founded and co-chaired, with K. M. Nicholas, the Southwest Organometallic Chemistry Workshops held annually the last weekend in May in Norman. He also served on the scientific committee for the first three International Symposium on the Relationship of Tin Upon Malignant Cell Growth.

Professor Zuckerman's research interests were directed toward organometallic chemistry of the fourth-group elements and their compounds. His particular interest was with tin-containing compounds and their possible medicinal and industrial applications. Spectroscopic and structural methods, tin-119m Mossbauer spectroscopy, were his foremost specialty so he was considered an expert in the field. His research was supported by numerous institutions including the National Institutes of Health (NIH), National Cancer Institute, National Science Foundation (NSF), Office of Naval Research, and North Atlantic Treaty Organization (NATO), to name a few.

Dr. Zuckerman's lists of academic and literary accomplishments are as impressive as they are extensive. In nearly 30 years of chemistry, Professor Zuckerman managed to do more than the average chemist and for good reason — he was much above average in his profession. His over 200 speaking invitations and numerous consulting trips are just another indication of his ability. It was Dr. Zuckerman's ambition and desire for knowledge both in and out of chemistry that was the driving force behind his immense success. He had a powerful addiction to learning and forward progress; his intensity in his projects and endeavors was surpassed by few. The list of accomplishments Zuckerman had amassed is a feat in itself and is further complimented when the short time is considered. He had a dedication to his profession, college, group, and foremost to his family. He always prided himself by, " . . . never saying no because it is easier that way." Obviously, a thought worth noting.

Professor Zuckerman has left science with knowledge and advancement that will not be forgotten. He managed to instill his confidence into those with whom he had contact. It is always a tragedy to lose a person of such value and stature, but what Dr. Zuckerman has contributed will be used to build further the foundation of science. Dr. Zuckerman was a class "A" man with a class "A" act that should be a model for many to follow.

Larry R. Sherman
Chemistry Department
The University of Akron

CONTRIBUTORS

M. M. Amini
Department of Chemistry
College of Science
University of Notre Dame
Notre Dame, Indiana

Yasuaki Arakawa
Visiting Professor
Department of Anesthesiology
University of Utah School of Medicine
Salt Lake City, Utah

K. R. Simon Ascher
Head
Department of Toxicology
ARO, The Volcani Center
Bet Dagan, Israel

S. B. Bhonde
Junior Assistant
Department of Entomology
National Chemical Laboratory
Pune, Maharashtra, India

Nathan F. Cardarelli
Professor
Engineering and Science Division
University of Akron
Akron, Ohio

Ludo De Clercq
Chemical Engineer
Free University of Brussels V.U.B.
Brussels, Belgium

Marcel Gielen
Professor of Chemistry
Department of General and Chemistry
Free University of Brussels V.U.B.
Brussels, Belgium

Friedo Huber
Professor of Inorganic Chemistry
Department of Chemistry
University of Dortmund
Dortmund, West Germany

Eddie Joosen
Engineer in Chemistry and Agronomy
Department of General and Organic
  Chemistry
Free University of Brussels V.U.B.
Brussels, Belgium

Hans Jörnvall
Professor
Department of Physiological Chemistry
Karolinska Institute
Stockholm, Sweden

Attallah Kappas
Fairchild Professor and Physician-in-Chief
Department of Metabolism—Pharmacology
The Rockefeller University Hospital
New York, New York

Baldwin King
Professor and Chair of Chemistry
Department of Chemistry
Drew University
Madison, New Jersey

Thomas P. Lockhart
Consultant
Eniricerche S.P.A.
Milan, Italy

Afework A. Mascio
Associate Professor and Chairman
Department of Biological Sciences
Drew University
Madison, New Jersey

Grant Mauk
Associate Professor
Department of Biochemistry
University of British Columbia
Vancouver, British Columbia, Canada

Christine E. McDermott
Assistant Professor
Department of Biology
University of Scranton
Scranton, Pennsylvania

Jacov Meisner
Researcher
Department of Toxicology
ARO, The Volcani Center
Bet Dagan, Israel

D. Amy Montelius
Graduate Student (Ph.D. Program)
Department of Toxicology and Pharmacology
University of Connecticut
Storrs, Connecticut

Ven L. Narayanan
Chief, Drug Synthesis and Chemistry Branch
National Cancer Institute
Health and Human Services
National Institutes of Health
Bethesda, Maryland

Mohamed Nasr
Acting Head
Surveillance, Reports, and Inquiries Section
Developmental Therapeutics Branch,
 AIDS Program
National Institute of Allergy and
 Infectious Diseases
Health and Human Services
National Institutes of Health
Bethesda, Maryland

Paul E. Neumann
Research Chemist
Department of Research
Kellogg Company
Battle Creek, Michigan

Kenneth D. Paull
Acting Deputy Branch Chief
Information Technology Branch
National Cancer Institute
Health and Human Services
National Institutes of Health
Bethesda, Maryland

Robert C. Poller
Department of Chemistry
King's College, Kensington
London, England

Robert Reichhart
Professor
Department of Biochemistry
University of the Saarlands
Saarbrücken, West Germany

A. L. Rheingold
Department of Chemistry
University of Delaware
Newark, Delaware

Daniel W. Rosenberg
Assistant Professor
Department of Metabolism—Pharmacology
The Rockerfeller University Hospital
New York, New York

Anil Kumar Saxena
Doctor
Department of Chemistry
University of Dortmund
Dortmund, West Germany

Ravindranath N. Sharma
Head, Scientist-in-Charge
Department of Entomology
National Chemical Laboratory
Pune, Maharashtra, India

Kevin R. Siebenlist
Assistant Professor and Scientist
Hemostasis Research
Department of Medicine
University of Wisconsin
Milwaukee, Wisconsin

Fumito C. Taketa
Professor and Vice Chairman
Department of Biochemistry
Medical College of Wisconsin
Milwaukee, Wisconsin

Vrushali Tare
Senior Scientific Assistant
Department of Entomology
National Chemical Laboratory
Pune, Maharashtra, India

R. W. Taylor
Department of Chemistry
University of Oklahoma
Norman, Oklahoma

Osamu Wada
Professor
Faculty of Medicine
Department of Hygiene and Preventive
  Medicine
University of Tokyo
Hongo, Tokyo, Japan

Rudolph Willem
Assistant
Department of General and Organic
  Chemistry
Free University of Brussels V.U.B.
Brussels, Belgium

Michael Zeppezauer
Professor
Department of Biochemistry
University of the Saarlands
Saarbrücken, West Germany

M. R. Zimmerman
Professor
Department of Pathology and Laboratory
  Medicine
Hahnemann University
Philadelphia, Pennsylvania

J. J. Zuckerman
Deceased
Professor
Department of Chemistry
University of Oklahoma
Norman, Oklahoma

TABLE OF CONTENTS

Chapter 1
Tin as a Vital Nutrient: Environmental Ubiquity...1
Nate F. Cardarelli

Chapter 2
The Scarcity of Tumors in Antiquity..29
Michael R. Zimmerman

Chapter 3
The Importance of Hydrogen Bonding of Organotins in Water... 33
M. M. Amini, R. W. Taylor, J. J. Zuckerman, and A. L. Rheingold

Chapter 4
New Developments in Antitumor-Active Organotin Compounds.......................39
Marcel Gielen, Ludo De Clercq, Rudolph Willem, and Eddie Joosen

Chapter 5
Synthesis and Characterization of Organotin Steroids 47
Anil Saxena and Friedo Huber

Chapter 6
Tin Steroids as Anticancer Agents...53
Nate F. Cardarelli

Chapter 7
Chemistry and Biology of Organotin Derivatives of Carbohydrates 59
Robert C. Poller

Chapter 8
Application of Solid State NMR to Problems in Structural Organotin Chemistry... 73
Thomas P. Lockhart

Chapter 9
Suppression of Cell Proliferation by Certain Organotin Compounds... 83
Yasuaki Arakawa and Osamu Wada

Chapter 10
Interaction of Triethyltin Bromide with Cat Hemoglobin... 107
F. Taketa, K. R. Siebenlist, and A. G. Mauk

Chapter 11
Triethyltin Bromide and Protein Phosphorylation in Subcellular Fractions from Rat and Rabbit Brain..117
F. Taketa and P. E. Neumann

Chapter 12
Toxicological Properties of Organic Derivatives of Tin: Production of Marked Alterations of Hepatic and Extra-Hepatic Heme Metabolism.......................125
Daniel W. Rosenberg and Attallah Kappas

Chapter 13
The Immune Functions of the Thymus and Their Alteration by Toxic Chemicals and
Radius... 137
Christine E. McDermott

Chapter 14
Homeostatic Thymic Hormone: Chemical Properties and Biological Action... 155
M. Zeppezauer, R. Reichhart, and H. Jörnvall

Chapter 15
Refinement and Evaluation of the Crown-Gall Tumor Disc Bioassay as a Primary Screen
for Diorganotin Compounds with Antitumor Activity...................................171
A. A. Mascio, A. D. Montelius, and A. King

Chapter 16
Organotins as Insect Chemosterilants... 179
K. R. S. Ascher and J. Meisner

Chapter 17
Bioactivity of Some Organotin Compounds on Insects..................................201
Rn. N. Sharma, Vrushali Tare, and S. B. Bhonde

Chapter 18
Computer-Assisted Structure—Anticancer Activity Correlations of Organotin
Compounds... 211
Mohamed Nasr, Kenneth D. Paull, and V. L. Narayanan

Index... 227

Chapter 1

TIN AS A VITAL NUTRIENT: ENVIRONMENTAL UBIQUITY

Nate F. Cardarelli

TABLE OF CONTENTS

I.	Introduction	2
II.	Background	2
III.	Tin in the Geosphere	3
	A. Meteoritic Tin	4
	B. Tin Ores	4
	C. Soil Tin	5
IV.	Tin in The Hydrosphere	6
V.	Atmospheric Tin	7
VI.	The Problem of Environmental Contamination	7
VII.	Analytical Procedures	8
VIII.	Tin in the Biosphere	9
	A. Fossil Fuels and Sediments	9
	B. Marine Plants	9
	C. Land Plants	9
	D. Tin in Food Plants	10
IX.	Is Tin Essential for Plant Growth?	12
X.	Tin in Animal Tissue	13
	A. Marine Animals	13
	B. Tin in Terrestrial Animals	13
XI.	Tin in the Human Body	15
	A. Tin in Milk	17
	B. Tin in the Human Lymphatic System	18
XII.	Discussion and Conclusion	18
	References	19

I. INTRODUCTION

A vital nutrient is defined as an element or compound essential to the life processes of a given species. When present in the appropriate chemical form and in the proper concentration, health and well-being are promoted. In contrast, an insufficient amount is detrimental to health, and if the lack is severe, death often ensues. One class of vital nutrients is the trace metals. Iron, copper, cobalt, manganese, magnesium, nickel, zinc, chromium, and molybdenum are considered essential to man. Deficiency diseases arise from either lack of quantity or the inability of the body to properly utilize the substance. A number of severe pathological conditions are known to arise from lack of iron, copper, and zinc in the human body.[1] The role of trace metals in animal and plant nutrition has been described elsewhere.[2,3]

The criterion for recognition of a given trace metal is based upon the results of deprivation. When intake is insufficient, a dramatic impairment of physiological function is observed. An organism isolated from access to the trace metal will display such impairment once body reserves are depleted. The symptomatology is reversible upon adding the element to the diet, with the provision that such addition occurs prior to the point where a vital process has not been completely disrupted.

Certain characteristics distinguish a vital trace metal. It obviously cannot be toxic at use levels. It must be readily available to the organism. This report focuses on the latter. Physiological usage of any trace metal leads to its excretion as a metabolic by-product. Thus, there is a continual, although usually very slow, drop in whole-body concentration. Consequently, the organism relies upon a continual intake of trace metals to replace such losses and maintain homeostasis (the tendency for stability in the body's internal environment).

In fetal life the developing organism relies upon the mother's trace metal supply. Inadequacies of such supply can lead to severe and permanent damage. For instance, lack of iodine in the human mother results in cretinism in the offspring. After parturition, the young rely on receiving trace metals through the mother's milk, at least in the very early stages of life. After weaning, the infant receives nourishment from various environmental sources. Foodstuffs and/or water must contain an adequate supply. Trace metals enter the body from edible vegetation and animal food sources for the most part, although water intake can also serve as an important source. Inadequacies in the quantity of trace metal intake lead to a deficiency in the consuming organism. Consequently, the general health of a given population will depend upon environmental availability of a given trace metal. The vital nutrient must be ubiquitous in nature and able to enter the food chain readily.

The thesis advanced here (and elsewhere[4]) is that tin is a vital trace nutrient. This report is keyed to providing evidence of the ubiquity of tin in the human environment. It is meant to both extend and compliment several earlier reports.[4,5]

II. BACKGROUND

Schwarz et al. reported in 1970 that rats deprived of dietary tin showed extremely poor growth, hair loss, seborrhea (excess secretion of oily fluids by the skin), toxicity, and a distinct lack of enery.[6] Symptomatology was in evidence within 1 to 2 weeks. The syndrome was reversed when tin, in organic or inorganic form, was added to the diet. A growth enhancement as high as 53% was noted with 2 ppm of tin (IV) sulfate in the diet. The claim was then put forward that tin is a vital trace nutrient, at least in rats.[6,7] It was further stated that the coordination chemistry of tin made it possible for this element to contribute to the tertiary structure of proteins and nucleic acid and to function at the active site of metalloenzymes.[8] This work has never been confirmed, although others have cited it, usually stating that tin is an essential nutrient of unknown function.[2,3,9]

Analysis of mouse tissue indicated that the thymus gland was the primary repository for tin.[10] In experimental studies using first ^{14}C labeled organotin and later with ^{113}Sn, it was observed that exogenous tin accumulates in the thymus and after a short dwelling time moves into lymphatic circulation.[4,5,11] The propensity of the thymus to accumulate tin has been noted by others.[12-15]

In 1972 Brown reported that triphenyltin acetate shows antitumor activity in mice.[16] From 1980 to the present a number of authors have noted that a wide range of tin compounds displays some degree of antitumor activity.[17-22] A time profile study of ^{113}Sn in various mice strains indicated that tin accumulated in the thymus gland of the noncancer prone cesarean-originated, barrier-sustained (COBS)s outbred albino mice, originally germ-free (supplied by the Charles River Breeding Laboratories, Wilmington, Ma.) outbred mice while by-passing the thymus of the two cancer-prone strains examined.[4,5,23] Thus a tin-thymus-anticancer axis appeared to exist. In a tentative hypothesis advanced by the author, this axis was linked to the vital trace-element zinc and the aging process.[4] Based upon this hypothesis and the known existence of an antiproliferative thymic steroid hormone, a series of tin steroids was synthesized.[4,24] Tests against mouse adenocarcinoma in vivo, P-388 mouse leukemia in vitro, and human KB epidermoid tumor in vitro showed a high degree of anticancer activity without gross toxicity when administered orally.[25]

The tin-thymus linkage can be illustrated by noting that the symptoms of tin deprivation are quite similar to the results of neonatal thymectomy (surgical removal of the thymus) in rats.[4]

The author thus hypothesizes that tin serves a vital function in the organisms defense against oncogenesis and that this factor is generated by the thymus gland and possibly other elements of the immune system. This report serves as an initial step in offering evidence that tin is an ubiquitous element thus meeting one of the prime requisites for a vital trace metal.

III. TIN IN THE GEOSPHERE

The analytical determination of tin in most environmental compartments is subject to two challenges — the sensitivity and accuracy of the methods used, and the inescapable fact that man has disseminated tin from mining focii over large areas of the world. Consequently, the thesis advanced that tin is ubiquitous must reasonably consider these factors.

Tin has been mined since prehistoric times. Early Bronze Age man processed both stream tin and vein ores in a number of near-eastern locales. Possibly the ancient mines of the Caucasian Mountains were the earliest. Tin from Cornwall entered the Mediterranean trade prior to the Roman era. During Roman times, mines in Cornwall, Spain, and Brittany were active. Probably millions of tons of tin were extracted from the major ones in Spain over the period 500 B.C. to 250 A.D. under Roman exploitation.[26] The major usages were the manufacture of bronze and pewter. Tin artifacts flowed readily through the channels of commerce which extended not only throughout the empire, but beyond to India, central Africa, and barbarian northern Europe. The widespread usage of the "tin can" in the later years of the 19th century, and the advent of organotin stabilizers for plastics and pesticides in the 20th, led to further diffusion of the element. Certain components of the environment would, of course, show greater contamination than others. Rock and volcanic and meteoritic tin could be presumed to be of natural occurrence and not subject to artifactural input. Deep sediments, isolated land and water areas, and the contents of environmental isolates, such as entombed objects sealed prior to about 2000 B.C. and the like, ought to show a relatively slight degree of contamination. Values for soil tin from agricultural areas would add less credence to the thesis than data from areas never farmed. The values found for atmospheric tin content probably have little relevance to this subject.

A. Meteoritic Tin

The cosmic abundance of tin has been estimated at 1.33 to 4.22 atoms per 10^6 atoms of silicon.[27] The analysis of meteors for tin content seems to be of relatively recent practice.[28-30] Using the dithiol method, Winchester and Aten determined the tin content in eight iron meteorites.[29] Values ranged from 20.2 to less than 0.8 ppm, with a weighted average of 6.7 ppm. In 1957, Onishi and Sandell published meteorite tin concentrations as high as 1600 ppm.[30] More recently, DeLaeter and Jeffrey, using the isotope dilution method (mass spectrometry), detected 0.1 to 7.6 ppm tin in 20 different iron meteorites, 0.1 to 0.2 ppm in stony-iron types, and <0.1 to 9 ppm in chondrites.[31] Hamaguchi and Kuroda reported in 1978 the following:[32]

- Iron meteorites — 0—20 ppm (2 of 56 specimens had 0 tin)
- Stony iron meteorites — <1—0.8 ppm (10 specimens)
- Chondrites — 0.02—2.4 ppm (47 specimens)
- Tektites — 0.77—0.95 ppm (3 specimens)
- Lunar rocks — 0.19—1.2ppm
- Lunar soil — 0.7 ppm

Cosmic materials obviously would not have an "exogenous" tin input, although one could argue contamination arising from the conditions of handling, storage, and analysis.

B. Tin Ores

There are a relatively small number of minerals known to contain tin in any appreciable quantity. Hamaguchi and Kuroda list 25 such minerals.[33] The major tin ore is cassiterite, SnO. Others are Berndtite, SnS_2; Nordenskioldite, $CaSn(8O_3)_2$; Pabstite, $BaSn(Si_3O_9)$; Stokesite, $CaSn(Si_3O_9) \cdot 2H_2O$; Stannite, Cu_2FeSnS_4; Kusterite, $Cu_2(Zn_{0.77}Fe_{0.23})SnS_4$; Herzenbergite, SnS; Teallite, $PbSnS_2$; and Colusite, $Cu_{12}(As,Sn,V)_4S_{13}$.[34]

There are tin mining areas in Malaya, Thailand, China, Australia, and Bolivia.

Commercial tin ores were found in the Bauchi plateau of Nigeria in 1885 and mining operations commenced in 1906,[35] with production from 1 ton in 1906 to over 10,000 tons per annum in the 1940s. Usable tin ores have been found in California, although in most locales rock content is less than 5 ppm.[36] Fairly high lodes were noted in Plumas and Trinity Counties in 1884,[37] and were mined in Riverside County in 1897.[38,39] Discoveries were also made in San Diego County[40] and other areas.[41] Tin ores have been found in North and South Carolina,[42,43] Virginia,[44] Idaho,[45] in the Black Hills of South Dakota,[46,47] New Mexico,[48] and Washington State[49] prior to 1940. The loss of foreign tin sources during World War II gave impetus to further U.S. exploration. Tin deposits were found in the mountains of New Mexico,[50] Nevada,[51,52] and Oregon.[53] Harrison and Allen noted that wet-chemical methods were inadequate to measure tin in rocks, whereas spectrochemical analysis disclosed tin contents in Oregon rocks as high as 0.005%.[53]

Stream tin was noted in Alaska as early as 1908[54-56] and was commercially mined.[57,58] In Canada, tin lodes were found in Ontario and Manitoba,[59] Nova Scotia,[60,61] and British Columbia.[62] Tin has been discovered in Mexico[63] and in Finland, Germany, and France.[64]

The purpose of this report is not to provide a comprehensive guide to tin deposits, but rather to note that they are indeed widespread. In general, when man has sought tin, he has found it, although usually in concentrations of much less than 1000 ppm and thus not commercially viable.

Trace metal analyses have been performed on various rock types around the world. Most of the earlier studies relied on wet chemical methods or spectroscopy. The former lacked sensitivity below about 100 ppm and the latter below about 5 ppm.[65,66] It is generally recognized that small amounts of tin are present in most rock classifications.[67-69] Table 1 provides a representative sampling of the tin content in rock.

Table 1
TIN CONTENT OF ROCK

Rock type	Location of sampling	Tin conc (ppm)	Ref.
Igneous (general)	—	2.49	70
		<5—440	30
		2.0—2.5	70
Silicic (general)	—	3.9—4.0	31
	Colorado, Ireland, Rhode Island	1.3—4.3	71
	Finland	3.8	72
Carbonatites	Uganda, Zaire	<5	66
Limestone	Uganda, Zaire	5—10	66
Shale (general)	—	3.5—4.2	70
Granites	—	3	30
	—	1.5	73
	Cornwall	15—45	74
Sandstone		0.1—1.0	70
		1.6	73
Sedimentary (general)		0—80	30
Adamellite	Cornwall	15—45	74
Oliverian magma	New Hampshire	100	75
Olivine basalts	Ireland	5—20	76
Basaltic	Hawaii	0.92—3.5	71
	—	1.5	30
Gneissen	Various in mining areas	800—8000	30
Ultramafic	—	0.5	30
	—	0.6—0.9	31
	Washington, California	0.74—0.80	71
Carbonates	—	0.1—4	70
	—	30	72
Mafic (general)	—	0.9—1.8	31
Grabbos	Greenland	Present	77

Tin abundances in sedimentary domains have been reported as 2.24 ppm (Continental shield), 2.47 ppm (Mobile-belt shelf), 2.20 ppm (Hemipelagic), and 2.12 ppm (Pelagic).[70] Oceanic carbonates contain about 0.4 ppm[70] and marine phosphates 10 to 15 ppm tin.[78]

In comparing the trace element content in standard rocks, it is of note that the tin content is usually greater than that of selenium, iodine, and cobalt, and sometimes higher than the boron and molybdenum concentration; all are recognized as vital trace nutrients.[70,79,80] Variations in tin content in the same general type of mineral can be high. The tin concentration in seven different micas was measured as 3.13 to 1166 ppm.[81]

C. Soil Tin

Cassiterite, the most common tin mineral, has a high density (6.95 g/cm^3) and considerable resistance to weathering.[82] Thus, enrichment is noted in alluvial deposits, with concentrations as high as 5% as in commercial ores. As rock slowly converts to soil the trace element content can show considerable variation.[83] In general, soils have less tin than their rock substrate,[73,74,84] although there are contrary indications.[85]

Table 2 summarizes a number of reports on soil-tin content. Where available the tin content of the underlying rock is also reported. Reports prior to about 1945 used analytical methods incapable of detecting tin to less than 10 ppm.[86-88]

It is noted that soil-tin content is almost always greater than that of the vital nutrients cobalt, molybdenum, selenium, and iodine.[91]

Table 2
TIN CONTENT IN SOILS

Soil type	Tin conc (ppm)	Tin conc rock substrate (ppm)	Ref.
Oceanic clay	1.5—55	—	70
Soil (not typed)	3.0—4.6	34—180	72
Clay	15—30	15—45	74
	Present	—	89
	19	—	90
Soil (not typed)	200 max	—	88, 96
	0.1—10	—	91
	4 (av)	—	92
	1—11	—	93
	10 (av)	—	94
	10—47	—	95
	250 max	—	97
	1.3—3	—	98
	<2—6	—	99
	0.4 max	—	100

IV. TIN IN THE HYDROSPHERE

Relatively few studies of the tin content of sea water could be located. Values show a relatively wide variation. Tin, as inorganic tin, has been reported as 0.18 ppb,[27] 0.008 to 0.033 ppb,[71] <5 ppm,[101] 0.3 to 62 ppm (pollution being the suspected origin for the higher values),[102] 0.3 to 1.22 ppb,[103] 2.5 ppm,[104] 1.8 ppb,[105] and 0.02 ppb.[106] Estuarine, harbor, and bay inorganic tin values are comparably higher: 2.2 to 3.9 ppb,[104] 50.1 ppb,[107] 2.1 to 38 ppb,[108] 0 to 0.57 ppb,[102] and 1 to 4 ppb.[109]

Fresh water inorganic tin also shows wide variation. Stream waters in tin mining areas have reported Sn concentrations of <1 to 17 ppb which are more likely due to stannite and other minerals and not the relatively hydrolytically stable cassiterite.[104] The Tejo River (Portugal) shows an average 0.94 ppb Sn as dissolved tin and 0.36 ppm in suspended matter; the higher figure may arise from organotin contaminants being absorbed by suspended particulates.[109] Tin contents of 1.3 ppb (Apalachicola River, Fla.), 1.4 ppb (Mobile River), and 2.1 ppb (Nelson River, Manitoba) have been reported.[110] River water values as high as 3100 ppm have been detected in the vicinity of industrial manufacture and usage of tin and tin chemicals.[111]

Tin in reservoir waters was sought, but not detected in a study covering the water supplies of 100 large U.S. cities.[112] An earlier study indicated reservoir tin content ranging from 0 to 0.1 ppm, with 22 of 24 sources positive.[113] Impoundment waters reportedly vary from 0 to 1.1 ppb.[114] Maguire et al. detected 0.73 ppb inorganic tin in Lake Superior.[107] Isolated lakes far from sources of industrial pollution also have varying tin content ranging from 0.49 ppb to 500 ppm.[107,115] However, Kleinkopf, who examined trace metals in some 439 water samples from remote Maine lakes, noted that 336 of the total had no detectable tin.[115]

Considerable quantities of methyltin and *n*-butyltin species have been measured in lakes and marine harbors.[102,107] Presumably, the lower alkyl tins are anthropogenic in origin, probably being degradation products of antifouling paints. Organotins tend to concentrate in the surface layer.[107] Hodge et al. measured a tin content of 0.49 ppm at a 10-m depth and 0.084 ppb at 62m at Grand Haven Harbor, Lake Michigan.[108] It should be noted that values of other trace metals, especially zinc, nickel, and manganese, show lower values in fresh water than that reported for tin.[110,113]

Pepin et al. measured tin values ranging from <2 to 14 ppm in mineral waters.[116] Inorganic tin in rain water has been reported in part-per-trillion concentrations.[102,117]

Shimizu and Ogata analyzed table salt derived from marine sources and found a soluble tin content of 5.6 to 32.5 ppb, and insoluble tin from 10.0 to 410 ppb.[105]

V. ATMOSPHERIC TIN

Tin has an appreciable concentration in air. Values reported range from 12×10^{-9} to about 800×10^{-9} g/m^3.[92,118-122] Concentrations are continuously present, though variable at any given test site.[118,120] High values are found generally in the air of manufacturing cities.[118,120,121] Input arises from a number of sources. Oana reports that volcanic emissions contain 1 to 4 ppb of tin.[123] Lantzy and Mackenzie estimate that atmospheric emissions of tin from volcanic activity are 2.4×10^8 g/year in dust and 5×10^5 g/year as gas.[124] Other sources of emission are industrial particulates (400×10^8 g/year), fossil fuels (30×10^8 g/year), and continental dust (50×10^8 g/year).[124] In a later paper Byrd and Andrea provide much higher estimates.[125] Anthropogenic inputs are given as 3245×10^{12} g/year (coal burning), 1600×10^{12} g/year (oil burning), 1320×10^{12} g/year (wood burning), 540×10^{12} g/year (waste incineration), and 1220×10^{12} g/year (iron and steel production); while metallic tin production accounts for only 0.24×10^{12} g/year and organotin production and use about 0.008×10^{12} g/year. The much lower natural inputs are estimated at 1000 (sea spray), 800 (soil dust), 25 (volcanism), and 320×10^2 g/year (forest fires).[125]

As early as 1967 Smith and Schwarz noted that the trace elements in atmospheric dust could provide rats with the necessary vital amounts needed.[126] Rodents on an amino acid diet isolated from atmospheric dust showed wasting disease, while those on the same diet but exposed to nonfiltered air did not.

VI. THE PROBLEM OF ENVIRONMENTAL CONTAMINATION

Assessment of endogenous tin in surface soils, water, and living materials is difficult owing to long-term anthropogenic input and wide-scale distribution of tin alloys and organotins. It is widely believed that such input skews the results of those trying to determine natural tin content.

Organic tin input is relatively recent. Compounds were used to stabilize chlorinated oils as early as 1932.[127] Their use as thermostabilizers was extended to poly(vinylchloride) plastics and later urethane elastomers.[127-129] Widespread usage as agricultural insecticides and miticides and as the antifoulant in marine paints occurred in the early 1960s.[130,131] Environmental use is generally restricted to the lower alkyls, cyclics, and aryl compounds. Degradation processes are of both a chemical and a physical nature. Hydrolytic cleavage occurs in the aqueous environment[132-137] with the formation of relatively stable cations.[132]

In use, organotins are readily absorbed on particulates in water and vegetation. Freundlich isotherms are very high for lower alkyltin-soil systems, and thus little mobilization would be expected.[133,134,138] A small (0.02 ppm) organotin background in soil has been reported.[138] Photochemical degradation is extensive when materials such as agricultural pesticide are exposed to solar UV radiation.[134,139] Microbiol degradation in soil is a major detoxifying factor.[133,139-143] The end result of a degradation series appears to be inorganic tin as SnO or SnO_2.[139,140,143,144] Consequently, human input of tin alloys and organic tin compounds would eventually show up as a few stable, relatively insoluble, inorganic tin materials.

Anthropomorphic addition of tin compounds arise from mining operations, but how much is unknown. However, simple calculations show that to uniformly raise the natural tin background in the top cubic meter of soil and water on the planet by 1 ppb would require an elemental tin input in excess of 1×10^{12} g (1×10^6 tons) (assumes the Earth's surface area is 5.1×10^8 km and that the average density at the surface is 2 g/cm³). An increase of 1 ppm in surface tin would correspondingly require an input of one *billion* tons. The author thus opines that the total surface tin content, as measured in the studies cited, is far beyond the value that would arise exogenously from human activities.

VII. ANALYTICAL PROCEDURES

The claim that tin is ubiquitous in nature can be challenged, though with some difficulty, by pointing to the universal anthropomorphic input and, more pointedly, by questioning the analytical procedures used. Early wet chemical methods were hardly sensitive to tin levels below 100 ppm. However, titration with dithiol (4-methyl-1,2-dimercaptobenzene) has been extensively used to detect tin in biological materials and was so recommended as recently as 1940.[145]

Flame spectroscopy was much used during the 1920s and 1930s to detect metals in biological substances. Unfortunately the preliminary drying procedures at elevated temperatures would lead to the volatilization of tin.[146] Even well-known experts such as Ramage had great difficulty in quantitatively assessing animal and plant tissues for tin.[147,148] Relatively large sample aliquots were necessary, and even so values for tin below about 50 ppm would be doubtful.[149] The 3175.02-Å line was generally used as the tin reference.[90] Cholak's 1935 report aptly illustrates the difficulties encountered,[150] although he and Story were successful to a limited degree in determining tissue tin.[151] Through elaborate clean-up techniques, tin could be concentrated prior to spectrographic analysis.[95] Emission spectrography[152] and cathode layer arc spectroscopy[101] techniques were used in the 1950s. However, tin values below about 5 ppm remain dubious.

X-ray fluorescence techniques based on the 3.6-Å Sn line have been used to advantage.[153,154] Precision at 5 μg appears possible[155] at a sensitivity limit of 20 to 30 ppb.[153]

Atomic absorption techniques were applied in the 1960s usually based on the 2246.05-Å Sn line.[156] A sensitivity of 1 ppm and a 0.1-ppm detection limit for tin in water were noted.[156] Improvements in instrumentation and techniques extended the detection limit to the low nanogram region.[102,108,157,158]

Gas chromatography with photometric detection is a current useful tool not only to determine tin concentration in the sub-ppb range, but also to allow speciation of organotin compounds.[159-161] Chromatography in tandem with atomic absorption and/or mass spectrometry hold promise that rapid speciation of tin compounds in biological tissue may be performed.[162,163] Improvements have also been made in chemical methods of tin analysis.[164] The catechol violet method was recommended in 1967,[165] and appears to be useful down to about 5 ppm tin concentration.[166] Spectrophotometric quantization using phenylfluorene was successfully used to determine tin in the low parts-per-million range in the 1950s.[167] Recoveries of 90% or better on doped samples have been reported.[168] Detection in the low parts-per-billion range is possible with a preliminary removal of interfering ions such as Ge^{2+}, Mo^{6+}, etc. and concentration.[105] Color development is in accordance with Beer's law over the critical 0.03- to 3.0-μg range.[169] The method has been aptly used in determining tin in plant tissue.[170] Color development can be enhanced using xylenol orange and cetylpyridinium bromide.[171] Detection in the submicrogram range has been reported.[172] The Quercetin (3,5,7,3′,4′-pentahydroxy-flavone) spectrophotometric method has been used to analyze tin in food.[164] 3,4′,7 Trihydroxyflavone is possibly more sensitive, and a detection limit of 7×10^{-9} has been reported.[173]

Polarographic methods are well known and have for several decades been used to assist in the characterization of tin compounds as well as to detect tin down to levels of 1 ppm.[164,174]

Probably the greatest accuracy and lowest detection limit can be achieved by physical, rather than chemical, methods. Tin has ten stable isotopes between mass numbers 112 and

124, the most of any element.[175] Relative abundances are well known. In 1964 Hamaguchi et al. demonstrated that neutron activation analysis would allow detection of tin in the sub-ppm range in marine biomaterials.[103] The method was applied to the detection of trace metals in human tissue, both normal and pathological.[176-178] The advantages of first removing major elements such as sodium and potassium has been described.[177] By 1971 the tin detection limit was asserted to be 0.014 ppm, which is adequate for the measurement of this element in almost all biological materials.[178] Conceptually, one ought to be able to measure tin content in the sub-ppb range with extreme accuracy using modern activation, detection, and discrimination instrumentation.

The speciation of natural tin compounds in trace amounts remains quite complex. To date speciation in the sub-ppm area has only been done for the lower alkyltins in water. The nature of the tin materials found in animal and plant tissue remains unknown.

VIII. TIN IN THE BIOSPHERE

A. Fossil Fuels and Sediments

Crude oil contains approximately 0.01 ppm tin,[124,179] while coal contains about 1 ppm.[124,180,181] However, the tin content of coal ash averages 0.02% with a maximum of 0.05% noted.[182] Flue dust from coal contains tin.[183]

Lake sediments reflect the impact of fossil fuel combustion. Goldberg et al. measured tin content in sediment cores from Lake Michigan.[184] The core depth can be approximately related to the date of settling, the greater depth being the earlier. At 50 and 55 cm depth, corresponding to the years 1840 and 1855, tin content was 2 ppm. This is prior to much coal combustion in the area, and wood was the primary fuel. The tin content increased only to 2.5 and 3 ppm, respectively, for 1880 and 1900. By 1940 it was 6 ppm; 8 ppm in 1950; and 26 ppm in 1960; then dropping to 20 ppm in 1968 with the placement of emission control devices on coal- and oil-burning plants. The situation is similar in ocean waters. Pre-1900 sediments ranged from 1 to 6 ppm (84 to 39 cm depth), while post-1900 values increased steadily to 20 ppm at the 1-cm depth.[108]

Tin in peat ash varied from 50 to 300 ppm, with all of 50 samples of Finnish peats being positive for Sn.[185] Tin also appears to accumulate in humus.[85]

B. Marine Plants

Cornec was the first to spectroscopically detect tin in marine algae, although he could not quantify it.[186] In 1939 LaGrange et al. found tin in a different algal species.[187] Black and Mitchell examined a number of algae species using cathode-layer arc spectroscopy.[101] Tin concentration, by dry weight, varied from 0.08 to 1.8 ppm. No bioaccumulation of tin was observed. Importantly, these reserachers noted that the trace elements are not removed by washing with tap water (pH not stated) and thus appear to be in an insoluble form. Also, they report a seasonal variation in tin content of *Laminaria digitata* (brown algae) frond (leaf). Single-cell green algae contained 0.03 to 3.8 ppm of Sn based on dry weight.[101] Values are in accordance with Maher: 0.34 to 1.11 ppm,[158] 0.10 to 0.65 ppm,[71] 1.5 to 3.5 ppm,[106] and 0.03 to 1.06 ppm.[108]

Algae reportedly concentrated tin with a factor as high as 10^5.[188] Organotin compounds are also found in algae, the amount varying with the degree of pollution.[189]

Marine and fresh water plankton in general have ash-tin content of 4 to 7 ppm.[157]

C. Land Plants

Tin content in terrestrial plants varies widely. It has been suggested that average plant ash tin is 0.3 ppm.[124,191] Whether plants accumulate tin or need tin as a nutrient remains unanswered. Peterson et al. noted that plants growing in soil uncontaminated with cassiterite ore had 1.5 to 32 ppm dry weight tin content, whereas those same species growing in tin-mining areas showed a 16-fold increase in tin content.[170] Sedges (tufted marsh plants) and mosses are said to be the best accumulators.[192] A number of authors have noted tin accumulation in land plants;[100,193,194] however, others find no appreciable difference between plant tissue tin and the tin content of the underlying soil.[195] In some instances soil tin has been reported as being much higher than plant tin.[88] Millman indicates that plant tissue tin is not related to soil tin in any direct fashion.[97] Hunter found the tin content in the leaf of bracken to be fairly constant.[100] He also notes far higher tin content than that of molybdenum, a known vital nutrient. The extensive data of Sainsbury et al. from the Lost River tin district of Alaska indicate that plant tin-to-soil tin ratios are above 1 when the tin-soil content is below 100 ppm; and below 1 when soil tin is over 150 ppm.[196]

It is not unusual to find that the plant species will accumulate vital trace metals such as cobalt,[197] magnesium,[198] and zinc.[199] The discovery of the vital trace metals was brought about, in most cases, through noting the ubiquity of the element throughout the plant or animal kingdom. For instance, the ubiquity of manganese was found prior to its discovered need in plants and animals.[200,201]

In the study of tin in plants, average values are difficult to determine since trace metal content varies with the organ examined,[100,104,201] although much of the tin remains in the roots[92,202] and is dependent upon the plant or organ age,[201,203,204] species,[205,206] and season.[205,207]

The literature indicates that tin was found in plant tissue prior to the advent of the tin can and far before organotin compounds entered commerce,[208] thus indicating that environmental contamination does not play a role.

Table 3 presents a compendium of Sn concentration found in various plant species and plant organs.

Grain and hay mixtures used as animal feed show 0.1 to 0.5 ppm tin in the ash.[220] Tin is found in various fertilizers ranging from 0.2 to 15 ppm.[92]

D. Tin in Food Plants

Tin enters the animal by ingestion and possibly through respiration, at least with the higher life forms. Studies concerning tin in foodstuffs were generally concerned with tin entering the consumable from contact with alloys of tin. As early as 1777 Gmelin noted that a mild form of food poisoning arose from cooking vegetables in tin ware.[221] Orfila briefly touched on the subject,[222] and Hall reported that the acetic, tarataric, and citric acids from canned vegetables will slowly dissolve tin plate and tin foil, thus contaminating the foodstuff.[223] Others noted a high tin content in canned foods[4,224] and that at high enough levels, poisoning resulted.[225-229] Tin in canned cherries at the 7300-ppm level caused nausea and collapse.[226] At least one death from inorganic tin poisoning has been reported.[228] Importantly, health concerns prompted scientists to examine canned foods. Obviously, one cannot report on the degree of contamination arising from the can unless the natural tin background is known. Therefore, a series of studies beginning in the late 19th century have examined the tin content in foodstuffs. Weber noted natural tin was present in mushrooms, blackberries, blueberries, peas, peaches, sweet potatos, string beans, pineapple, etc.[227] Others reported the presence of tin in a variety of vegetable, fruit, and meat products.[127,174,229-234] Table 4 presents a few of the tin values found for untreated foods.

Zook et al., in examining 11 wheats and 20 different flours, all of which contain tin, point out that tin content is not related to the geographical origin of the sample.[236] It is also noted in this report that tin content in wheat and flours is greater than that of the vital nutrients manganese, copper, nickel, chromium, and selenium, and about the same as that of zinc.

Although little used, neutron activities appear to be the premier method of analysis of foods.[237] Any method requiring high temperature would mean volatilization losses.[238] Even wet-ashing techniques give at best an 80% organic tin recovery.[168,239]

Table 3
TIN IN PLANTS

Plant					
Common name	Species name	Organ	Sn content (ppm)	Type	Ref.
Lichens	—	—	30—100	Ash	72
Mosses	—	—	10—30	Ash	72
Ferns	—	—	10—60	Ash	72
Herbs	—	—	3.0—4.4	Ash	72
Grasses	—	—	3.0—38	Ash	72
Mixed pasture grasses	—	—	0.4	Ash	84
Red clover	—	—	0.2	Ash	84
Corn	—	Leaves	0.3	Ash	90
Grass, scirpus	—	—	0.3	Ash	95
Pasture grass	—	—	0.39—0.46	Ash	95
Beech	*Fagus* spp.	Leaves	0.14	Dry	97
Birch	*Betulla* spp.	Leaves	0.08—1.20	Dry	97
		Twigs	0.36	Dry	97
Oak	*Quercus* spp.	Leaves	0.17—1.40	Dry	97
		Twigs	0.90	Dry	97
Willow	—	Leaves	0.13	Dry	97
Tea	*Camellia sinensis*	Leaves	2—2.8	Dry	98
Bracken	—	Frond	0.8—7.2	Dry	100
		Rhizome	2.8—3.9	Dry	100
Mangrove	—	Leaves	3.8—6.5	Dry	104
		Twigs	3.9—5.1	Dry	104
Corn	*Zea mays*	Leaves, young	0.69—1.66	Dry	204
		Leaves, tasseling	1.06—1.80	Dry	204
		Leaves, mature	0.30—1.56	Dry	204
		Stalks, mature	0.70	Dry	204
		Grain, mature	2.84	Dry	204
		Cobs	6.79	Dry	204
		Husks	1.11	Dry	204
Ragweed	*Ambrosia Artemisi folia*	Tops	0.33—0.83	Dry	204
Various	—	—	46	Ash	209
			5—10	Dry	209
Fern	*Gleichenia linearis*	—	32	Dry	170
Tea		Leaves	Present	Dry	210
Herb	*Silene cucubates*	—	20	Dry	211
Tobacco	—	Not specified	Present	Dry	212
Potato	—	Not specified	Present	Dry	212
Persimmon	—	Not specified	Present	Dry	212
Camelia	—	Not specified	Present	Dry	212
Cherry tree	—	Not specified	Present	Dry	212
Range grasses	—	Blade tops	0.2—1.9	Dry	213
Oak	*Quercus* spp.	Twigs	17.0	Dry	214
Ornamentals	(13 species)	Foliage	0.1—1.6	Dry	215
Vegetable plants	(14 species)	All parts	0.62—9.92	Dry	216
Hardwood	—	—	(0.01—0.05%)	Ash	217
Citris plants	—	Fruit juice	Present	Ash	218
Sugar beets	—	—	Present	Ash	219

Table 4
TIN CONTENT IN FOOD PLANTS AND PROCESSED FOODS

Foodstuff	Tin content (ppm)	Ref.
Black-eyed peas	6—8.7	174
Beets	2.1	174
Green peas	0	174
Prunes	21—24	174
16 vegetables, 7 grains	0.07—9.0	234
Flour	0.6—1.8	235
Bran	0.2—3.4	235
Wheat germ	0.3—0.5	235
Whole wheat	0.3—2.5	235
20 flours' ash	3.3—8.0	236
11 wheats' ash	3.7—32.2	236
25 bread products' ash	4.1—10.5	236

IX. IS TIN ESSENTIAL FOR PLANT GROWTH?

It is reasonable to assume that most, if not all soils contain tin. Beeson et al. examined about 900 soil samples and found all of them to contain tin, with 1% having over 10 ppm.[238]

Tin minerals are well known, and the most likely form of tin in soil would be as SnO_2. The influx into plant life ought to proceed at a very slow rate due to the highly insoluble nature of this material. Indeed, tin accumulations are higher in the roots of food plants than in the above-ground parts.[202] However, there is transport and accumulation at favored sites. More tin is found in the cell metabolic structures (plastids) than in the sap of fruit trees and potato vines.[240] It has been speculated that accumulator plants may need the element accumulated.[211] The high tin concentrations seen in tree leaves etc. would indicate reasonably rapid transport, and thus one would expect the transporting compounds to be water soluble, i.e., biochemical processing occurs within the plant wherein inorganic tin is converted from an insoluble to a soluble form.

The processed form is obviously not toxic to plants and certainly not toxic to the higher individuals in the food chain.

In general, insoluble inorganic tin salts and oxides are nontoxic to plants or animals.[241-245] However, specific soluble salts such as the halides and certain hydrates can be moderately toxic.[224,231,244,246] It is possible, perhaps even likely, that the processed tin compound(s) is in organic form. Tin-protein complexes are highly insoluble and would not be expected.[247,248] In so far as known, the in vivo tin species in plants have never been characterized.

Tin salts applied as a fertilizer stimulate growth in some plants. Micheels, in the first report of its kind, found that colloidal tin metal stimulated plant-root growth by a factor of $5 \times$.[249] Tin-chloride supplement of the soil resulted in the enhanced growth of timothy[250] and parsley, soy beans, cow peas, beans (4 species), peas, corn, clover, and the weeds sesbania and beggarweed.[251] Other plants, 24 species in all, showed no effect when treated with tin (IV) chloride at 26.3 lb/acre. Turnip growth, however, was retarded.[251] The general concensus before 1970 was that natural environmental tin is neither harmful nor beneficial to plants.[82] There are contrary indications to the above reports. For instance, Vanselow applied tin (II) chloride at 150 ppm (tin) to the soil around orange tree seedlings and spectrographically found no tin in the leaves.[252]

Are there natural *organotin* compounds in vegetation? Of course, humans add considerable agricultural organotin to the environment.[4,253] It has been stated that one organotin agricultural pesticide, triphenyltin acetate, does not penetrate celery foliage or roots, but slowly degrades in the soil or on the foliage.[254] The behavior of tripropyltin chloride is quite different. It interacts with *Escherichia coli* by binding with phospholipids and phosphate compounds in the cell membrane,[255] and mediates a chloride-hydroxide exchange across the thylakoid membrane of the chloroplasts.[256] That is, at least one organotin alters plant cell membrane permeability. Tin (II) chloride greatly enhanced chlorophyl content in several algae and thus enhanced growth rate.[250]

The last piece of evidence to be presented is the report of Curtin et al.[257] who found 23 to 80 ppm tin in the ashed residue of the vapor transpired from coniferous trees.[257] There was very little tin in the A (ground cover) and B (top soil) horizons of the soil involved, whereas twig ash contained 6 to 40 ppm tin, with very little tin in the needles. Curtin et al. thus indicate that (1) tin is accumulated, (2) the site of accumulation is the leaf, and (3) reasonably volatile tin compound(s) are transpired by the leaf.[257] Whatever is leaving the leaf is almost certainly not tin oxide and probably not any inorganic tin form known to exist as a mineral. It is thus suggested that the tin content in plant life is in organic form.

X. TIN IN ANIMAL TISSUE

A. Marine Animals

Tin concentrations in marine species have been determined by a number of investigators. Table 5 is a compendium of such values.

Tin content in marine organisms appears to be at a higher level than molybdenum and cobalt, known trace nutrients.[27] Since ocean water tin content is probably less than 0.01 ppm and a number of marine organisms show very high concentrations, especially echinodermata,[190] it is obvious that some of animals are accumulators. Smith estimates the biomagnification to be as high as 10^6.[106]

Skeletal fish debris from pelagic deposits show tin concentrations ranging from 500 to 1500 ppm.[267] Tong et al. reports that the tin content in lake trout significantly decreases with age, whereas other trace metals (chromium, cobalt, manganese, etc.) tend to increase with age.[268]

B. Tin in Terrestrial Animals

With the exception of the human species, very little analytical work has been performed on the tin content of mammals and other land animals. Data on birds is almost completely lacking so far; the author is only aware of data on the chicken egg shell (2.9 ppm tin content).[102]

The major scientific interest in the tin content of meat products arose from concern over contamination from packaging in tin cans.[230,269-271] Prior to the middle 1930s the spectroscopic detection of tin in animal tissue below about 10 ppm was difficult,[272] owing primarily to losses occurring during the preliminary tissue drying at elevated temperatures, insufficient flame intensity, and interference by other trace metals.[273]

Bertrand and Ciurea, in 1931, were the first to provide a reasonable analysis of tin content in meats (cow, horse, and sheep).[274] Organs examined were the pancreas (3.03 to 3.92 ppm Sn), stomach (0.4 to 1.64), large intestine (0.68 to 0.92), lung (0.98 to 2.04), muscle (1.54 to 1.86), kidney (1.12 to 1.78), blood (1.25 to 1.64), heart (1.47 to 2.42), brain (2.4 to 3.0), spleen (2.4 to 3.09), small intestine (2.85 to 3.66), skin (6.2 to 9.48), and liver (2.14 to 3.73).

In 1952 some 245 rib eye steaks from as many cows were examined. In all cases tin was detected, but at unusually low levels since the investigators ashed their samples at 500°C for 2 hr in a muffle furnace.[275] Even so, tin concentration was reported as higher than that of cobalt and chromium, both vital trace metals.

Table 5
TIN IN MARINE ORGANISMS

Type	Common name	Type tissue	Prepn (weight)	Tin conc (ppm)	Ref.
General	—	—	—	8	27
Mollusca	(General)	Whole body	Dry	0.23—0.71	71
—	Coral	Shell	Ash	0.73	102
—	Sea shells	Shell	Ash	0.59	102
Coelenterata	—	Whole body	Dry	1.2	106
Crustacea	2 spp.	Whole body	Dry	0.38—3.0	106
	2 spp.	Eggs	Dry	0.06	106
Mollusca	5 spp.	Shell	Dry	0.03—0.09	106
		Flesh	Dry	00.03—1.2	106
Cephalopoda	Octopus, 2 spp.	Muscle	Dry	0.21—0.29	106
		Liver	Dry	0.4—1.6	106
Echinodermata	Starfish, 3 spp.	Whole body	Dry	0.07—0.96	106
Tunicata	5 spp.	Whole body	Dry	2.3—3.4	106
		Internal organs	Dry	0.7—15.0	106
Pisces	Fish (general)	Whole body	Wet	<1	111
Mollusca	Oyster	Shell	Dry	<0.01	158
		Viscera	Dry	1.25	158
		Muscle	Dry	0.03	158
Pisces	Fish (4 spp.)	Muscle	Dry	<0.01—0.023	158
General	Marine plankton (general)	Whole body	Ash	4—7	190
Mollusca	Snail	Whole body	Ash	<1—20	190
Arthropods	—	Whole body	Ash	<1—50	190
Tunicata	—	Whole body	Ash	8	190
Echinodermata		Whole body	Ash	Up to 800	190
Fish (fertilizer)		—	Ash	Positive	250
Dysidea Etheria	Sponge	Whole body	Dry	7	258
Chondrilla Nucula	Sponge	Whole body	Dry	4	258
Terpios Zeteki	Sponge	Whole body	Dry	50	258
Mollusca	Snail	Whole body	Dry	<8.4 × 10^{-8} mol/kg	259
	Oyster	Whole body	Dry		259
Coelenterata	Sponge	Whole body	Ash	4	260
Ctenophora	—	Whole body	Ash	7	260
Mollusca	Snail	Whole body	Ash	<1—20	260
Cephalopoda		Whole body	Ash	3	260
Copepoda		Whole body	Ash	<1—90	260
Chaetognatha		Whole body	Ash	20	260
Tunicata		Whole body	Ash	8	260
Cyanea capillata		Whole body	Dry	32	261
Mollusca	Oyster	Whole body	Dry	10—55	262
Pisces	Fish	Bone	Ash	Present	263
	Fish	Muscle	Ash	Present	264
	Fish	Muscle	Ash	Present	265
Gastropoda (6 spp.)	Snail	Whole body	Ash	250—1500	266
Lamellibronchiata (2 spp.)		Whole body	Ash	Not detected	266
Echinodermata (5 spp.)	Starfish	Whole body	Ash	800	266
Lapadogaster govani (1 spp.)	Fish	Whole body	Ash	Not detected	266

Table 5 (continued)
TIN IN MARINE ORGANISMS

Type	Common name	Type tissue	Prepn (weight)	Tin conc (ppm)	Ref.
Urochordata (1 spp.)		Whole body	Ash	Not detected	266
Crustacea (1 spp.)		Whole body	Ash	200	266
Nemertea (1 spp.)		Whole body	Ash	200	266
Polychaeta (1 spp.)		Whole body	Ash	Not detected	266

Tin has been detected in dog and rat teeth,[276] and indeed as Milne et al. have pointed out, rats deprived of tin have dental defects.[277] Dingle and Sheldon in 1938 reported no tin present in bovine milk,[278] while in 1946, Godar and Alexander found 0.4 ppm.[274] It has been noted that the lymph nodes of the cow are repository sites for tin.[279]

Russoff et al. noted that all adult rats contain a small amount of tin.[280] Recent work has shown that the laboratory rat and mouse have a tin content in all organs examined, except the blood and certain endocrine organs, with the major repository site being the thymus gland.[4,282-284]

XI. TIN IN THE HUMAN BODY

A number of studies have been performed in which the trace metal content of human tissue has been determined. A detailed description has been provided elsewhere.[4] Table 6 is a compendium of human tissue tin data taken from a number of observers. Values are for "natural" tissue i.e., not exposed to unusual levels of environmental tin such as would be the case with tin miners, etc. All values are based on wet weight unless otherwise noted. The "0" values noted in the earlier reports reflect only the instrumental limitations of the technique.[151,233] The most thorough and recent report which summarizes much of the literature is provided by Anspaugh et al.[286-288]

In 1964 Tipton and Shafer examined tin in tissue, emphasizing the lungs, from autopsies of 200 victims of instantaneous accidental death.[296] They note that 137 out of 140 individuals had <5 to 920 μg of tin per gram of lung tissue ash. Tin was found in the aorta, brain, heart, kidney, liver, muscle, ovary, pancreas, spleen, stomach, testes, and uterus. Oddly, none was found in the thyroid of any victim, while the prostrate, which usually shows no other trace element, had tin. It was further noted that tin levels do not vary statistically with geographical areas, age, or sex.

Table 7 is taken from Tipton and Cook,[297] who examined 29 different tissues from 150 adult victims of instantaneous accidental death. They report a 5- to 72-ppm range and 23-ppm average tissue tin (ash weight) content for the human body. Tin was found in 3/4 or more of all tissues examined, except the brain and muscle.

Few have examined tin content of the human fetus. Misk finds a trace in the fetal heart and spleen with a higher level in the liver.[285] Schroeder et al. report no tin in stillborns.[234]

In an early paper, Datta reports that rats excrete 89 to 92% of the tin input in feces and 5.5 to 6.2% in urine.[300] He concluded that about 2% of the tin input is stored. The general view was that exogenous tin in humans was a contaminant from ingesting canned foods. Perry and Perry examined urine from U.S. residents of various ages, races, and sexes and found approximately 7 to 17 μg of tin per liter.[301] Africans, supposedly never exposed to the tin can, had an average of 10.7 ppb tin in their urine. Interestingly, tin was found in all

Table 6
TIN CONTENT IN HUMAN TISSUE

Organ	Tin (ppm)	Ref.
Brain	5.9	151
	0	233
	1.02	285
	0.06	286
	0—105 (ash)	293
Kidney	3.3	151
	15	233
	Present	285
	5—5.5	286
	12.5	290
	0.2	291
	20	292
	5—70 (ash)	293
Heart	15.7	185
	15	151
	0	233
	1.64	286
	3.9	287
	22	292
	10—130 (ash)	293
Lungs	25.9	285
	55	151
	1.2	286
	0.8	291
	45	292
	15—420 (ash)	293
Teeth	Present	276
	120 (enamel)	294
	93 (dentine)	294
Stomach membrane	20	151
	3.5—4.3	286
	0—70 (ash)	293
Liver	30	151
	Present	233
	6.5—9.6	286
	15.4	290
	0.4	291
	60	292
Spleen	20	151
	Present	233
	1.7—2.4	286
	10—50 (ash)	293
Small intestine	25	151
	30 (ash)	293
Skin	15	151
	2.9—3.7	186
Colon	25	151
Blood	0	151
	4.7	286
	0	290
	0.005	291
Urinary bladder	10	151
	2.34	286
Gall bladder	0	151

Table 6 (continued)
TIN CONTENT IN HUMAN TISSUE

Organ	Tin (ppm)	Ref.
Muscle	0	151
	0	233
	1.2	286
	0.07	291
	11	292
Rib	0	151
Femur	0	151
	1.8—3	287
	4.1	291
	8	292
	10 (ash)	293
Spinal fluid	0	151
	Trace	295
Pancreas	Present	151
	1.75	286
	10—105 (ash)	293
Adrenal gland	2.5—3.6	286
Diaphragm	1.76	286
Esophagus	4.55	286
	20 (ash)	293
Ovary	5.4	286
	2.1	287
	0.3	291
Testes	1.87	286
	3.3	287
	0.3	291
	0	293
Large intestine	9 (ash)	286
	10 (ash)	293
Rectum	1.5—4.2	286
Sigmoid Colon	2.2—6.8	286
Larynx	5.3	286
Omentum	1.2—1.25	286
Prostate	2.1	286
	0—250 (ash)	293
Thyroid	2.3—3.2	286
	5—15 (ash)	293
Trachae	6.08	286
Uterus	2.2	286
Aorta	3.7	286
	Present	289

urine samples examined. Calloway and McMullen reported that all the tin ingested is promptly secreted in the feces.[302] In contrast, the studies of Tipton et al. indicate that when a human intake is 1.31×10^{-3} g/day for 30 days, about 0.10×10^{-3} g is retained by the body with the remainder excreted.[303] In another experimental study, Hamilton et al. found that a 5-week-old infant retains 0.36 mg/day when on an 11.23-mg/day tin diet[304]

A. Tin in Milk

Tin does not cross the placental barrier in rodents[4,22] nor humans.[234] Infant mice receive tin in the mothers' milk.[4,281] Although Dingle and Shelden were unable to detect tin in human or bovine milk in 1938,[278] Mallinckrodt and Pooth reported tin in human milk,[290] and others found it present in cows' milk.[304]

Table 7
TIN IN HUMAN TISSUE: FREQUENCY AND CONCENTRATION[297]

Organ	No. examined	No. positive for tin	Approximate tin content (ppm, ash weight)
Adrenal gland	15	14	10
Thyroid	21	16	8
Pancreus	139	73	15
Testes	72	54	5
Ovaries	16	13	10
Liver	150	144	25
Spleen	143	120	5
Intestine	109	107	40
Aorta	105	96	8
Brain	129	7	Trace
Skin	22	21	10
Stomach	131	111	12
Muscle	137	26	5
Lung	140	137	35
Kidney	145	140	10
Heart	140	84	20
Uterus	32	24	4

B. Tin in the Human Lymphatic System

The accumulation of tin in the thymus gland of mice, as reported by Cardarelli et al., served as the initial impetus for a series of studies.[4,11] Other studies have been confirmatory.[283,284,305] High tin levels are also noted in the lymph nodes,[291] spleen,[305] and bone.[281,291,292] Tin accumulation in the lymph nodes has also been reported.[5,279]

XII. DISCUSSION AND CONCLUSION

The data reviewed in this article clearly support the contention that tin is ubiquitous. Indeed, wherever researched, using methods that avoid the volatility problem and are sufficiently sensitive below 10 ppm levels, tin has been found.

In 1964 the late and highly respected H. A. Schroeder felt that tin was an abnormal trace element with no vital function.[234] This conclusion was based essentially upon a perceived lack of environmental ubiquity, lack of tin in the newborn, and no proven biological effect. The question of ubiquity hopefully has been addressed here. There is as yet no conclusive data regarding lack of tissue tin in infancy, although the theory previously advanced by Cardarelli will simply handle either condition without modification.[4]

At this time there is no proven vital effect of tin in humans. Certainly it can be reasonably asserted that tin is essential to proper dentition in rodents and possibly in humans.[276,277,284,306-308] The work of Schwarz and colleagues showed that dietary tin was vital to growth in rats.[6-8] The linkage between tin, the thymus gland, and oncogenesis is discussed in Chapter 6 and elsewhere.[4,5]

In addition to being ubiquitous, tin possesses a number of properties common to vital trace metals. It is bioaccumulated. Schroeder et al. note that of the 30 common trace metals, tin is 21st in the cosmos, 17th in the geosphere, 12th in the hydrosphere (probably 10th in the plant kingdom — *author*), and 8th in the human body.[234] Carried still further into the microcosm, tin appears to be 5th in the lymphatic system and 3rd in the thymus, superceded only by iron and zinc.[305] Inorganic tin is capable of entering into biological activity at saline pH,[137,308] and it is far less toxic than other known vital trace elements such as copper and cobalt.[4] Human tissue tin appears not to vary with age.[234,289] The average concentration of tin in human cells is 10^6 to 10^8 atoms — the same range as cobalt, iodine, chromium, and selenium, known vital nutrients.[310]

The biochemical tin compounds, presuming they exist, would almost certainly be low molecular weight, fat-soluble organic tin materials.[238]

REFERENCES

1. **Prasad, A. S. Ed.**, *Trace Elements in Human Health and Disease,* Vol. 1, Academic Press, New York, 1976.
2. **Underwood, E. J.**, *Trace Elements in Human and Animal Nutrition,* Academic Press, New York, 1977.
3. **Pendias, A. K. and Pendias, H.**, *Trace Elements in Soils and Plants,* CRC Press, Boca Raton, Fla., 1984.
4. **Cardarelli, N. F., Ed.**, *Tin as a Vital Nutrient: Implications in Cancer Prophylaxis and Other Physiological Processes,* CRC Press, Boca Raton, Fla., 1985.
5. **Cardarelli, N. F., Cardarelli, B. M., and Marioneaux, M.**, Tin as a vital trace nutrient, *J. Nutr. Growth Cancer,.* 1, 181, 1984.
6. **Schwarz, K., Milne, D. B., and Vinyard, E.**, Growth effects of tin compounds in rats maintained in a trace elements controlled environment, *Biochem. Biophys. Res. Commun.,* 40, 22, 1970.
7. **Schwarz, K.**, Tin as an essential growth factor for rats, in *Newer Trace Elements in Nutrition,* Mertz, W. and Cornatzer, W. E., Eds., Marcel Dekker, New York, 1971, 313.
8. **Schwarz, K.**, Recent dietary trace element research exemplified by tin, fluorine, and silicon, *Fed. Proc. Fed. Am. Soc. Exp. Biol.,* 33, 1748, 1974.
9. **Freiden, R.**, The chemical elements of life, *Sci. Am.,* 227, 52, 1972.
10. **Cardarelli, N. F., Quitter, B. M., Allen, A., Dobbins, E., Libby, E. P., Hager, P., and Sherman, L.**, Organotin implications in anticarcinogenesis: background and thymus involvement, *Aust. J. Exp. Biol. Med. Sci.,* 62, 199, 1984.
11. **Ege, G. N. and Warbick, A.**, Lymphoscintography: a comparison of anitimary sulfide colloid and ^{99m}Tc stannous phytate, *Br. J. Radiol.,* 52, 124, 1979.
12. **Shofran, B.**, Effect of a tin free diet on COBS mice, unpublished, Department of Chemistry, Scranton University, Pennsylvania.
13. **Keefer, T.**, Radioactive Sn-113 in COBS and A/KI mice, unpublished, Department of Chemistry, Scranton University, Pennsylvania.
14. **Sherman, L. R., Bilgicer, K. I., and Cardarelli, N. F.**, Analysis of tin in mice and human organs, *J. Nutr. Growth Cancer,* 2, 107, 1985.
15. **Bilgicer, K. I.**, Analysis of Tin in Mouse and Human Organs, Thesis, University of Scranton, Scranton, Pa., 1983.
16. **Brown, N. M.**, The Effect of Two Organotin Compounds on C3H-Strain Mice, Ph.D. thesis, Clemson University, Clemson, S.C., 1972.
17. **Crowe, A. J. and Smith, P. J.**, Dialkyltin dihalide complexes: a new class of metallic derivatives exhibiting anti-tumor activity, *Chem. Ind. (London),* 200, 1980.
18. **Crowe, A. J.**, Synthesis and Studies on Some Biologically Active Organotin Compounds, Ph.D. thesis, University of London, London, 1980.
19. **Crowe, A. J., Smith, P. J., and Atassi, G.**, Investigations into the antitumor activity of organotin compounds. I. Diorganotin dihalide and dipseudohalide complexes, *Chem. Biol. Interact.,* 32, 171, 1980.
20. **Gielen, M., Jurkschat, K., and Atassi, G.**, Bis(halophenylstannyl)methanes: new organotin compounds exhibiting anti-tumor activity, *Bull. Soc. Chim. Belg.,* 93, 153, 1984.
21. **Barbieri, R., Pellerito, L., Ruisi, G., LoGiudice, M. T., Huber, F., and Atassi, G.**, The antitumor activity of diorganotin (IV) complexes with adenine and glycylglycine, *Inorg. Chim. Acta,* 66, L39, 1982.
22. **Cardarelli, N. F., Cardarelli, B., Libby, E. P., and Dobbins, E.**, Organotin implications in anticarcinogenesis: effect of several organotins on tumor growth rate in mice, *Aust. J. Exp. Biol. Med. Sci.,* 62, 209, 1984.

23. **Cardarelli, N. and Cardarelli, B.**, Method and Composition for the Detection of a Precancerous or Leukemic Condition in Mammals, U.S. Patent 4511551, April 16, 1985.
24. **Cardarelli, N. F. and Kanakkanatt, S. V.**, Tin Steroids and Their Use as Antineoplastic Agents, U.S. Patent 518,073, 1985.
25. **Cardarelli, N. F.**, Tin steroids as anticancer agents, in *Tin and Malignant Cell Growth*, Zuckerman, J. J., Ed., CRC Press, Boca Raton, 1988, chap. 6.
26. **Forbes, R. J.**, Metallurgy, in *A History of Technology*, Singer, C., Holmyard, E. J., Hall, A. R., and Williams, T. I., Eds., Oxford University Press, New York, 1956, 41.
27. **Wedepohl, K. H.**, *Geochemistry*, Holt, Reinhart, & Winston, New York, 1971.
28. **Goldberg, E., Uchiyania, A., and Brown, H.**, The distribution of nickel, cobalt, gallium, palladium, and gold in iron meteorites, *Geochim. Cosmochim. Acta*, 2, 1, 1951.
29. **Winchester, J. W. and Aten, A. H. W.**, The content of tin in iron meteorites, *Geochim. Cosmochim. Acta*, 12, 57, 1957.
30. **Onishi, H. and Sandell, H. B.**, Meteoritic and terrestrial abundance of tin, *Geochim. Cosmochim. Acta*, 12, 262, 1957.
31. **DeLaeter, J. R. and Jeffrey, P. M.**, Tin: its isotopic and elemental abundance, *Geochim. Cosmochim. Acta*, 31, 969, 1967.
32. **Hamaguchi, H. and Kuroda, R.**, Tin: SOC. Abundance in meteorities, tektites, cosmos and lunar materials, in *Handbook of Geochemistry*, Springer-Verlag, Berlin, 1978, 50C1.
33. **Hamaguchi, H. and Kuroda, R.**, Tin: abundance in rock forming minerals, in *Handbook of Geochemistry*, Springer-Verlag, Berlin, 1978, 50D1.
34. **Bergerhoff, G.**, Tin: crystal chemistry, in *Handbook of Geochemistry*, Springer-Verlag, Berlin, 1969, 50A1.
35. **Duggan, A. J.**, A survey of sleeping sickness in northern Nigeria from the earliest times to the present day, *Trans. R. Soc. Trop. Med. Hyg.*, 55, 439, 1962.
36. **Nockolds, S. R. and Allen, R.**, The geochemistry of some igneous rock series, *Geochim. Cosmochim. Acta*, 4, 105, 1953.
37. **Hanks, H. G.**, Tin in Plumas and Trinity Counties, California State Minerologists Report No. 4, 410, 1884.
38. **Fairbanks, J. W.**, The tin deposits at Temescal, Southern California, *Am. J. Sci.*, 4, 39, 1897.
39. **Dudley, P. H.**, Geology of a portion of the Perris Block, Southern California, *Can. J. Mines Ged.*, 31, 481, 1935.
40. **Penfield, S. L. and Ford, W. E.**, On stibiotantalite, *Am. J. Sci.*, 22, 61, 1906.
41. **Pabst, A.**, Minerals of California, Division of Mines Bull. No. 113, California Department of Natural Resources, 1938.
42. **St. Clair, S.**, Commercial tin in (North) Carolina, *Min. Metall.*, 16, 302, 1935.
43. **Haney, M.**, The tin deposits of the carolinas, *Eng. Min. J.*, 126, 1023, 1928.
44. **Ferguson, H. G.**, Tin deposits near Irish Creek, Virginia, *Va. Geol. Surv. Bull.*, 15-A, 1918.
45. **Livingston, D. C.**, Tungsten, cinnabar, manganese, molybdenum and tin deposits of Idaho, *Idaho Univ. Sch. Mines Bull.*, 14(2), 1919.
46. **Hess, F. L.**, Tin, tungsten and tantalum deposits of South Dakota, *U.S. Geol. Surv. Bull.*, 380, 131, 1909.
47. **Darton, N. G. and Paige, S.**, Description of the Central Black Hills, in Geol. Atlas, U.S. Central Black Hills Folio No. 129, U.S. Geological Survey, Alexandria, Va., 1925.
48. **Hill, J. M.**, The Taylor Creek tin deposits, New Mexico, *U.S. Geol. Surv. Bull.*, 725, 347, 1920.
49. **Fernquist, C. O.**, Tin found near Spokane, Washington, *Mineralogist*, 3, 14, 1935.
50. **Fries, C.**, Tin deposits of the Black Range, Catron and Sierra Counties, New Mexico, *U.S. Geol. Surv. Bull.*, 922-M, 1940.
51. **Fries, C.**, Tin deposits of northern Lander County, Nevada, *U.S. Geol. Surv. Bull.*, 931-L, 1942.
52. **Smith, W. C. and Gianella, V. P.**, Tin deposits at Majuba Hill, Pershing County, Nevada, *U.S. Geol. Surv. Bull.*, 931-C, 1942.
53. **Harrison, H. C. and Allen, J. E.**, An investigation of the reported occurrence of tin at Juniper Ridge, Oregon, *Ore. Dep. Geol. Miner. Ind. Bull.*, No. 23, 1942.
54. **Knopf, A.**, Geology of the Seward Peninsula tin deposits, *U.S. Geol. Surv. Bull.*, 358, 1, 1908.
55. **Waters, A. E.**, Placer concentrates of the Ramparts and Hot Springs Districts, Alaska, *U.S. Geol. Surv. Bull.*, 844, 227, 1934.
56. **Johnson, B. L.**, Occurrence of wolframite and cassiterite in the gold placers of Deadwood Creek, Birch Creek District, Alaska, *U.S. Geol. Surv. Bull.*, 442, 246, 1910.
57. **Harrington, G. L.**, Tin mining in Seward Peninsula, *U.S. Geol. Surv. Bull.*, 692, 353, 1919.
58. **Chapin, P.**, Tin deposits of the Ruby District (Alaska), *U.S. Geol. Surv. Bull.*, 692, 331, 1919.
59. **DeLury, J. S.**, An occurrence of tin near the Ontario-Manitoba boundary, *Can. Min. J.*, 41, 520, 1920.
60. **Davidson, E. H.**, Tin Lodes in Nova Scotia, Annu. Rep. on Mines, Nova Scotia Department of Public Works and Mines, 1932, 211.

61. **Messervey, J. P.,** Tin in Nova Scotia, Annu. Rep. on Mines, Nova Scotia Department of Public Works and Mines, 1932, 227.
62. **Gunning, H. C.,** A tin-silver vein at Snowflake Mine, British Columbia, *Econ. Geol.,* 26, 215, 1931.
63. **Sampson, S.,** Some tin placer deposits of Mexico, *Eng. Min. J.,* 124, 137, 1927.
64. **Lindgren, W.,** *Mineral Deposits,* McGraw-Hill, New York, 1928.
65. **Higazy, R. A.,** The distribution and significance of the trace elements in the Braefoot Outer Sill, Fife, *Trans. Edinburgh Geol. Soc.,* 15, 150, 1952.
66. **Higazy, R. A.,** Trace elements of volcanic ultrabasic potassic rocks of southwestern Uganda and adjoining parts of the Belgium Congo, *Bull. Geol. Soc. Am.,* 65, 39, 1954.
67. **Goldschmidt, V. M.,** The geochemical background of minor-element distribution, *Soil Sci.,* 60, 1, 1945.
68. **Connor, J. J. and Shacklette, H. T.,** Background geochemistry of some rocks, soils, plants, and vegetables in the coterminous United States, *U.S. Geol. Surv. Prof. Pap.,* 574F, 168, 1975.
69. **Griffitts, W. R. and Milne, D. B.,** Tin, in *Geochemistry and the Environment,* Vol. 2, Beeson, K. C., Ed., National Academy of Sciences, Washington, D.C., 1977, 88.
70. **Horn, M. K. and Adams, J. A. S.,** Computer-derived geochemical balances and element abundances, *Geochim. Cosmochim. Acta,* 30, 279, 1966.
71. **Smith, J. D. and Burton, J. D.,** The occurrence and distribution of tin with particular reference to marine environments, *Geochim. Cosmochim. Acta,* 36, 621, 1972.
72. **Lounamaa, J.,** Trace elements in plants growing wild on different rocks in Finland, *Ann. Bot. Soc. Zool. Bot. Fenn.* Vanamo, 29, 1, 1956.
73. **Ure, A. M. and Bacon, J. R.,** Comprehensive analysis of soils and rocks by spark source mass spectrometry, *Analyst (London),* 103, 807, 1978.
74. **Butler, J. R.,** The geochemistry and mineralogy of rock weathering. I. The Lizard area, Cornwall, *Geochim. Cosmochim. Acta,* 4, 157, 1953.
75. **Billings, M. P. and Rabbitt, J. C.,** Chemical analysis and calculated modes of the Oliverian Magma Series, Mt. Washington Quadrangle, New Hampshire, *Bull. Geol. Soc. Am.,* 58, 573, 1947.
76. **Patterson, E. M.,** A petrochemical study of the tertiary lavas of North-East Ireland, *Geochim. Cosmochim. Acta,* 2, 283, 1952.
77. **Wager, L. R. and Mitchell, R. L.,** Preliminary observations on the distribution of trace elements in the rocks of the Skaergaard Intrusion, Greenland, *Mineral. Mag.,* 26, 283, 1943.
78. **Tooms, J. S., Summerhayes, C. P., and Cronan, D. S.,** Geochemistry of marine phosphate and manganese deposits, *Oceanogr. Mar. Biol. Annu. Rev.,* 7, 49, 1969.
79. **Fleischer, M.,** Summary of new data on rock samples G-1 and W-1, 1962—1965, *Geochim. Cosmochim. Acta,* 29, 1263, 1965.
80. **Fleischer, M.,** U.S. geological survey standards. I. Additional data on rocks G-1 and W-1, 1965—1967, *Geochim. Cosmochim. Acta,* 33, 65, 1969.
81. **Johansen, O. and Steinnes, E.,** Determination of tin in geological material by neutron activation analysis, *Analyst,* 94, 976, 1969.
82. **Wallihan, E. F.,** Tin, in *Diagnostic Criteria for Plants and Soils,* Chapman, H. D., Ed., University of California Press, Riverside, 1966, 476.
83. **Butler, J. R.,** The geochemistry and mineralogy of rock weathering. II. The Nordmarka area, Oslo, *Geochim. Cosmochim. Acta,* 6, 268, 1955.
84. **Mitchell, R. L.,** Application of spectrographic analysis to soil investigations, *Analyst (London),* 71, 361, 1946.
85. **Present, E. W.,** Geochemistry of iron, magnesium, lead, copper, zinc, antimony, silver, tin, and cadmium in the soils of the Bathurst area, New Brunswick *Geol. Surv. Can. Bull.,* 174, 1971.
86. **Allison, R. V. and Gaddum, L. W.,** The trace element content of some important soils. A comparison, *Proc. Soil Sci. Soc. Fla.,* 2, 68, 1940.
87. **Carrigan, R. A. and Rogers, L. H.,** The trace element content of certain Florida soils and related plant materials, *Proc. Soil Sci. Soc. Fla.,* 2, 92, 1940.
88. **Mitchell, R. L.,** The Spectrographic Analysis of Soils, Plants, and Related Materials, Tech. Comm. No. 44, Commonwealth Bureau of Soil Science, Harpenden, Engl., 1948.
89. **Ahrens, L. H.,** Trace elements in clay, *S. Afr. J. Sci.,* 41, 152, 1945.
90. **Shimp, N. F., Conner, J., Prince, A. L., and Bear, F. E.,** Spectrochemical analysis of soils and biological materials, *Soil Sci.,* 83, 51, 1957.
91. **Shacklette, H. T. and Boerngen, J. G.,** Element concentrations in soils and other surficial materials of the coterminous United States, *U.S. Geol. Surv. Prof. Pap.,* 1270, 1984.
92. **Pendias, A. K. and Pendias, H.,** *Trace Elements in Soils and Plants,* CRC Press, Boca Raton, Fla., 1984.
93. **Prince, A. L.,** Trace-element delivery capacity of the New Jersey soil types as measured by spectrographic analysis of soils and mature corn leaves, *Soil Sci.,* 84, 413, 1957.

94. **Rose, A. W., Hawkes, H. E., and Webb, S. S.,** *Geochemistry in Mineral Exploration*, Academic Press, London, 1979.
95. **Mitchell, R. L. and Scott, R. O.,** Concentration methods in spectrographic analysis. II. Recovery of trace constituents in plant materials and soil extracts by mixed organic reagents, *J. Soc. Chem. Ind.*, 66, 330, 1947.
96. **Mitchell, R. L.,** The distribution of trace elements in soils and grasses, *Proc. Nutr. Soc.*, 1, 183, 1944.
97. **Millman, A. P.,** Biogeochemical investigations in areas of copper-tin mineralization in Southwest England, *Geochim. Cosmochim. Acta*, 12, 85, 1957.
98. **Laycock, D. H.,** The mineral content of some Nyasaland tea leaves and tea soils, *J. Sci. Food Agric.*, 5, 266, 1954.
99. **Kick, H., Burger, H., and Sommer, K.,** Gesanthalte an Pb, Zn, Sn, As, Cd, Hg, Cu, Ni, Cr und Co in Landwirtschaftlich und Gartnerish Genutzen Boden Nordrhein-Westfalens, *Landwirtsch. Forsch.*, 33, 12, 1980.
100. **Hunter, J. G.,** The composition of bracken. Some major and trace element constituents, *J. Sci. Food Agric.*, 4, 10, 1953.
101. **Black, W. A. P. and Mitchell, R. L.,** Trace elements in the uncommon brown algae and in sea water, *J. Mar. Biol. Assoc. U.K.*, 30, 575, 1952.
102. **Braman, R. S. and Tompkins, M. A.,** Separation and determination of nanogram amounts of inorganic tin and methyltin compounds in the environment, *Anal. Chem.*, 51, 12, 1979.
103. **Hamaguchi, H., Kawabuchi, K., Onuma, N., and Kuroda, R.,** Determination of trace quantities of tin by neutron activation analysis, *Anal. Chim. Acta*, 30, 335, 1964.
104. **Peterson, P. J., Burton, M. A. S., Gregson, M., Nye, S. M., and Porter, E. K.,** Accumulation of tin by mangrove species in West Malaysia, *Sci. Total Environ.*, 11, 213, 1979.
105. **Shimizu, K. and Ogata, N.,** Determination of tin in common salt with phenylfluorone, *Jpn. Anal.*, 12, 526, 1963.
106. **Smith, J. D.,** Tin in organisms and water in the Gulf of Naples, *Nature (London)*, 225, 103, 1970.
107. **Maguire, R. J., Chau, Y. K., Bengert, G. A., Hale, E. J., Wong, P. T. S., and Kramer, O.,** Occurrence of organotin compounds in Ontario lakes and rivers, *Environ. Sci. Technol.*, 16, 698, 1982.
108. **Hodge, V. F., Seidel, S. L., and Goldberg, E. D.,** Determination of tin (IV) and organotin compounds in natural waters. Coastal sediments and macro algae by atomic absorption spectrometry, *Anal. Chem.*, 51, 1256, 1979.
109. **Andreae, M., Byrd, J. T., and Froehlich, P. N.,** Arsenic, antimony, germanium, and tin in the Tejo Estuary, Portugal: modeling a polluted estuary, *Environ. Sci. Technol.*, 17, 731, 1983.
110. **Durum, W. H. and Haffity, J.,** Occurrence of minor elements in water, Geol. Surv. Circ. 445, U.S. Geological Survey, Washington, D.C., 1961, 1.
111. **Schramel, P., Samsahl, K., and Pavlu, J.,** Some determinations of Hg, As, Se, Sb, Sn, and Br in water plants, sediments, and fishes in Bavarian rivers, *Int. J. Environ. Stud.*, 5, 37, 1973.
112. **Durfor, C. N. and Becker, E.,** Selected data on public supplies of the 100 largest cities in the United States, *J. Am. Water Works Assoc.*, 56, 237, 1964.
113. **Braidech, M. M. and Emery, F. H.,** The spectrographic determination of minor chemical constituents in various water supplies in the United States, *J. Am. Water Works Assoc.*, 27, 557, 1935.
114. **Bond, R. G. and Staub, C. P.,** *Handbook of Environmental Control*, Vol 3, CRC Press, Boca Raton, Fla., 1973, 23.
115. **Kleinkopf, M. D.,** Spectrographic determination of trace elements in lake waters of northern Maine, *Geol. Soc. Am. Bull.*, 71, 1231, 1960.
116. **Pepin, D., Gardes, A., and Petit, J.,** Etude spectrographique des elements-traces des eaux minerales, *Analusis*, 2, 549, 1973.
117. **Braman, R. S. and Tompkins, M. A.,** Separation and determination of nanogram amounts of inorganic tin and methyltin compounds in the environment, *Anal. Chem.*, 51, 12, 1974.
118. **Bogen, J.,** Trace elements in atmospheric aerosol in the Heidelberg area, measured by instrumental neutron activation analysis, *Atmos. Environ.*, 7, 1117, 1973.
119. **Dittrich, T. and Cothern, C. R.,** Analysis of trace metal particulates in atmospheric samples using X-ray fluorescence, *J. Air Pollut. Control Assoc.*, 21, 716, 1971.
120. **Laamanen, A., Lofgren, A., and Partanen, T. J.,** Some trace metals in particulates in the air of Helsinki and Turku, 1964—1969, *Work Environ. Health*, 8, 63, 1971.
121. **Lee, E. E., Goranson, S. S., Enrione, R. E., and Morgan, G. B.,** National Air Surveillance Cascade Impactor Network. II. Size distribution measurements of trace metal components, *Environ. Sci. Technol.*, 6, 1025, 1972.
122. **Tabor, E. C. and Warren, W. V.,** Distribution of certain metals in the atmosphere of some American cities, *AMA Arch. Ind. Health*, 17, 145, 1958.
123. **Oana, S.,** Volcanic gases and sublimates from Showashinzan, *Bull. Volcanol.*, 24, 49, 1962.

124. **Lantzy, R. J. and Mackenzie, F. T.,** Atmospheric trace metals: global cycles and assessment of man's impact, *Geochim. Cosmochim. Acta,* 43, 511, 1979.
125. **Byrd, J. T. and Andrea, M. O.,** Tin and methyltin species in sea water: concentration and fluxes, *Science,* 218, 565, 1982.
126. **Smith, J. C. and Schwarz, K.,** A controlled environmental system for new trace element deficiencies, *J. Nutr.,* 93, 182, 1967.
127. **Piver, W. T.,** Organotin compounds: industrial application and biological investigation, *Environ. Health Perspect.,* 4, 61, 1973.
128. **Yngve, V.,** Stabilized Vinyl Resins, U.S. Patent 2219463, 1940.
129. **Yngve, V.,** Stabilized Artificial Resins, U.S. Patent 2307092, 1943.
130. **Russell, J. F.,** Antifouling Uses of Organotins (1960—1981), Libr. Bibliogr. No. 8, International Tin Research Institute, Greenford, U.K., September 1981.
131. **Zedlar, R. J. and Beiter, C. B.,** Organotins: Biological Activity and Uses Soap and Chemical Specialities, International Tin Research Institute, Greenford, U.K., March 1962.
132. **Tobias, R. S.,** Bonded organometallic cations in aqueous solutions and crystals, *Organomet. Chem. Rev.,* 1, 93, 1966.
133. **Blunden, S. J. and Chapman, A. H.,** The environmental degradation of organotin compounds — a review, *Environ. Tech. Lett.,* 3, 267, 1982.
134. **Blunden, S. J. and Chapman, A. H.,** A Review of the Degradation of Organotin Compounds in the Environment and Their Determination in Water, Int. Tin Res. Inst. Rep. No. 626, International Tin Research Institute, Greenford, U.K., 1983.
135. **Pettine, M., Millero, F. J., and Macchi, G.,** Hydrolysis of tin (II) in aqueous solutions, *Anal. Chem.,* 53, 1039, 1981.
136. **Plazzogna, G., Peruzzo, V., and Rossetto, G.,** The acid cleavage of mixed alkyltin (IV) compounds, *Inorg. Chim. Acta Lett.,* 31, L395, 1978.
137. **Tobias, R. S.,** Organotin (IV) ions in aqueous media, in Proc. Organotin Workshop, Good, M., Ed., New Orleans, La., February 17 to 19, 1978.
138. **Slesinger, A. E.,** The Safe Disposal of Organotins in Soils, M & T Chemicals, Rahway, N.J., 1979.
139. **Barnes, R. D., Bull, A. T., and Poller, R. C.,** Studies on the persistence of the organotin fungicide fentin acetate (triphenyltin acetate) in the soil and surfaces exposed to light, *Pestic. Sci.,* 4, 305, 1973.
140. **Cardarelli, N. F.,** *Controlled Releases Molluscicides,* University of Akron, Akron, Ohio, May 1977.
141. **Barug, D. and Vonk, J. W.,** Studies on the degradation of bis(tributyltin) oxide in soil, *Pestic. Sci.,* 11, 77, 1980.
142. **Orsler, R. J. and Holland, G. E.,** Degradation of tributyltin oxide by fungal culture filtrates, *Int. Biodeterior. Bull.,* 18, 95, 1982.
143. **Olson, G. J., Iverson, W. P., and Brinckman, F. E.,** Biodetermination of Standard Reference Materials, Bur. Stand. Doc. No. NBSIR 81-2246, National Bureau of Standards, Washington, D.C., April 1981.
144. **Sherman, L. R. and Jackson, J. C.,** Tri-n-butyltin fluoride as a controlled-release mosquito larvicide, in *Controlled Release of Pesticides and Pharmaceuticals,* Lewis, D. H., Ed., Plenum Press, New York, 1981, 287.
145. **DeGiacomo, R.,** The determination of tin in foodstuffs by means of Dithiol, *Analyst (London),* 65, 216, 1940.
146. **Fox, H. M. and Ramage, H.,** A spectrographic analysis of animal tissue, *Proc. R. Soc. Ser. B,* 108, 157, 1931.
147. **Fox, H. M. and Ramage, H.,** Spectrographic analysis of animal tissue, *Nature,* 126, 682, 1930.
148. **Fox, H. M. and Ramage, H.,** Elements present in animal tissue, *Nature,* 126, 883, 1930.
149. **Ramage, H.,** Spectrographic chemical analysis, *Nature,* 123, 601, 1929.
150. **Cholak, J.,** Quantitative spectrographique determination of lead in biological material, *Ind. Eng. Chem. Anal. Ed.,* 1, 287, 1935.
151. **Cholak, J. and Story, R. V.,** Spectrographic analysis of biological materials — lead, tin, aluminum, copper, and silver, *Ind. Eng. Chem.,* 10, 619, 1938.
152. **Butt, E. M., Nusbaum, R. E., Gilmour, T. C., and DiDio, S. L.,** Use of emission spectrograph for study of inorganic elements in human tissue, *Am. J. Clin. Pathol.,* 24, 385, 1954.
153. **Blasius, M. B., Kerkhoff, S. J., Wright, R. S., and Cothern, C. R.,** Use of X-ray fluorescence to determine trace metals in water resources, *Water Resour. Bull.,* 8, 704, 1972.
154. **Gofman, J. W., de Lalla, O. F., Kovich, E. L., Lowe, O., Martin, W., Piluso, D. L., Tandy, R. K., and Upham, B. S.,** Chemical elements of the blood of man, *Arch. Environ. Health,* 8, 105, 1964.
155. **Chamberlain, B. R. and Leech, R. J.,** Determination of microgram quantities of tin (IV) by a combined ion exchange/X-ray fluorescence technique, *Talanta,* 14, 597, 1967.
156. **Capacho-Delgado, L. and Manning, D. C.,** Determination of tin by atomic absorption spectroscopy, *Spectrochim. Acta,* 22, 1505, 1966.

157. **Dogan, S. and Haerdi, W.,** Determination of total tin in environmental biological and water samples by atomic absorption spectrometry with graphite furnace, *Int. J. Environ. Anal. Chem.*, 8, 249, 1980.
158. **Maher, W.,** Measurement of total tin in marine organisms by stannane generation and atomic absorption spectrometry, *Anal. Chim. Acta*, 138, 365, 1982.
159. **Maguire, R. J. and Huneault, H.,** Determination of butyltin species in water by gas chromatography with flame photometric detection, *J. Chromatogr.*, 109, 458, 1981.
160. **Jackson, J. A., Blair, W. R., Brinckman, F. E., and Iverson, W. P.,** Gas-chromatographic speciation of methylstannanes in the Chesapeake Bay using purge and trap sampling with tin-selective detector, *Environ. Sci. Technol.*, 16, 110, 1982.
161. **Kompulainen, J. and Koivistoinen, P.,** Advances in tin compound analysis with special reference to organotin pesticide residues, *Residue Rev.*, 66, 1, 1977.
162. **Blair, W. R., Parris, G. E., Iverson, W. P., and Brinckman, F. E.,** Advances in the speciation of trace organotin compounds in aqueous environments, in Proc. Int. Controlled Release Symp., Cardarelli, N. F., Ed., University of Akron, Akron Ohio, September 13 to 15, 1976, 8.
163. **Brinckman, F. E., Blair, W. R., and Parks, S. J.,** Current practice and prospects for speciation of trace organotins in aqueous media, in Organotin Workshop Rep., Good, M., Ed., New Orleans, La., February 17 to 19, 1978.
164. **Horwitz, W.,** Commonly used methods of analysis for tin in foods, *J. Assoc. Off. Anal. Chem.*, 62, 1251, 1979.
165. **Analytical Methods Committee,** The determination of small amounts of tin in organic matter, *Analyst (London)*, 92, 320, 1967.
166. **Lowry, R. R. and Tinsley, I. J.,** Determination of tin salts in fats, *J. Am. Oil Chem. Soc.*, 49, 508, 1972.
167. **Bennett, R. L. and Smith, H. A.,** Spectrophotometric determination of tin with phenylfluorene, *Anal. Chem.*, 31, 1441, 1959.
168. **Thompson, M. H. and McClellan, G.,** Residues in food. The determination of microgram quantities of tin in foods, *J. Assoc. Off. Anal. Chem.*, 45, 979, 1962.
169. **Smith, J. D.,** The spectrophotometric determination of microgram amounts of tin with phenylfluorene, *Analyst (London)*, 95, 347, 1970.
170. **Peterson, P. J., Burton, M. A. S., Gregson, M., Nye, S. M., and Porter, E. K.,** Tin in plants and surface waters in Malaysian ecosystems, in *Trace Substances in Environmental Health*, Vol. 10, Hemphill, D. D., Ed., University of Missouri, Columbia Press, 1976, 123.
171. **Svoboda, V. and Chromy, V.,** Reactions of metallchronic indicators on micelles. III. Spectrophotometric determination of minute amounts of lanthanum with xylenol orange, *Talanta*, 13, 237, 1966.
172. **Kulkarni, W. H. and Good, M. L.,** Phenylfluorene method for the determination of tin in submicrogram levels with cetyltrimethylammonium bromide, *Anal. Chem.*, 50, 973, 1978.
173. **Filer, T. D.,** Fluorometric determination of submicrogram quantities of tin, *Anal. Chem.*, 43, 1753, 1971.
174. **Godar, E. M. and Alexander, O. R.,** Polarographic determination of tin in foods and biological materials, *Ind. Eng. Chem. Anal. Ed.*, 18, 681, 1946.
175. **Hamaguchi, H. and Kuroda, R.,** Tin: isotopes in nature, in *Handbook of Geochemistry*, Springer-Verlag, Berlin, 1969, 50B-1.
176. **Danielson, A. and Steinnes, E.,** A study of some selected trace elements in normal and cancerous tissue by neutron activation analysis, *J. Nucl. Med.*, 11, 260, 1970.
177. **Maletskos, C. J. and Tang, C. W.,** Multiple element trace analysis of human tissues by neutron activation after removal of ^{24}Na and ^{42}K, *Phys. Med. Biol.*, 15, 155, 1970.
178. **Leddicotte, G. W.,** Activation analysis of the biological trace elements, *Methods Biochem. Anal.*, 19, 345, 1971.
179. **Bertine, K. K. and Goldberg, E. D.,** Fossil fuel combustion and major sedimentary cycle, *Science*, 173, 233, 1971.
180. **Zubovic, P., Stadnichenko, T., and Sheffey, N.,** Geochemistry of minor elements in coals of the northern Great Plains coal province, *U.S. Geol. Surv. Bull.*, 1117-A, 1961.
181. **Zubovic, P., Stadnichenko, T., and Sheffey, N. B.,** Distribution of minor elements in coal beds of the eastern Interior Region, *U.S. Geol. Surv. Bull.*, 1117-B, 1964.
182. **Goldschmidt, V. M.,** Rare elements in coal ashes, *Ind. Eng. Chem.*, 27, 1100, 1935.
183. **Jorissen, A.,** Sur la presence du molybdene, du selenium, du bismuth, etc., *Ann. Soc. Geol. Belg.*, 23, 101, 1895/1896.
184. **Goldberg, E. D., Hodge, V. F., Griffin, J. J., and Koide, M.,** Impact of fossil fuel combustion on the sediments of Lake Michigan, *Environ. Sci. Technol.*, 15, 466, 1981.
185. **Gordon, M.,** Trace elements in peat, *Torfnachrichten*, 3, 12, 1953.
186. **Cornec, E.,** Etude spectrographique des cendres de plantes marines, *C. R. Acad. Sci.*, 168, 513, 1919.
187. **LaGrange, R. and Tchakirian, A.,** Sur la determination spectrographique de quelques elements existant en traces dans certaines alques calcaires (*Lithothamnium calcareum*), *C. R. Acad. Sci.*, 209, 58, 1939.

188. **Smith, J. D. and Burton, J. D.,** The occurrence and distribution of tin with particular reference to marine environments, *Geochim. Cosmochim. Acta,* 36, 621, 1972.
189. **Ishii, T.,** Tin in marine algae, *Bull. Jpn. Soc. Sci. Fish.,* 48, 1609, 1982.
190. **Hamaguchi, H. and Kuroda, R.,** Tin: biogeochemistry, in *Handbook of Geochemistry,* Wedepohl, K. H., Ed., Springer-Verlag, Berlin, 1969, 50L-1.
191. **Bowen, J. M.,** *Trace Elements in Biochemistry,* Academic Press, New York, 1966, 241.
192. **Bardyuk, V. V. and Ivashov, P. V.,** The accumulation of trace elements in plants on a tin ore deposit in the southern part of the Soviet Far East, *Tr. Buryat. Inst. Estestv. Nauk, Buryat, Fil. Sib. Otd. Akad. Nauk SSSR,* 2, 83, 1969.
193. **Sarosiek, J. and Klys, B.,.** Badania and zawartoscle cyny w roslinach i glebie Sudetow, *Acta Soc. Bot. Pol.,* 31, 737, 1962.
194. **Dubrovolskii, V. V.,** Distribution of trace elements between the soil forming ground layer, soil, and vegetation under conditions of the Moscow region, *Nauchn. Dokl. Vyssh. Shk. Biol. Nauki,* 3, 193, 1963.
195. **Glazovskaya, M. A.,** Biological cycle of elements in various landscape zones of the Urals, *Fiz. Khim. Biol. Miner. Pochv. SSSR,* p. 148, 1964; *Chem. Abstr.,* 62, 4562.
196. **Sainsbury, C. L., Hamilton, J. C., and Huffman, C.,** Geochemical cycle of selected trace elements in the tin-tungsten-beryllium district, western Seward Peninsula, Alaska, A reconnaissance study, *U.S. Geol. Surv. Bull.,* 1242-F, 1968.
197. **Lazar, V. A. and Beeson, K. G.,** Mineral nutrients in native vegetation on Atlantic Coastal Plain soil types, *J. Agric. Food Chem.,* 4, 439, 1956.
198. **Rao, A. L. S.,** Distribution of trace elements in biological material, *J. Indian Chem. Soc.,* 17, 351, 1940.
199. **Robinson, W. O. and Edgington, G.,** Minor elements in plants and some accumulator plants, *Soil Sci.,* 60, 15, 1945.
200. **Bertrand, G. and Medigreceanu, F.,** Recherches sur la presence du manganese dans la serie animale, *Ann. Inst. Pasteur,* 27, 282, 1913.
201. **Warren, H. V., Delavault, R. E., and Irish, R. I.,** Biogeochemical investigations in the Pacific Northwest, *Bull. Geol. Soc. Am.,* 63, 435, 1952.
202. **Bertrand, G. and Medigreceanu, F.,** Recherches sur la presence et al repartition du manganese dans les organes des animaux, *Bull Soc. Chim. (Paris),* 2, 857, 1912.
203. **Wallihan, E. F.,** Chemical composition of leaves in different parts of sugar maple trees, *J. For.,* 42, 684, 1944.
204. **Prince, A. L.,** Influence of soil types on the mineral composition of corn tissues as determined spectrographically, *Soil Sci.,* 83, 599, 1957.
205. **McHargue, J. S. and Roy, W. R.,** Mineral and nitrogen content of the leaves of some forest trees at different times in the growing season, *Bot. Gaz.,* 94, 381, 1932.
206. **Hou, H. and Merkle, F. G.,** Chemical composition of certain calcifugous and calcicolous plants, *Soil Sci.,* 69, 471, 1950.
207. **Bradford, G. R. and Harding, R. B.,** A survey of microelements in leaves of forty-three high producing orange orchards in southern California, *Proc. Am. Soc. Hortic. Sci.,* 70, 252, 1957.
208. **Forchhammer, J. G.,** Ueber den Einfluss des Kochsalzes auf die Bildung der Mineralien, *Ann. Phys. U. Chem.,* 95, 60, 1855.
209. **Sarosiek, J. and Klys, B.,** Observations on the tin content of the plants and soils of the Sudetes, *Acta Soc. Bot. Pol.,* 31, 737, 1962.
210. **Nagata, M.,** Spectrochemical analysis of minute quantities of metals in plant materials. II, *J. Chem. Soc. Jpn.,* 72, 344, 1951.
211. **Peterson, P. J.,** Unusual accumulation of elements by plants and animals, *Sci. Prog. (Oxford),* 59, 505, 1971.
212. **Nagata, M.,** Spectrographic analysis of minute quantities of metals in plant materials. I, *J. Chem. Soc. Jpn.,* 70, 410, 1949.
213. **Mitchell, R. L.,** Trace elements in some constituent species of moorland grazing, *J. Br. Grassl. Soc.,* 9, 301, 1954.
214. **Harbough, J. W.,** Biogeochemical investigations in the Tri-State district, *Econ. Geol.,* 45, 548, 1950.
215. **Hanna, W. J. and Grant, C. L.,** Spectrochemical analysis of the foliage of certain trees and ornamentals for 23 elements, *Bull. Torrey Bot. Club,* 89, 293, 1962.
216. **Hadzimicev, P.,** Natural content of heavy metals (copper, zinc, tin) in foods from the vegetable belt around Sofia, Khranit, *Khranitelna Promishlenost,* 20, 18, 1971.
217. **Gaddum, L. W. and Rogers, L. H.,** A Study of Some Trace Elements in Fertilizer Materials, Rep. Fla. Agric. Exp. Stn., No. 290, University of Florida, Gainesville, 1936, 13.
218. **Roberts, J. A. and Gaddum, L. W.,** Citrus fruit juices, *Ind. Eng. Chem.,* 29, 574, 1937.
219. **Brechpott, R.,** Determination spectrographique de certains elements mineurs dans la betterave sucriere, *Agricultura,* 38, 115, 1936.

220. **Hodgekiss, W. S. and Errington, B. J.**, Spectrographic investigations of minor elements in hay and grain mixtures, *Trans. Ky. Acad. Sci.*, 9, 17, 1941.
221. **Gmelin, J. F.**, *Allgemeine Geschichte der Pflanzengifte*, Vol. 3, Gabriel Nicohaus Raspe Publishing, Nurnberg, 1777, 151.
222. **Orfila, M.**, *Traite des Poisons*, Vol. 2, Chez Crochard, Paris, 1826, 720.
223. **Hall, F. P.**, On the action of certain vegetable acids on lead and tin, *Am. Chem. J.*, 4, 440, 1878.
224. **Henner, O.**, On the occurrence of tin in articles of food and drink, and on the physiological action of tin compounds, *Analyst (London)*, p. 218, 1880.
225. **Sedgewick, L. W.**, Noxious salts of tin in fruits prepared in tin vessels, *Lancet*, 1, 1129, 1888.
226. **Luff, A. P. and Metcalf, J. H.**, Four cases of tin poisoning caused by tinned cherries, *Br. Med. J.*, 1, 833, 1890.
227. **Weber, H. A.**, On the occurrence of tin in canned foods, *J. Am. Chem. Soc.*, 13, 200, 1891.
228. **Campbell, W. A.**, Tin poisoning, *Ther. Gaz.*, 9, 152, 1893.
229. **Warburton, S., Udler, W., Ewerts, R. M., and Haynes, W. S.**, Outbreak of foodborne illness attributed to tin, *Public Health Rep. (Washington)*, 77, 798, 1962.
230. **Lehman, K. B.**, Untersuchungen uber die Hygienische Bedeutung des Zinns, Insbesondere in Konserven, *Arch. Hyg. (München)*, 45, 88, 1902.
231. **Calvary, H. O.**, Trace elements in food, *Food Res.*, 7, 313, 1942.
232. **Duke, J. A.**, Ethnobotanical observations on the Choco' Indians, *Econ. Bot.*, 23, 344, 1970.
233. **Boyd, T. C. and De, N. K.**, Some applications of the spectroscope in medical research, *Indian J. Med. Res.*, 20, 789, 1933.
234. **Schroeder, H. A., Balassa, J. J., and Tipton, I. H.**, Abnormal trace metals in man: tin, *J. Chronic Dis.*, 17, 483, 1964.
235. **Kent, N. L.**, The occurrence of lead, tin, and silver in wheat and its milling products, *J. Soc. Chem. Ind.*, 61, 183, 1942.
236. **Zook, E. G., Greene, F. E., and Morris, E. R.**, Nutrient composition of selected wheats and wheat products. VI. Distribution of manganese, copper, nickel, zinc, magnesium, lead, tin, cadmium, chromium, and selenium as determined by absorption spectroscopy and colorimetry, *Cereal Chem.*, 47, 720, 1970.
237. **Chisaka, H., Tanizaki, Y., and Nagatsuka, S.**, Studies on determination of tin and poisonous trace elements in canned juices by neutron activation analysis, *Radioisotopes*, 22, 247, 1973.
238. **Beeson, K. C., Griffitts, W. R., and Milne, D. B.**, Tin, in *Geochemistry and the Environment*, Vol. 2, National Academy of Sciences, Washington, D. C., 1977, 88.
239. **Hutner, S. H.**, Inorganic nutrition, *Annu. Rev. Microbiol.*, 26, 313, 1972.
240. **Porutskii, G. E., Golovchenko, V. P., and Cherednichenko, S. V.**, Content of trace elements in various plant organs, *Dokl Akad. Nauk SSSR*, 146, 1223, 1962.
241. **De Groot, A. P., Feron, V. J., and Till, H. P.**, Short term toxicity studies on some salts and oxides of tin in rats, *Food Cosmet. Toxicol.*, 11, 19, 1973.
242. **Wong, P. T. S., Chau, Y. K., Dramar, O., and Bengert, C. A.**, Structure-toxicity relationship of tin compounds on algae, *Can. J. Fish. Aquat. Sci.*, 39, 483, 1982.
243. **Dack, G. M.**, *Food Poisoning*, University of Chicago Press, Chicago, 1965.
244. **Orfila, M.**, *Traite Des Poisons*, Vol. 1, 3rd ed., Gabon & Crockard, Paris, 1826, 551.
245. **Gough, L. P., Shacklette, H. T., and Case, A. A.**, Element concentrations toxic to plants, animals and man, *U.S. Geol. Surv. Bull.*, 1466, 80, 1979.
246. **Pedley, F. G.**, Chronic poisoning by tin and its salts, *J. Ind. Hyg.*, 9, 43, 1927.
247. **Goss, B. C.**, Absorption of tin by proteins and its relation to the solution of tin by canned foods, *J. Ind. Eng. Chem.*, 9, 144, 1917.
248. **Goss, B. C.**, Inhibition of digestion of proteins by absorbed tin, *J. Biol. Chem.*, 30, 53, 1917.
249. **Micheels, H.**, Etudes diverses sur le stimulants de la nutrition chez les plantes, *Rev. Sci. (Paris)*, 5, 427, 1906.
250. **Young, R. S.**, Certain Rarer Elements in Soils and Fertilizers, and Their Rate in Plant Growth, Cornell Univ. Agric. Exp. Stn., Memoir 174, April 1935, 3.
251. **Allison, R. V., Bryan, O. C., and Hunter, J. H.**, The stimulation of plant response on the raw peat soils of the Florida Everglades through the use of copper sulfate and other chemicals, *Fla. Agric. Exp. Stn. Bull.*, 190, 33, 1927.
252. **Vanselow, A. P.**, Unpublished results; cited in Wallihan, E. F., Tin, in *Diagnostic Criteria for Plants and Soils*, University of California Press, Riverside, 1966, 476.
253. **Dostal, A.**, The occurrence of tin in various constituents of living environment, *Cs. Hyg.*, 23, 231, 1978.
254. **Kroller, E.**, Triphenyzinnverbindungen im Pflanzenschutz und ihre Ruckstands-bestimmung, *Dtsch. Lebensm. Rundsch.*, 56, 190, 1960.
255. **Yamada, J., Tatsuguchi, K., and Watanabe, T.**, Uptake of tripropyltin chloride by *Escherichia coli*, *Agric. Biol. Chem.*, 42, 1867, 1978.

256. **Watling, A. S., and Selwyn, M. J.,** Effect of some organometallic compounds on the permeability of chloroplast membranes, *FEBS Lett.*, 10, 139, 1970.
257. **Curtin, G. C., King, H. D., and Mosier, E. L.,** Movement of elements into the atmosphere from coniferous trees in subalpine forests of Colorado and Idaho, *J. Geochem. Explor.*, 3, 245, 1974.
258. **Bowen, V. T. and Sutton, D.,** Mineral constituents of marine sponges. I. The genera *Dysidea Chondrilla Terplos, J. Mar. Res.*, 10, 153, 1951.
259. **Maher, W.,** Measurement of total tin in marine organisms by stannane generation and atomic absorption spectrometry, *Anal. Chim. Acta*, 138, 365, 1982.
260. **Nichols, C. D., Curl, H., and Bowen, V. T.,** Spectrographic analysis of marine plankton, *Limnol. Oceanogr.*, 4m 472, 1959.
261. **Noddack, I. and Noddack, W.,** Der Haufigkeiten der Schwermetalle in Meerestieren, *Ark. Zool.*, 32A, 1, 1939.
262. **Orton, J. H.,** An Account of Investigations into the Cause or Causes of the Unusual Mortality Among Oysters in English Oyster Beds During 1920 and 1921, *Fish. Invest.*, 6, Rep. No. 3, 1924.
263. **Petkovich, T. A.,** Elemental chemical composition of bone tissue of Black Sea plankton-feeding and benthos-feeding fishes, *Dopov. Akad. Nauk Ukr. RSR Ser. B*, 2, 142, 1967.
264. **Petkovich, T. A.,** On the chemical elemental composition of the plankton-eating fish of the Black Sea, *Gidrobiol. Zh.*, 1, 53, 1965.
265. **Zore, V. A. and Tichonova, E. I.,** Simultaneous spectral determination of lead, copper, and tin in fresh fish and some preserves, *Gig. Sanit.*, 28, 58, 1963.
266. **Webb, D. A.,** Studies on the ultimate composition of biological materials. II. Spectrographic analysis of marine vertibrates with special reference to the chemical composition of the environment, *Sci. Proc. R. Dublin Soc.*, 21, 505, 1937.
267. **Arrhenius, G., Bramlette, M. N., and Picciotto, E.,** Localization of radioactive and stable heavy metal nuclides in ocean sediments, *Nature*, 180, 85, 1957.
268. **Tong, S. S. C., Youngs, W. D., Gutenmann, W. H., and Lisk, D. J.,** Trace metals in Lake Cayuga lake trout *Salvelinus mamaycush* in relation to age, *J. Fish. Res. Board Can.*, 31, 238, 1974.
269. **Menke, A.,** Tin in canned food, *Chem. News*, 38, 971, 1878.
270. **Gunther, T.,** Kurzere mittheilung aus der Praxis, *Z. Unter. Nahr. Genussm.*, 2, 915, 1899.
271. **Wirthle, F.,** Ueber den Zinngehalt von Fleisch-conserven, wie einige Bemerkungen uber die Zinnbestimmung uber die Verbindungsform in welcher das Zinn in Fleisch-conserven verkommen kann, *Chem. Ztg.*, 24, 263, 1900.
272. **Fox, H. M. and Ramage, H.,** Elements present in animal tissue, *Nature*, 126, 883, 1930.
273. **Fox, H. M. and Ramage, H.,** A spectrographic analysis of animal tissue, *Proc. R. Soc. Ser. B.*, 108, 157, 1931.
274. **Bertrand, G. and Ciurea, V.,** L'etain dans l'organisms des animaux, *C. R. Acad. Sci.*, 192, 780, 1931.
275. **Mitteldorf, A. J. and Landon, D. O.,** spectrochemical determinations of mineral element of beef, *Anal. Chem.*, 24, 469, 1952.
276. **Lowater, F. and Murray, M. M.,** Chemical composition of teeth. V. Spectrographic analysis, *Biochem. J.*, 31, 837, 1937.
277. **Milne, D. B., Schwarz, K., and Sognnaes, R. F.,** Effect of newer essential trace elements on rat incisor pigmentation, *Fed. Proc. Fed. Am. Soc. Exp. Biol.*, 31, 700, 1972.
278. **Dingle, H. and Sheldon, J. H.,** Spectrographic examination of the mineral content of human and other milk, *Biochem. J.*, 32, 1078, 1938.
279. **Herok, J. and Gotte, H.,** Radiometric analysis of triphenyltin acetate in the metabolism of plants and animals, *Int. J. Appl. Radiat. Isot.*, 14, 461, 1963.
280. **Russoff, L. L. and Gaddum, L. W.,** Trace element content of the new born rat as determined spectroscopically, *J. Nutr.*, 15, 169, 1938.
281. **Flinn, F. B. and Inouye, J. M.,** Metals in our foods, *J.A.M.A.*, 90, 1010, 1928.
282. **Masters, J. and Sherman, L. R.,** Determining the Difference in Tin Concentrations between New York Medical College and University of Scranton Rats and Mice, unpublished, 1984.
283. **Masters, J. G.,** Tin-Time profile in the Thymus Gland, B.S. thesis, University of Scranton, Scranton, Pa., February 10, 1985.
284. **Bilgicer, K. I.,** Analysis of Tin in Mouse and Human Organs, B.S. thesis, University of Scranton, Scranton, Pa., June 1983.
285. **Misk, E.,** L'etain dans l'organisme humain, *C.R. Seances Acad. Sci.*, 176, 138, 1923.
286. **Anspaugh, L. R., Robinson, W. C., Martin, W. H., and Lowe, E. A.,** Compilation of Published Information on Elemental Concentrations in Human Organs in Both Normal and Diseased States, Rep. UCRL 51013, Part 2, Lawrence Livermore Laboratory, University of California, Livermore, 1971.
287. **Anspaugh, L. R., Robinson, W. C., Martin, S. H., and Lowe, O. A.,** Compilation of Published Information on Elemental Concentrations in Human Organs in Both Normal and Diseased States, Rep. UCRL 51013, Part 3, Lawrence Livermore Laboratory, University of California, Livermore, 1971.

288. **Anspaugh, L. R., Robinson, W. C., Martin, W. H., and Lowe, O. A.**, Compilation of Published Information on Elemental Concentrations in Human Organs in Both Normal and Diseased States, Rep. UCRL 51013, Part 1, Lawrence Livermore Laboratory, University of California, Livermore, 1971.
289. **Avtandilov, G. G.**, Trace element content in normal and atherosclerotic portions of the human aorta in connection with age, *Arch. Pathol.*, 29, 40, 1967.
290. **Geldmacher-von Mallinckrodt, M. and Pooth, M.**, Spontaneous determination of 25 metals and metalloids in biological materials, *Arch. Toxicol.*, 25, 5, 1969.
291. **Hamilton, E. I., Minski, M. J., and Cleary, J. J.**, The concentration and distribution of some stable elements in healthy human tissues from the United Kingdom. An environmental study, *Sci. Total Environ.*, 1, 341, 1972/1973.
292. **Kehoe, R. A., Cholak, J., and Story, R. V.**, A spectrochemical study of the normal ranges of concentration of certain trace metals in biological materials, *J. Nutr.*, 19, 579, 1940.
293. **Koch, H. J., Smith, E. R., Shimp, N. F., and Connor, J.**, Analysis of trace elements in human tissue. I. Normal tissue, *Cancer*, 9, 499, 1956.
294. **Pearlman, R. S., Hefferren, J. J., and Lyon, H. W.**, Determination of tin in enamel and dentine by atomic absorption spectroscopy, *J. Dent. Res.*, 49, 1437, 1970.
295. **Scott, G. H. and McMillan, J. H.**, Spectrographic analysis of human spinal fluid, *Proc. Soc. Exp. Biol. (N.Y.)*, 35, 287, 1938.
296. **Tipton, I. H. and Shafer, J. J.**, Statistical analysis of lung trace element levels, *Arch. Environ. Health*, 8, 59, 1964.
297. **Tipton, I. H. and Cook, M. J.**, Trace elements in human tissue. II. Adult subjects from the United States, *Health Phys.*, 99, 103, 1963.
298. **Schryver, S. B.**, Some investigations on the toxicology of tin, with special reference to the metallic contamination of canned food, *J. Hyg.*, 9, 253, 1909.
299. **Lunde, G. and Mathiesen, E.**, The nutritive value of canned foods, *Tidskr. Hermetikinol.*, 7/8, 1, 1937.
300. **Datta, M. C.**, Metallic contamination of foodstuffs, *Indian J. Med. Res.*, 28, 451, 1940.
301. **Perry, H. M. and Perry, E. F.**, Normal concentration of some trace metals in human urine: changes produced by ethylene diamine tetraacetate, *J. Clin. Invest.*, 38, 1452, 1959.
302. **Calloway, D. H. and McMullen, J. J.**, Fecal excretion of iron and tin by men fed stored canned foods, *Am. J. Clin. Nutr.*, 18, 1, 1966.
303. **Tipton, I. H., Stewart, P. L., and Martin, P. G.**, Trace elements in diets and excretia, *Health Phys.*, 12, 1683, 1966.
304. **Hamilton, E. I., Minski, M. J., Cleary, J. J., and Halsey, V. S.**, Comments upon the chemical elements present in evaporated milk for consumption by babies, *Sci. Total Environ.*, 1, 205, 1972.
305. **Sherman, L. R., Bilgicer, K. I., and Cardarelli, N. F.**, Analysis of tin in mouse and human organs, *J. Nutr. Growth Cancer*, 2, 107, 1985.
306. **Myers, H. M.**, A hypothesis concerning the caries-preventative mechanism of tin, *J. Am. Dent. Assoc.*, 77, 1308, 1968.
307. **Bowes, J. H. and Murray, M. M.**, The chemical composition of teeth. II. The composition of human enamel and dentine, *Biochem. J.*, 29, 2722, 1935.
308. **Thompson, J. A. J., Sheffer, M. G., Pierce, R. C., Chav, Y. K., Cooney, J. J., Cullen, W. R., and Maguire, R. J.**, Organotin Compounds in the Aquatic Environment: Scientific Criteria for Assessing Their Effects on Environmental Quality, Rep. NRCC No. 22494, National Research Council of Canada, Ottawa, 1985.
309. **Nielsen, F. H. and Sandstead, H. H.**, Are nickel, vanadium, silicon, fluorine and tin essential for man? a Review, *Am. J. Clin. Nutr.*, 27, 515, 1974.
310. **Hutchinson, G. E.**, The influence of the environment, *Proc. Natl. Acad. Sci. U.S.A.*, 54, 930, 1964.

Chapter 2

THE SCARCITY OF TUMORS IN ANTIQUITY

Michael R. Zimmerman

The discussion of the paleopathologic evidence of cancer is best initiated with a series of definitions. Neoplasm, from *neo,* new, and *plasia,* growth, is a general term for a tissue proliferation, either benign or malignant. The word tumor has come to be synonymous with neoplasm, but formerly meant any swelling, a fact that must be kept in mind when reading the older medical literature. Benign tumors are localized, with no potential for infiltration into surrounding tissues or metastasis, the spread to distant organs. Damage by benign tumors is due to either local pressure effects or, occasionally, the production of hormones. Malignant tumors, cancers, have the potential of metastasis or can kill by rapid local growth and replacement of normal structures. Cancers are subdivided into carcinomas, of epithelial origin (tissues covering the body or lining hollow organs), and sarcomas, of soft tissue origin, including bone. Physicians use a variety of synonyms and euphemisms for cancer, such as malignancy, tumor, mitotic lesion, CA, etc. and avoid the use of the word cancer. Perhaps the mechanism operating here is the same as the ancient Egyptian concept that the word has the same characteristics as the entity itself.

Almost all paleopathologic diagnoses of tumors are gross diagnoses of lesions in skeletal material, and most of these have been benign. An early example is that of a proliferative lesion present on the femur of the 300,000-year-old-type specimen of *Homo erectus* discovered by Dubois in Java in 1891 to 1892. This lesion has been interpreted as either myositis ossificans (a reaction to trauma, with bleeding into and calcification of muscle around the bone) or an osteophyte due to excessive fluorine ingestion,[1] in neither case a true neoplasm. Brothwell[2] describes and illustrates a number of skeletal defects and proliferative lesions, primarily from ancient Egypt and medieval Europe, considered to represent a variety of neoplasms, both benign and malignant. However, he considers his diagnoses "very tentative", with the differential diagnosis primarily consisting of infectious processes. Strouhal,[3] in his studies of Egyptian material dating to the third to fourth centuries A.D., has described a calcified pelvic mass in a middle aged woman, interpreted as a calcified leiomyoma (a benign smooth muscle tumor) of the uterus and a skull with a large central defect, diagnosed as a result of a carcinoma of the posterior nasal cavity. Metastatic malignant melanoma has been diagnosed in a group of ancient Peruvian skeletons,[4] but the authors were unable to confirm the diagnosis by histologic studies.

Only a few microscopic diagnoses of tumors have been in mummified tissues. Two benign tumors were found in Egyptian mummies, Sandison[5] reporting a small squamous papilloma (a skin tag) of the hand and Zimmerman[6] a fibrous histiocytoma (a skin tumor) of the heel. Gerszten[7] has recently demonstrated lipoma (a benign fat tumor) and rhabdomyosarcoma (a malignant tumor of muscle) in two Peruvian mummies. No other tumors, benign or malignant, have been diagnosed histologically, although many other diseases have been described in the hundreds of mummies examined in the 20th century.[8]

There are few references in the literature to the antiquity of cancer. Tumors mentioned in Egyptian papyri have been interpreted as neoplasms by one author,[9] but simply as swellings[4] or possibly varicose veins[10] by others. The ancient Greeks noted the crab-like nature of malignant tumors in the second century A.D.,[11] but the first reports of certain cancers have only been in the relatively recent past. These include cancer of the nasal passages in snuff users in 1761,[12] Hodgkin's disease in 1832,[13] multiple myeloma in 1840,[14] and a variety of occupational tumors in the 18th, 19th and 20th centuries.[15] The late description of these tumors, which have distinctive clinical and/or pathologic features, suggests infrequency of occurrence until the recent past.

Several explanations have been offered for the scarcity of tumors in ancient remains. As noted above, cancer may be a relatively recent disease. Another possible explanation is the early death of individuals in ancient populations, but this statistical construct is influenced by high infant mortality. Many individuals in antiquity did live to an advanced age, developing other diseases of the aged. Atherosclerosis has been demonstrated in Egyptian[16,17] and Alaskan[18] mummies. Paget's disease, a thickening of the bone of obscure etiology found in the elderly, has also been described in an Egyptian mummy,[26] and degenerative joint disease is an almost ubiquitous paleopathologic diagnosis. In addition, it must be remembered that, at least in modern populations, diseases such as leukemia and osteosarcoma (malignant primary bone tumors) occur primarily in the young.

The suggestion has been offered that mummified tumors are not well-enough preserved to allow diagnosis. Certainly the inherent problems of diagnosis are immensely magnified in examining ancient material. Artifacts of decomposition do produce difficulties even in the recognition of normal tissues,[19,20] and diagnosis of cancer is on another level of difficulty. Mummified tissue is rehydrated using Ruffer's solution (water, alcohol, and sodium carbonate).[21] While the rehydrated tissue is processed in the same fashion as fresh tissue, the artifacts of rehydration may be compounded upon those of decomposition and desiccation.

As an approach to these problems, I undertook an experimental study of the effects of mummification on the histology of malignant tumors.[22] The tissues examined were obtained from adult human cadavers undergoing postmortem examination, all within 24 hr after death. Small specimens were selected from tumors, bisected, and one half immediately fixed and processed. The other halves were oven dried at 40°C (104°F) for 7 to 14 days, rehydrated, and processed for microscopic examination, using the standard hematoxylin and eosin stain and a number of special stains. To limit observer bias, the slides were numerically coded and not examined for several weeks to months. The slides of the mummified tissues were examined first, diagnosed, and then compared to the control, fresh tissue slides.

Both primary and metastatic tumors were found to be quite well preserved. One of the most common tumors in modern industrial populations is carcinoma of the lung. A mummified small cell carcinoma showed excellent preservation of the typical darkly stained nuclei and the pattern of replacement of the lung. Carcinoma of the breast showed preservation of the classic infiltrating pattern, although glandular areas were no longer seen. Other tumors included in this study, such as carcinoid tumor and lymphoma, were also well preserved.

Of particular interest, metastatic tumors were often better preserved than the adjacent normal tissues. Examples were malignancies metastatic to the liver from the intestinal tract and an ovarian carcinoma metastatic to the diaphragm in which the characteristic psammoma bodies (microscopic calcified nodules) were easily seen.

This experimental approach produces changes similar to those seen in the tissues of actual mummies. Mummies are not as well preserved, probably because of slower or more erratic desiccation and contamination by microorganisms. The results of this study do permit some general and specific comments and extrapolations to actual mummies.

In general, it can be said that the pattern of replacement of normal structures by tumor, upon which the pathologist depends to a great extent for diagnosis, is well preserved under these conditions of mummification. The nuclei of malignant cells are larger and darker staining than those of normal cells and retain this distinction after mummification and rehydration. Thus, the criteria of malignancy are preserved by mummification, and the paleopathologist should be able to diagnose cancer in mummies. The results of the experimental study would indicate that the virtual absence of reports of cancer in mummies is not owing to any technical difficulty. Such lesions in ancient tissues should be, if anything, better preserved than normal tissues.

In an ancient population, lacking recourse to surgical intervention, pathologic evidence of cancer should be present at death in essentially all cancer cases. Recent statistics indicate that approximately 17% of deaths recorded in the U.S. are attributed to cancer and suggest that the chance of developing cancer over a lifetime is on the order of 25%.[23] The virtual absence of malignancies in ancient tissues can only be interpreted as indicating their extreme rarity in antiquity. It has been estimated, on epidemiologic considerations, that up to 75% of human cancers are related to environmental factors.[24] Paleopathologic studies suggest that such factors are limited to the modern world.

REFERENCES

1. **Soriano, M.,** The fluoric origin of the bone lesion in the *Pithecanthropus erectus* femur, *Am. J. Phys. Anthropol.,* 32, 49, 1970.
2. **Brothwell, D.,** The evidence for neoplasms, in *Diseases in Antiquity,* Brothwell, D. and Sandison, A. T., Eds., Charles C Thomas, Springfield, Ill., 1967, 320.
3. **Strouhal, E.,** Tumors in the remains of ancient Egyptians, *Am. J. Phys. Anthropol.,* 45, 613, 1976.
4. **Urteaga, O. and Pack, G. T.,** On the antiquity of melanoma, *Cancer,* 19, 607, 1966.
5. **Sandison, A. T.,** Diseases of the skin, in *Diseases in Antiquity,* Brothwell, D. and Sandison, A. T., Eds., Charles C Thomas, Springfield, Ill., 1967, 449.
6. **Zimmerman, M. R.,** A possible histiocytoma in an Egyptian mummy, *Arch. Dermatol.,* 117, 364, 1981.
7. **Gerszten, E.,** personal communication, 1984.
8. **Zimmerman, M. R.,** Annotated bibliography of paleopathology, *Trans. Stud. Coll. Physicians Philadelphia,* 2, 41, 112, 187, 289, 1980.
9. **Butterfield, W. C.,** Tumor treatment, 3000 B.C., *Surgery,* 60, 476, 1966.
10. **Majno, G.,** *The Healing Hand: Man and Wound in the Ancient World,* Harvard University Press, Cambridge, Mass., 1975.
11. **Krook, J.,** Man's early challenge to neoplasms, *Minn. Med.,* 52, 1159, 1969.
12. **Redmond, E. D.,** Tobacco and cancer — the first clinical report, 1761, *N. Engl. J. Med.,* 282, 18, 1970.
13. **Holleb, A. I.,** Classics in oncology: Thomas Hodgkin (1798—1866), *Cancer,* 23, 52, 1973.
14. **Clamp, J. R.,** Some aspects of the first recorded case of multiple myeloma, *Lancet,* 2, 1354, 1967.
15. **Shimkin, M. D.,** Some historical landmarks in cancer epidemiology, in *Cancer Epidemiology and Prevention: Current Concepts,* Schottenfeld, D., Ed., Charles C Thomas, Springfield, Ill., 1975, 3.
16. **Shattock, G. S.,** Report on the pathology of King Merneptah, *Lancet,* 1, 319, 1909.
17. **Zimmerman, M. R.,** The mummies of the tomb of Nebwenenef: paleopathology and archeology, *J. Am. Res. Cent. Egypt,* 14, 33, 1977.
18. **Zimmerman, M. R.,** Paleopathology in Alaskan mummies, *Am. Sci.,* 73, 20, 1985.
19. **Evans, W. E. D.,** Some histologic findings in spontaneously preserved bodies, *Med. Sci. Law,* 2, 155, 1962.
20. **Zimmerman, M. R.,** Histologic examination of experimentally mummified tissues, *Am. J. Phys. Anthropol.,* 37, 271, 1972.
21. **Ruffer, M. A.,** *Studies in the Paleopathology of Egypt,* University of Chicago Press, Chicago, 1921.
22. **Zimmerman, M. R.,** An experimental study of mummification pertinent to the antiquity of cancer, *Cancer,* 40, 1358, 1977.
23. **Shottenfeld, D.,** Introduction — the magnitude of cancer, in *Cancer Epidemiology and Prevention: Current Concepts,* Shottenfeld, D., Ed., Charles C Thomas, Springfield, Ill., 1975, 3.
24. **Lilienfeld, A. M., Pedersen, E. and Dowd, J. E.,** *Cancer Epidemiology: Methods of Study,* Johns Hopkins University Press, Baltimore, 1967.

Chapter 3

THE IMPORTANCE OF HYDROGEN BONDING OF ORGANOTINS IN WATER

M. M. Amini, R. W. Taylor, J. J. Zuckerman, and A. L. Rheingold

The importance of organometallics in living organisms[1,2] and in the environment[3-5] is beginning to be recognized. The main group-IV element compounds exhibit biological activity both as medicinals[6-8] and poisons,[9,10] and much interest lies in organotins as potential anticancer agents[11,12] as well as in trying to understand why triorganotin(IV) derivatives are so intensely biocidal.[12-16]

Biology is a watery province, but one that organometallic chemists are taught early to shun.[17] Hence, little information exists on the aqueous behavior of organometallics. Thus, chemical, spectroscopic, and structural data from organic-solvent solution and solid-state studies are often applied to the biological situation where they may be largely irrelevant.

We have been studying by X-ray crystallography the structures of selected organotin(IV) compounds in situations in which hydrogen bonding is possible, and we have noted a remarkable fact. When the potential for hydrogen bonding exists in an organotin(IV) crystal, it dominates the choice of structure. That is, the lattice adopts an arrangement in which hydrogen bonding is maximized, forcing the organotin(IV) moiety to accommodate itself as best it can. This can mean relinquishing a favored for a less-favored bonding partner,[18] adopting a lower coordination number at the tin atom than would otherwise be possible,[19,22] forming a lattice of discrete ions with their charges delocalized by hydrogen bonding rather than the expected, covalently bonded product of a condensation reaction,[20] or the habit of the crystal being determined by the axis of propagation of the hydrogen bonds rather than the axis of tin atom association,[18] or even an 18-crown-6 molecule in a crown-ether derivative adopting an unusual ring conformation with a higher energy sequence of torsional angles.[21,23] We communicate here the results of a direct experimental test of this concept.

Recently, we discovered a new environment for water in an organotin(IV) complex, $\{[(CH_3)_2SnCl_2 \cdot H_2O]_2 \cdot 18\text{-crown-6}\}_n$, **1**. In its formation, the tin moiety captures adventitious moisture to form a hydrogen-bonded lattice rather than coordinate directly to the crown ether. Hydrate formation is a feature of all tin(IV) crown-ether materials whose structures have been authenticated.[24-26] Coordination of the water oxygen atom to tin apparently enhances the propensity for hydrogen bonding, and the water molecules in our structure were found to be five-coordinated through unique, twin, three-center (doubly bifurcated) hydrogen bonds to the crown-ether oxygen atoms. The tin atoms are arranged in the conventionally preferred[27,28] Sn_2Cl_2 dimers through tin-chloride atom bridging.[21]

We now report the structures of two close analogs, $\{[(CH_3)_2SnCl_2 \cdot H_2O]_2 \cdot \text{dicyclohexano-18-crown-6}\}_n$, **2**, and $[(CH_3)_2SnCl_2 \cdot 2 H_2O \cdot 15\text{-crown-5}]_n$, **3**. The first, relative to **1**, has been subjected to a shear force as a result of a ring centroid-ring centroid slippage in the packing of the larger dicyclohexano crown-ether molecules, whereas in **1** the nearly planar rings are stacked in parallel over one another. The result is that the Sn_2Cl_2 dimeric unit in **2** is stretched beyond accepted donor-acceptor bonding distances, while, at the same time, the hydrogen bonding is enhanced (see Figure 1) as shown by a tightening of the contacts with the crown-ether oxygen atoms (see Table 1). The structure contains the second authenticated example of five-coordinated water molecules, and the crown-ether molecule is forced to adopt the same, higher energy ring conformation as in **1**.*

In **3** all semblance of the common[27,28] Sn_2Cl_2 dimer is gone in favor of the addition of a second molecule of water *cis*-coordinated to tin which is hydrogen bonded to a crown-ether ligand of a neighboring asymmetric unit to form an infinite chain of zig-zag units.**

Thus, the interactions with water oxygen atoms and the consequent enhancement of hydrogen bonding must be taken into account in discussing the role of organometallics in biology and the environment.

ACKNOWLEDGMENT

Our work is supported by the Office of Naval Research. Supplementary material available. Listings of atomic coordinates and temperature factors, bond lengths, bond angles, anisotropic temperature factors, and observed and calculated structure factors have been deposited.

---

* Dimethyltin(IV) dichloride crystallizes with dicyclohexano-18-crown-6 (perhydrodibenzo[b,k][1,4,7,10,13,16]hexaoxacyclooctadecane) as a monohydrate, mp 122 to 127°C, $\{[(CH_3)_2\text{-}SnCl_2 \cdot H_2O]_2 \cdot \text{dicyclohexano-18-crown-6}\}_n$, **2**, $C_{24}H_{52}Cl_4O_8Sn_2$, fw 847.96 daltons, in the triclinic space group P$\bar{1}$ with $a = 10.192(1)$, $b = 10.300(1)$, $c = 10.380(2)$ Å, $\alpha = 108.93(1)$, $\beta = 102.22(1)$, $\gamma = 111.25(1)°$, $V = 891.1(2)$ Å^3, $Z = 1$, $\rho_{calcd} = 1.580$ g cm^{-3} and was solved by direct methods (SHELXTL-SOLV) using 3250 unique reflections (5σ cutoff) from 4326 collected (4100 unique) on an R3 Nicolet automated diffractometer (MoKα, $\mu = 17.46$ cm^{-1}, $4° \leq 2\theta \leq 55°$; scan speed 3° min^{-1}) to a final, conventional R value of 5.42% and R_w of 5.33% at 23°C. Corrections for absorption (empirical) and secondary extinction were applied. The final refinement utilized anisotropic thermal parameters for all nonhydrogen atoms; remaining hydrogen atoms were treated as fixed, idealized isotropic contributions. The hydrogen atoms attached to oxygen and carbon were not located. Each water molecule makes four hydrogen-bonded contacts to the oxygen atoms of a crown ether. Each crown-ether molecule makes eight hydrogen-bonded contacts, four on each side. The central pair of oxygen atoms are hydrogen bonded on both sides of the ring. We view the geometry at tin as five coordinated, trigonal bipyramidal with the two methyl groups and one chlorine equatorial and the second chlorine and the water molecule axial. There are inversion centers at the centroid of the crown-ether ring and at the center of the vestigal Sn_2Cl_2 system.

** Dimethyltin(IV) dichloride crystallizes with 15-crown-5 (1,4,7,10,13-pentaoxacyclopentadecane) as a dihydrate, mp 103 to 109°C $\{(CH_3)_2SnCl_2 \cdot 2H_2O \cdot \text{15-crown-5}\}_n$, **3**, $C_{12}H_{30}Cl_2O_7Sn$, fw 475.96 daltons, in the monoclinic space group C2/c with $a = 9.313(2)$, $b = 17.266(3)$, $c = 13.525(3)$ Å, $\beta = 107.37(2)°$, $V = 2075.71$ Å^3, $Z = 4$, $\rho_{calcd} = 1.523$ g cm^{-1} and was solved by direct methods (SHELXTL-SOLV) using 2127 unique reflections (5σ cutoff) from 2565 collected (2386 unique) ($\mu = 16.18$ cm^{-1}) at the same settings and temperature as in Reference 26 to a final, conventional R value of 4.14% and R_w of 4.65%. The same corrections were applied and the same parameters refined as for **2**. The tin atom is six coordinated in a distorted octahedron with *trans*- dimethyltin, but *cis*-SnCl$_2$ and Sn(OH$_2$)$_2$ groups. The 15-crown-5 molecules are disordered; two equally occupied concentric and coplanar rings are staggered to produce ten equally spaced peripheral oxygen atoms with ten superimposed, or nearly superimposed, carbon atoms.

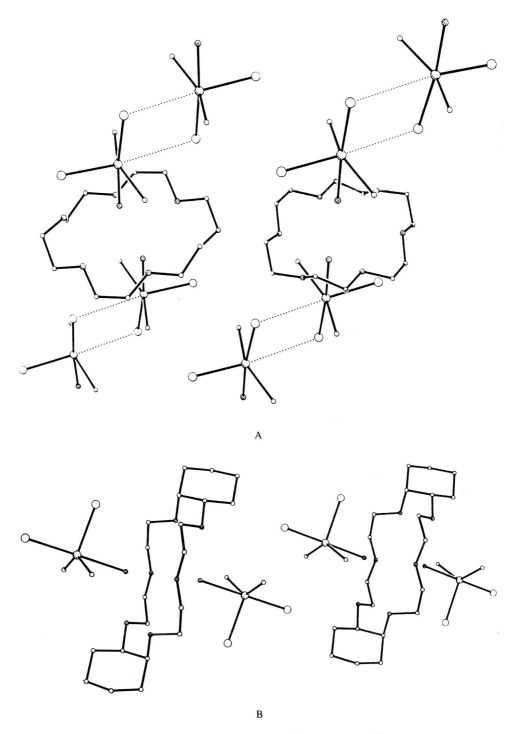

FIGURE 1. Portions of the three lattices (see text) showing in (A) how the network of hydrogen bonds is formed in layers for **1**, in (B) in stacks for **2**, and in (C) in zig-zag chains for **3**. **1** uses six-coordinated octahedral and **2** five-coordinated, trigonal bipyramidal tin monohydrates, while **3** uses an octahedral tin *cis*-dihydrate. In **1**, the octahedral geometry is achieved by long Sn . . . Cl interactions; in **2**, still longer Sn . . . Cl interactions produce very weakly associated Sn-dimer units related by an inversion center. In **3**, the octahedral *cis*-dihydrate structures are independent. Large shaded circles = Sn, large open circles = Cl, small shaded circles = O, and small open circles = C. All oxygen atoms on Sn represent molecules of water. The essential hydrogen bonding occurs between the H atoms of the water molecules and the adjacent ether-oxygen atoms.

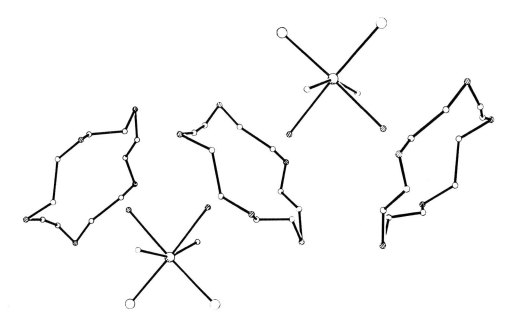

FIGURE 1C

Table 1
HYDROGEN BONDING O . . . O INTERNUCLEAR DISTANCES IN 1, 2, AND 3

18-Crown-6		Dicyclohexano-18-crown-6	
O(5). . .(3)	= 2.976(6)Å	O(1). . .O(3a)	= 2.869(5) Å
	2.950(4)[a]	. . .O(4)	= 2.903(5)
. . . O(4)	= 3.023(7)	. . .O(3)	= 3.087(5)
	2.959(4)[a]	. . .O(2a)	= 3.094(5)
O(6). . .O(1)	= 3.011(6)		
	2.971(3)[a]		
. . .O(2)	= 2.921(6)		
	2.881(4)[a]		

[a] Data collected at −120°C.

From Amini, M. M., Rheingold, A. L., Taylor, R. W., and Zuckerman, J. J., *J. Am. Chem. Soc.*, 106, 7289, 1984. With permission.

REFERENCES

1. **Thayer, J. S.**, *Organometallic Compounds and Living Organisms,* Academic Press, New York, 1984.
2. **Crowe, A. J.**, Organometallics in medicine, *Chem. Ind. (London),* 304, 1983.
3. **Craig, P. J.**, Environmental aspects of organometallic chemistry, in *Comprehensive Organometallic Chemistry,* Vol. 2, Wilkinson, G., Stone, F. G. A., and Abel, E. W., Eds., Pergamon Press, Oxford, 1982, 979.
4. **Zoller, W. H.**, Selenium biomethylation products from soil and sewer sludge, *Science,* 208, 500, 1980.

5. **Brinckman, F. E., Jr. and Bellama, J. M., Eds.,** *Organometals and Organometalloids. Occurrence and Fate in the Environment,* ACS Symp. Ser. No. 82, American Chemical Society, Washington, D.C., 1978.
6. **Zuckerman, J. J.,** Organotin chemistry: a brief primer with comments on organometallic chemotherapy, in *Tin as a Vital Trace Nutrient: Implications in Anticarcinogenesis and Other Physiological Processes,* Cardarelli, N., Ed., CRC Press, Boca Raton, Fla., 1986, ch. 24.
7. **Boschke, F. L., Ed.,** *Bioactive Organo-Silicon Compounds, Topics in Current Chemistry,* Vol. 84, Springer-Verlag, Berlin, 1979.
8. **Voronkov, M. G., Zelchan, G. E., and Lukevits, E. Ya.,** *Kremni i Zhizn* (Silicon and Life), 2nd ed., Zinatne, Riga, 1978.
9. **Ratclife, J. M.,** *Lead in Man and the Environment,* Halsted Press, New York, 1981.
10. **Nriagu, J. O., Ed.,** *Topics in Environmental Health, The Biogeochemistry of Lead,* Vol. 1 (Parts A and B), Ann Arbor Science Publishers, Ann Arbor, Mich., 1978.
11. **Cardarelli, N., Ed.,** *Tin as a Vital Trace Nutrient: Implications in Anticarcinogenesis and Other Physiological Processes,* CRC Press, Boca Raton, Fla., 1986.
12. **Zuckerman, J. J.,** *Tin and Malignant Cell Growth,* CRC Press, Boca Raton, Fla., in press.
13. **Brinckman, F. E., Jr.,** Environmental organotin chemistry today: experiences in the field and laboratory, *J. Organomet. Chem. Libr.,* 12, 343, 1981.
14. **Zuckerman, J. J., Reisdorf, R. P., Ellis, H. V., III, and Wilkinson, R. R.,** Organotins in biology and the environment, in *Organometals and Organometalloids. Occurrence and Fate in the Environment,* Brinckman, F. E., Jr. and Bellama, J. M., Eds., ACS Symp. Seer. No. 82, American Chemical Society, Washington, D.C., 1978, 388.
15. **Aldridge, W. N.,** The biological properties of organogermanium, -tin and -lead compounds, in *The Organometallic and Coordination Chemistry of Germanium, Tin and Lead, Rev. Si, Ge, Tin, Lead Compounds,* 4, 9, 1978.
16. **Zuckerman, J. J., Ed.,** *Organotin Compounds: New Chemistry and Applications,* Adv. Chem. Ser. No. 157, American Chemical Society, Washington, D.C., 1976.
17. **Rochow, E. G.,** Twenty years ago it was possible to state authoritatively, "...there are no organometallic compounds in nature, there seemingly being no mechanism for their formation..." in *Organometallic Chemistry,* Reinhold Publishing, New York, 1964.
18. **Ho, B. Y. K., Molloy, K. C., Zuckerman, J. J., Reidinger, F., and Zubieta, J. A.,** The crystal structure and variable-temperature ^{119}Sn Mössbauer study of trimethyltin glycinate, a one-dimensional, amino-bridged polymer, *J. Organomet. Chem.,* 187, 212, 1980.
19. **Nasser, F. A. K., Hossain, M. B., van der Helm, D., and Zuckerman, J. J.,** Oxy and thio phosphorus acid derivatives of tin. XIV. The crystal and molecular structure of the dimeric di-*O*, phenylmonothiophosphatodiphenyltin(IV) hydroxide, $[HO(C_6H_5)_2SnOP(S)\ (OC_6H_5)_2]_2$, *Inorg. Chem.,* 22, 3107, 1983.
20. **Nasser, F. A. K., Hossain, M. B., van der Helm, D., and Zuckerman, J. J.,** The crystal and molecular structure of dianthranilium amide dimethyltetrachlorotin(IV) dihydrate, $[2\text{-}H_3NC_6H_4\text{-}C(O)NH_2]_2^{2+}[(CH_3)_2SnCl_4]_2^-\mu\text{-}H_2O)_2$ at 138 K. A hydrogen-bonded network lattice, *Inorg. Chem.,* 23, 606, 1984.
21. **Amini, M. M., Rheingold, A. L., Taylor, R. W., and Zuckerman, J. J.,** A new environment for water. The first authenticated example of water molecules engaged in twin, three-center hydrogen bonds. The crystal and molecular structure of $\{[(CH_3)_2SnCl_2\cdot H_2O]_2\cdot 18\text{-crown-}6\}_n$, *J. Am. Chem. Soc.,* 106, 7289, 1984; **Anon.,** Water molecule found in new environment, *Chem. Eng. News,* p.30, November 19, 1984.
22. **Molloy, K. C., Purcell, T. G., Hahn, F. E., Schumann, H., and Zuckerman, J. J.,** Organotin biocides. IV. Crystal and molecular structure of tricyclohexylstannyl 3-indolylacetate, incorporating the first monodentate carboxylate group bonded to a triorganotin(IV), *Organometallics,* 5, 85, 1986.
23. **Dobler, M.,** 18-Krone-6: nur einfaches molekül?, *Chimia,* 38, 415, 1984.
24. **Cussak, P. A., Patel, B. N., and Smith, P. J.,** Synthetic and structural studies of tin(IV) complexes of crown ethers, *J. Chem. Soc. Dalton Trans.,* 1239, 1984.
25. **Valle, G., Cassol, A., and Russo, U.,** Synthesis and X-ray crystal structures of a tin(IV) tetrahalide adduct with a crown ether, *Inorg. Chim. Acta,* 82, 81, 1984.
26. **Valle, G., Ruisi, G., and Russo, U.,** Synthesis and X-ray crystal structure of a dimethyltin(IV) dithiocyanate bihydrate adduct with a crown ether, *Inorg. Chim. Acta,* 99, L21, 1985.
27. **Zubieta, J. A. and Zuckerman, J. J.,** Structural tin chemistry, *Prog. Inorg. Chem.,* 24, 251, 1978.
28. **Smith, P. M.,** A bibliography of X-ray crystal structures of organotin compounds, *J. Organomet. Chem. Libr.,* 12, 97, 1981.

Chapter 4

NEW DEVELOPMENTS IN ANTITUMOR-ACTIVE ORGANOTIN COMPOUNDS

Marcel Gielen, Ludo De Clercq, Rudolph Willem, and Eddie Joosen

TABLE OF CONTENTS

I.	Introduction	40
II.	More Active Organotin Antitumorals by Covalent Targeting?	41
III.	Antitumor Activity of Water-Soluble Organotin Compounds	41
IV.	Antitumor Activity of Cyclodextrin Organotin Inclusion Compounds	42
V.	Antitumor Activity of 1,3-Dioxa-2-Stannacyclo-Pentanes and Hexanes	42
VI.	Conclusion	45
	References	45

I. INTRODUCTION

Besides "*cis*-platin", Cl–Pt(NH$_3$)–NH$_3$ / Cl, several second-generation platinum coordination compounds have been prepared and tested in which either the two NH$_3$ ligands have been replaced by two amines (or by a diamine), or the chloro ligands by other anionic ones like malonato or sulfato or both. In any case, two strong *cis*-Pt–N bonds and two weaker *(cis-)* Pt–X (X = Cl, OR, etc.) bonds seem to be necessary to devise an active compound.[1] The loss of their labile ligands allows the metal subsequently to coordinate, with suitably oriented nitrogenous bases on DNA.[2] Indeed, the antitumor activity of such complexes, as well as that of the metallocene dichlorides, (n^5-C$_5$H$_5$)$_2$MCl$_2$ (with M = Ti, V, Nb, Mo),[3] seems to be dependent upon the Cl–M–Cl bond angle and hence upon the bite (the corresponding nonbonding chlorine-chlorine distance): only those compounds for which this angle is smaller than 95° (giving a bite size of less than 3.6 Å, the upper limit for DNA-metal cross-links) are active. The widespread success of those compounds in the clinical treatment of testicular or ovarian cancers, for instance, has stimulated research in the area of metal-based antitumor drugs and spurred the search for organometallic compounds with improved therapeutic properties. Hollis et al.[4] have prepared several stable platinum complexes of vitamin C, a new group of promising antitumor agents, like the *cis*-1,2-diaminocyclohexane compound (**1**),

1

which have shown good activity in a variety of preclinical antitumor screens, and in which the ascorbate ligand is coordinated to the metal through the C$_2$-carbon atom and the secondary O$_5$-oxygen atom (instead of the two oxygen-binding sites like in the malonates or sulfates).

In general, the organotin compounds of the type R$_2$SnX$_2$, tested until now against P388 lymphocytic leukemia in mice, showed only marginal activity,[5-7] even if almost 50% of the tested diorganotin dihalides do exhibit some activity.[8] However, a T/C value, i.e., the ratio of medium survival times of treated (T) and untreated (C) mice (expressed as a percentage) as high as 198 has been reported for diphenyltin chloride hydroxide,[9] other rather active compounds being the *ortho*-phenanthroline complexes of diethyltin diiodide (T/C = 184%), dibromide (T/C = 176%), and dichloride (T/C = 177%), the 2,2'-bipyridyl complex of (CH$_3$CH$_2$)$_2$Sn(NCS)$_2$ (T/C = 179%), the bis-pyridyl complex of diphenyltin dichloride (T/C = 180%), and the 3,4,7,8-tetramethyl-1,10-phenanthroline complex of diphenyltin dibromide (T/C = 177%). The structure/activity relationship for diorganotin-dihalide complexes is different from that of the metal dihalides in that the Cl–M–Cl bond angles of both active and inactive compounds are all of the same order of magnitude, and that the Sn–N bond lengths appear to determine the antitumor activity:[10] the more stable complexes exhibit lower activities. Those with an average Sn–N bond length larger than 2.39 Å show antitumor activity, whereas those with an average Sn–N bond length smaller than 2.39 Å are inactive. This implies that a predissociation of the (bidentate) nitrogenous ligand might be a crucial step in the formation of a tin-DNA complex.

II. MORE ACTIVE ORGANOTIN ANTITUMORALS BY COVALENT TARGETING?

Following Riess and LeBlanc's suggestion[11] to use perfluoro-chemicals as a vehicle to transport drugs to tumors (they cite the tendency of $C_8F_{17}Br$ to concentrate in the macrophages of malignant tumors as indicative for this), we prepared a series of organotin compounds of the type $[CF_3(CF_2)_5CH_2CH_2]_2SnX_2$ (with X = Cl or Br) and their 2,2'-bipyridyl- and ortho-phenanthroline complexes, using the classical scheme:[12]

$CF_3(CF_2)_5CH_2CH_2MgI - (C_6H_5)_2SnCl_2 / Et_2O \rightarrow$
$[CF_3(CF_2)_5CH_2CH_2]Sn(C_6H_5)_2 - X_2 / CH_3OH/C_6H_6 \rightarrow$
$[CF_3(CF_2)_5CH_2CH_2]SnX_2 - B$ (2,2'-bipyridyl or ortho-phenanthroline) $\rightarrow$
$[CF_3(CF_2)_5CH_2CH_2]SnX_2 \cdot B$

Their in vivo antitumor activity against P388 lymphocytic leukemia in CDF_1 mice was evaluated and showed to be quite low (T/C = 125%) for the uncomplexed dichloro compound, whereas the other compounds were found inactive.

III. ANTITUMOR ACTIVITY OF WATER-SOLUBLE ORGANOTIN COMPOUNDS

In his review paper on antitumor effects of silicon, germanium, tin, and lead compounds,[13] Atassi underlines the fact that all the organotin compounds tested up to now are poorly soluble in water and that this might be the major obstacle to the improvement of their carcinostatic effect. We have prepared some water-soluble organotin compounds,[14] among which are:

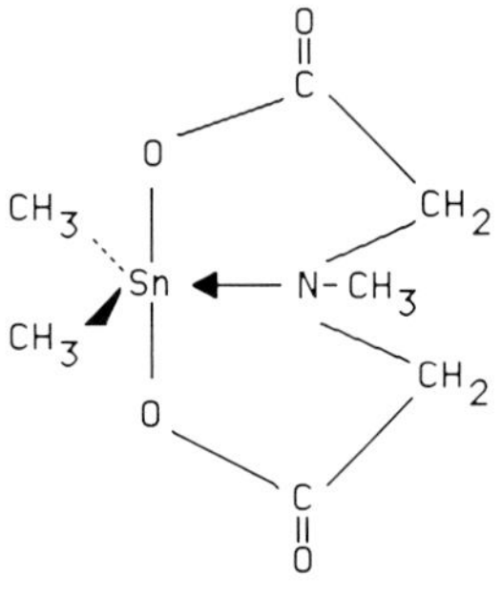

2 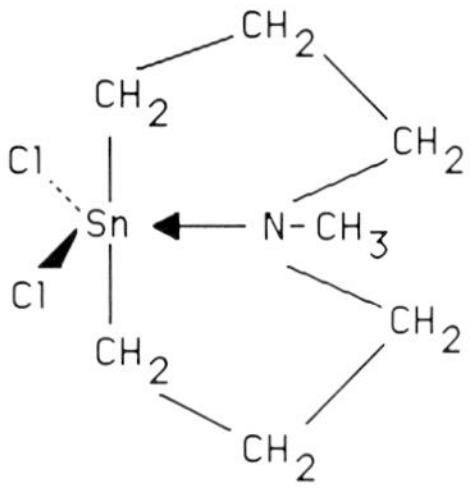   **3**

Unfortunately, for the dimethyl compound (**2**), a T/C value of 122% has been obtained for doses of 30 to 60 mg/kg, whereas the dichloro compound (**3**) showed no activity at all. Another water-soluble intramolecularly coordinated diorganotin dichloride (**4**) has been synthesized, too, and its antitumor activity is now being tested by G. Atassi at the Borget Institute, Brussels, Belgium.

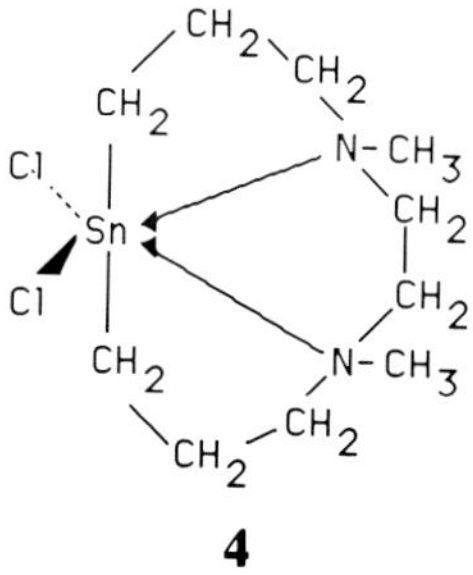

4

These results are somewhat discouraging. However, we are currently preparing other water-soluble diorganotin dihalides containing sugar residues bound to the tin atom, either via oxygen-tin bonds[15] or by a carbon-tin bond (**5**) (**6**) (see also Reference 16), as, for example:

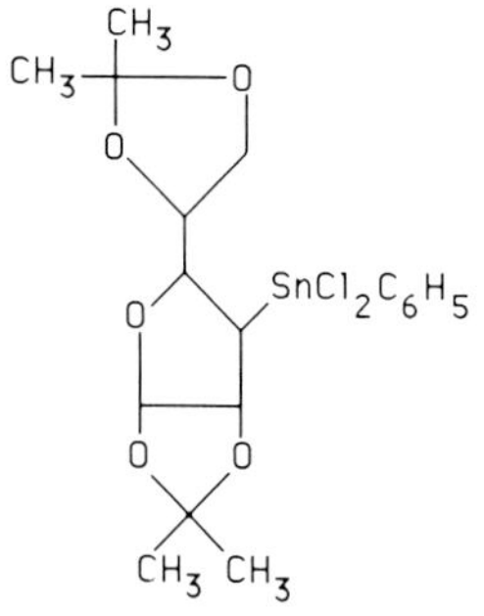

5 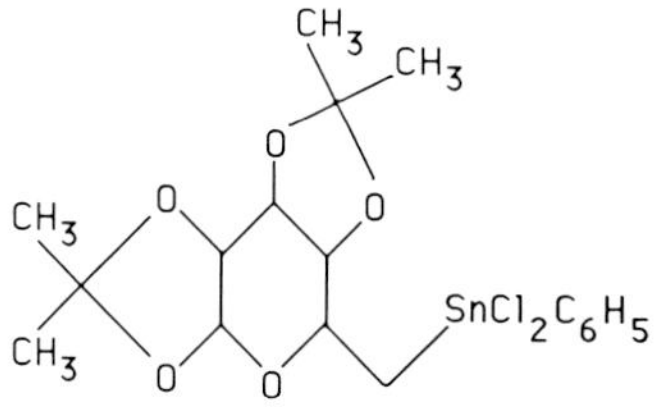   **6**

IV. ANTITUMOR ACTIVITY OF CYCLODEXTRIN ORGANOTIN INCLUSION COMPOUNDS

Another simple way to enhance the water solubility and the bioavailability of organotin compounds is to prepare their cyclodextrin inclusion complexes.[17] It is well known that cyclodextrins are highly resistant towards the usual starch-hydrolyzing enzymes, that the degree of toxicity of pure cyclodextrin is very low, and that 1:1 and even 1:2 complexes can be formed when the guest molecule is too large to find complete accommodation in one cavity and when its end is also amenable to complex formation (as is the case for prostaglandins, vitamin D3, indomethacin, etc.).[17]

The stability of the complex is an increasing function of the hydrophobic character of the substituents (methyl and ethyl groups increase the stability).

We have prepared some inclusion complexes of diorganotin dihalides in cyclodextrins (**7**):[18]

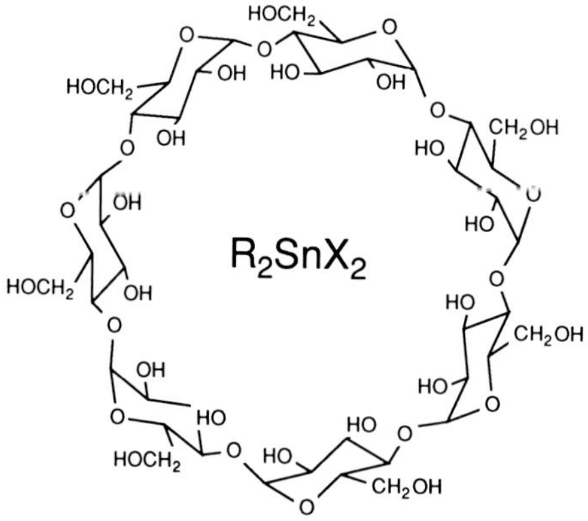

7

V. ANTITUMOR ACTIVITY OF 1,3-DIOXA-2-STANNACYCLO-PENTANES AND HEXANES

We have prepared a series of cyclic organotin compounds containing O–Sn–O fragments that can, for example, very easily be prepared from diorganotin oxides and diols.[16,19] The idea came from the relatively interesting antitumoral properties of some compounds with O–Sn–S bonds described recently by Huber et al.[6] Up to now, almost all our syntheses were undertaken with di-*n*-butyltin oxide because of the well known toxicology of *n*-butyltin compounds, but we are planning to prepare dimethyl, diphenyl, dibenzyl, and di-t-butyl compounds as well. One possible problem with the Sn–O bonds is their sensitivty towards hydrolysis; of course, the rate of hydrolysis will differ from one compound to the other, and it is clear that if they reach their target before hydrolyzing, this possible problem will be eluded, which means that not only an estimation of the rate of hydrolysis is necessary, but also their rate of resorption.

Di-*n*-butyltin derivatives of simple diols have already been described.[21-23] They are very easily prepared from the diol and di-*n*-butyltin oxide [see **8**] and can even react further with di-*n*-butyltin oxide to yield cyclic derivatives of oligomeric di-*n*-butyltin oxide (**9**):[24]

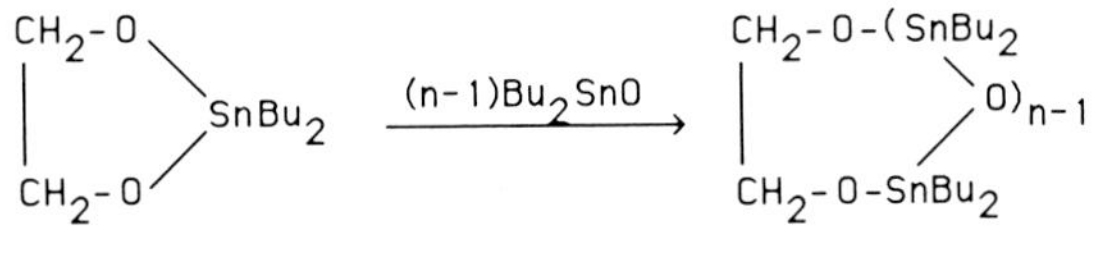

$$\begin{array}{c}CH_2-O\\ |\diagdown\\ SnBu_2\\ |\diagup\\ CH_2-O\end{array} \xrightarrow{(n-1)Bu_2SnO} \begin{array}{c}CH_2-O-(SnBu_2\\ |\diagdown\\ O)_{n-1}\\ |\diagup\\ CH_2-O-SnBu_2\end{array}$$

8   **9**

2,2-Di-*n*-butyl-1,3,2-dioxastannolan has been shown to be an infinite ribbon coordination polymer with six-coordinated tin,[25] similar to the di-*n*-butylstannylene derivative of propane-1,3-diol.[25]

Among the numerous 1,3-dioxa-2-stannacyclo-pentanes and hexanes we have prepared, the most promising ones are certainly the di-n-butyltin derivatives of pyridoxine (vitamin B6) (**10**), of riboflavin (vitamin B2), and of ascorbic acid (vitamin C) (**11**) being tested at the Bordet Institute, Brussels, Belgium.

We can also mention the di-*n*-butyltin derivatives of 7-(2,3-dihydroxypropyl)theophylline (**12**), of 3-morpholino- (**13**), 3-piperidino- and 3-(1-piperazinyl)-1,2-propanediol (**14**), of salicylic and 3,5-diiodosalicylic acid (**15**), of atropine sulfate (**16**) of citric acid, and of *N,N*-bis-(2-hydroxyethyl)-*p*-toluene sulfonamide (**17**) and tropic acid (**18**).

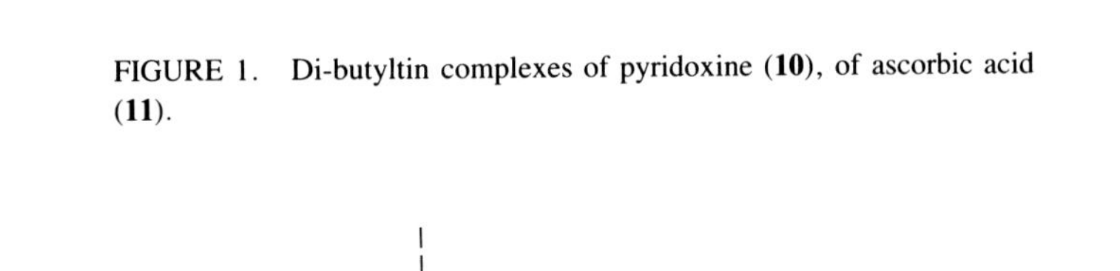

10   **11**

FIGURE 1. Di-butyltin complexes of pyridoxine (**10**), of ascorbic acid (**11**).

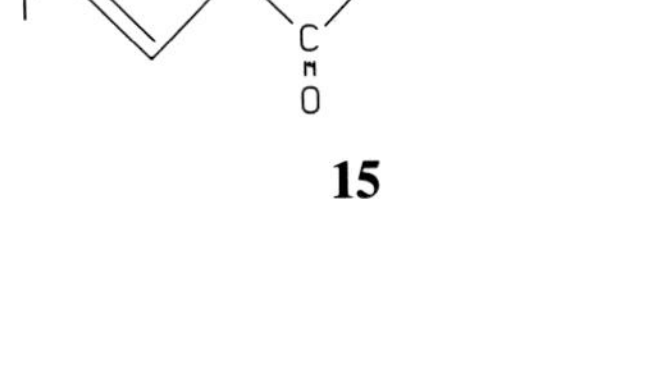

15

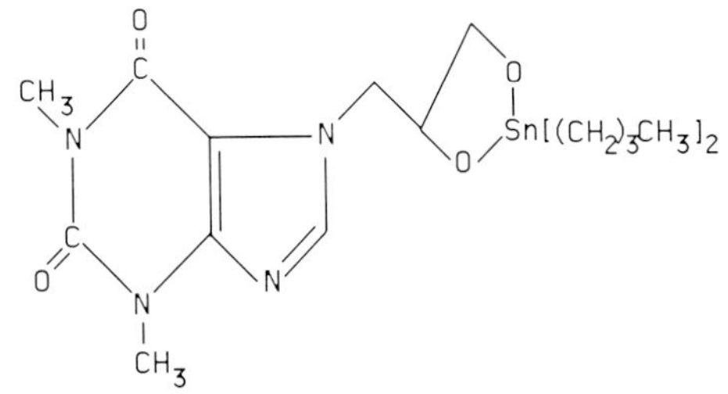

FIGURE 2. Di-*n*-butyltin complexes of atropine sulfate (**16**), of 7-(2,3-dihydroxypropyl)theophylline (**12**), 3,5-diiodosalicylic acid (**14**), tropic acid (**18**), *N,N*,-bis-(2-hydroxyethyl)-*p*-toluene sulfonamide (**17**), and 3-morpholino- (**13**) and 3-(1-piperazinyl)-1,2-propane diol (**14**).

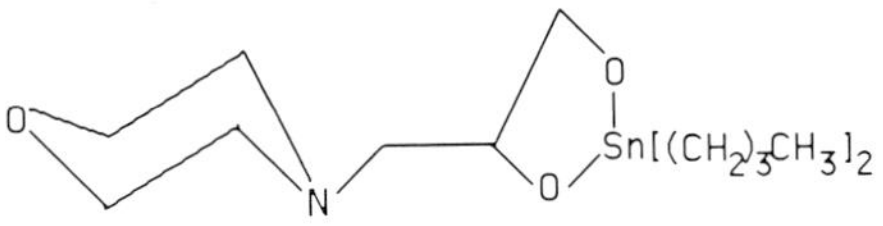

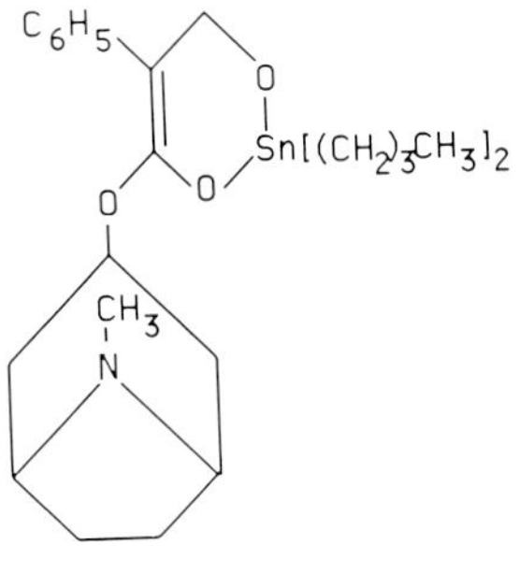

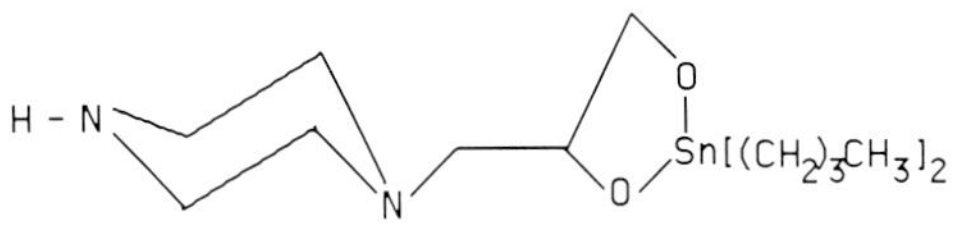

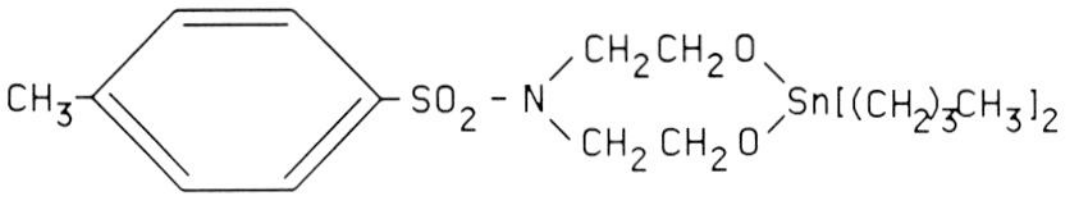

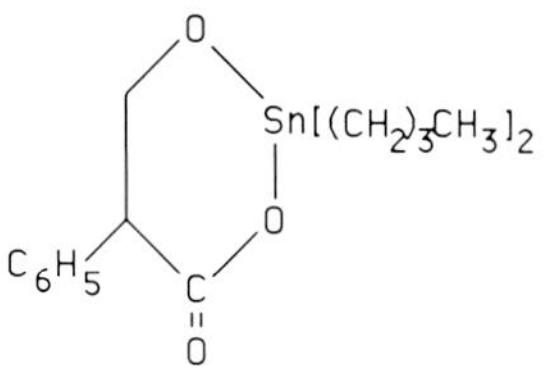

Di-*n*-butyltin derivatives of monosaccharides have also already been described,[27] and the structure of two di-*n*-butylstannylene-pyranosides has even been determined by X-ray diffraction: methyl 4,6-di-*O*-benzylidene-2,3-*O*-di-n-butylstannylene-alpha-D-glucopyranoside is a coordination dimer with five-coordinated tin atoms,[28] whereas the corresponding mannose compound is a coordination pentamer with five-coordinated tin atoms in the two terminal units and six-coordinated tin atoms in the three medial ones.[29] We have prepared some dibutyltin derivatives of sugars and related compounds like 2-deoxy-D-ribose or D-(+)-ribonic acid-gamma-lactone.

Organotin derivatives of nucleosides have also been described in the literature.[30,31] We have repeated the preparation of di-*n*-butyltin derivatives of adenosine (**19**) and of uridine (**20**):

19   **20**

VI. CONCLUSION

Organotin compounds seem to be very promising substrates for cancer chemotherapy. When one realizes that the first report on organotin compounds exhibiting antitumor activity appeared only 5 years ago,[32] then it becomes clear that much more research has to be performed in this area in order to find better active synthetic compounds that might prove more suitable than the organometallic compounds tested until now.

REFERENCES

1. **Camboli, D. and Besançon, J.**, Chimie de coordination et métallothérapie antitumorale, *L'Actual. Chim.*, 61, 37, 1985.
2. **Prestayko, A. W., Crooke, S. T., and Carter, S. K., Eds.**, *Cisplatin: Current Status and New Developments*, Academic Press, New York, 1980.
3. **Köpf, H. and Köpf-Maier, P.**, Tumor inhibition by metallocene dihalides of early transition metals: chemical and biological aspects, in *Platinum, Gold and Other Metal Chemotherapeutic Agents: Chemistry and Biochemistry*, Lippard, S. J., Ed., ACS Symp. Ser. No. 209, American Chemical Society, Washington, D.C., 1983, 315.
4. **Hollis, L. S., Amundsen, A. R., and Stern, E. W.**, Synthesis, structure and antitumor properties of platinum complexes of vitamin C, *J. Am. Chem. Soc.*, 107, 274, 1985.
5. **Gielen, M.**, Antitumor active organotin compounds, in *Tin as a Vital Nutrient: Implications in Cancer Prophylaxis and Other Physiological Processes*, Cardarelli, N. F., Ed., CRC Press, Boca Raton, Fla., 1986, 169.
6. **Huber, F., Roge, G., Carl, L., Atassi, G., Spreafico, F., Filippeschi, S., Barbieri, R., Silvestri, A., Rivarola, E., Ruisi, G., Di Bianca, F., and Alonzo, G.**, Studies on the antitumor activity of di- and tri-organotin(IV) complexes of aminoacids and related compounds, of mercaptoethanesulfonate and of purine-6-thiol, *J. Chem. Soc. Dalton Trans.*, 523, 1985.
7. **Gielen, M., Jurkschat, K., and Atassi, G.**, Bis-(halophenylstannyl)methanes; new organotin compounds exhibiting antitumor activity, *Bull. Soc. Chim. Belg.*, 93, 153, 1984.
8. **Narayanan, V. L.**, Strategy for the discovery and development of novel anticancer agents, in *Structure-Activity Relationships of Antitumor Agents*, Reinhoudt, D. N., Connors, T. A., Pinedo, H. M., and van de Poll, K. W., Eds., Martinus Nijhoff, The Hague, 1983, 5.
9. **Crowe, A. J., Smith, P. J., and Atassi, G.**, Investigations into the antitumor activity of organotin compounds. II. Diorganotin dihalide and dipseudohalide complexes, *Inorg. Chim. Acta*, 93, 179, 1984.
10. **Crowe, A. J., Smith, P. J., Cardin, C. J., Parge, H. E., and Smith, F. E.**, Possible predissociation of diorganotin dihalide complexes — relationship between antitumor activity and structure, *Cancer Lett.*, 24, 45, 1984.
11. **Riess, J. G. and Le Blanc, M.**, Solubility and transport phenomena in perfluorochemicals relevant to blood substitution and other medical applications, *Pure Appl. Chem.*, 54, 2383, 1982.

12. **De Clercq, L., Willen, R., Gielen, M., and Atassi, G.,** Synthesis, characterization and antitumor activity of bis(polyfluoroalkyl)tin dihalides, *Bull. Soc. Chim. Belg.,* 93, 1089, 1984.
13. **Atassi, G.,** Antitumor and toxic effects of silicon, germanium, tin and lead compounds, *Rev. Si, Ge, Sn, Pb Compd.,* 8, 219, 1986.
14. **Gielen, M., Willem, R., and Jurkschat, K.,** unpublished results, 1985.
15. **Crowe, A. J. and Smith, P. J.,** Synthesis of tributylstannyl ethers of carbohydrates, *J. Organomet. Chem.,* 110, C57, 1976.
16. **Patel, A. and Poller, R. C.,** Organotin derivatives of sugars, *Rev. Si, Ge, Sn, Pb Compd.,* 8, 263, 1986.
17. **Szejtli, J.,** *Cyclodextrins and Their Inclusion Complexes,* Akadémiai Kiadó, Budapest, 1982.
18. **Gielen, M., Joosen, E., and Willem, R.,** unpublished results, 1985.
19. **David, S. and Hanessian, S.,** Regioselective manipulation of hydroxyl groups via organotin derivatives, *Tetrahedron,* 41, 643, 1985.
21. **Davies, A. G. and Price, A. J.,** Five-coordinate complexes of 2,2-dibutyl-1,3,2-dioxastannolans, *J. Organomet. Chem.,* 258, 7, 1983.
22. **Mukaiyama, T., Tomioka, I., and Shimizu, M.,** Asymmetric acylation of meso-1,2-diols with d-ketopinic acid chloride, *Chem. Lett.,* 49, 1984.
23. **Shanzer, A., Libman, J., and Gottlieb, H. E.,** Optical enrichment of diols via their organotin complexes, *J. Org. Chem.,* 46, 4612, 1983.
24. **Davies, A. G., Hawari, J. A.-A., and Hua-do, P.,** Telomerization of poly(dialkyltin oxide) and alkane- or alkene-1,2-diols: the identification of cyclic derivatives of oligomeric dibutyltin oxide, *J. Organomet. Chem.,* 251, 203, 1983.
25. **Davies, A. G., Price, A. J., Dawes, H. M., and Hursthouse, M. B.,** The X-ray structure of 2,2-dibutyl-1,3,2-dioxastannolan, *J. Organomet. Chem.,* 270, C1, 1984.
26. **Pommier, J. C., Mendel, E., Valade, J., and Housty, J.,** Sur la structure du dibutylstannadioxa-2,6 cyclohexane, *J. Organomet. Chem.,* 55, C19, 1973.
27. **Munavu, R. M. and Szmant, H. H.,** Selective formation of 2 esters of some α-D-hexapyranosides via dibutylstannylene derivatives, *J. Org. Chem.,* 41, 1832, 1976.
28. **David, S., Pascard, C., and Cesario, M.,** The crystal and molecular structure of a carbohydrate-derived stannylene: a discussion of the regiospecific reactions of dialkyl derivatives of vicinal diols, *Nouveau J. Chim.,* 3, 63, 1979.
29. **Holzapfel, C. W., Koekemoer, J. M., Morris, C. F., Kruger, G. J., and Pretorius, J. A.,** *S. Afr. J. Chem.,* 35, 80, 1982.
30. **Wagner, D., Verheyden, J. V. H., and Moffatt, J. G.,** Preparation and synthetic utility of some organotin derivatives of nucleosides, *J. Org. Chem.,* 39, 24, 1974.
31. **Ikehara, M. and Maruyama, T.,** Studies of nucleosides and nucleotides. LXV, *Tetrahedron,* 31, 1369, 1975.
32. **Crowe, A. J. and Smith, P. J.,** Dialkyl dihalide tin complexes: a new class of metallic derivatives exhibiting antitumor activity, *Chem. Ind. (London),* 200, 1980.

Chapter 5

SYNTHESIS AND CHARACTERIZATION OF ORGANOTIN STEROIDS

Anil Saxena and Friedo Huber

During the First International Conference on Tin and Malignant Cell Growth, Professor Cardarelli presented the results of Kanakkanatt,[1] who obtained some phenyl and butyltin derivatives of steroids. The compounds, e.g., triphenyltin cholate and *n*-butyltin cholic anhydride, have been used for anticancer screening, but no structural characterization has been reported. Prior to the mentioning of $Me_3Sn(cholest)$ (Hcholest = cholestane) by Hudec[2] and a compound $Ph_3Pb(H_3chol)$ (H_4chol = cholic acid) by Pellerito et al.,[3] there seemed to be no detailed information on such compounds in the literature, though studies on adducts of organotin with steroids are underway in the laboratories of Pellerito.[4]

Due to lack of structural information, we proposed at the end of the first conference to start investigations on such compounds.

We synthesized methyl, ethyl, and phenyltin derivatives of H_4chol, Hcholest, and other steroids by different routes. The alkoxide method proved to be most favorable for preparation: reaction of, e.g., $R_2Sn(OMe)_2$ and cholic acid in methanol after some refluxing gave $R_2Sn(H_2chol)$ or $(R_2Sn)_3(Hchol)_2$ according to the stoichiometric ratio of the starting material in high yields as

$$R_2Sn(OMe)_2 + H_4chol \rightarrow (R_2Sn)(H_2chol)$$

$$3R_2Sn(OMe)_2 + 2H_4chol \rightarrow (R_2Sn)_3(Hchol)_2$$

Neutralization has also been used as in Reference 1, but to remove water of neutralization, we added 2,2-dimethoxypropane. By this method we obtained, e.g., $(Ph_3Sn)_n(H_{4-n}chol)$ (n = 1 to 4) according to

$$R_3SnOH + H_4chol \rightarrow [(R_3Sn)_n(H_{4-n}chol)] \qquad (n = 1 \text{ to } 4)$$

For synthesizing triorganotin compounds we reacted the appropriate triorganotin chlorides and steroids in ethereal medium in presence of triethylamine according to

$$R_3SnCl + Hcholest \rightarrow R_3Sn(cholest)$$

The compounds have been characterized by elemental analyses (Table 1), vibrational spectroscopy, ^1H, ^{13}C, ^{119}Sn NMR, and Mössbauer spectroscopy. Representative examples are given in Table 2. All compounds are highly soluble in common organic solvents and tend to dissociate in alcoholic media. Molecular weight measurements show about half of the calculated values (Table 1). The dimethyltin compounds are highly hydrolyzable in nature as compared to triphenyl and diphenyltin counterparts. They show sharp melting points (Table 1).

For recording the ^{119}Sn Mössbauer spectra the authors thank Dr. J. Pebler, Fachbereich Chemie der Philipps-Universität Marburg, West Germany, (compounds II and $\overline{N}$) and Professor Dr. L. Pellerito, Istituto di Clinica Generale, Universitá di Palermo, Italy (compound V). Anil Saxena would like to thank Alexander von Humboldt Stiftung for the award of a Postdoctoral Research Fellowship.

Table 1
ANALYTICAL, MOLECULAR WEIGHT, AND IR SPECTROSCOPIC DATA FOR ORGANOTIN STEROIDS

Compound	Analyses C found (calcd.)	Analyses H found (calcd.)	Mol wt found (calcd.)	mp (°C)	IR ν_{asym} COO	IR ν_{sym} COO	Raman Sn-C	Raman Sn-C
$[(C_{18}H_{15}Sn)(C_{24}H_{39}O_5)]$ (I)	65.40 (66.58)	7.20 (7.13)	390 (756.68)	98	1580, 1540	1430	—[b]	—
$[(C_{18}H_{15}Sn)_2(C_{24}H_{38}O_5)]$ (II)	64.60 (65.10)	6.60 (6.14)	563 (1105.36)	83	1725, 1637	1430	—[b]	—
$[(C_2H_6Sn)(C_{24}H_{38}O_5)]$ (III)	56.50 (56.21)	7.60 (7.92)	578 (554.68)	175—77	1735, 1570—1600	—	525	—
$[(C_2H_6Sn)_3(C_{24}H_{37}O_5)_2]$ (IV)	51.50 (51.55)	7.20 (7.32)	—	228	1610, 1560	—	520	—
$[(C_{18}H_{15}Sn)(C_{27}H_{45}O)]$ (V)	73.00 (73.47)	8.30 (8.16)	363[a] (734.68)	180	—	—	—	—
$[(C_2H_6Sn)(C_{24}H_{38}O_4)]$ (VI)	59.10 (57.91)	8.20 (8.16)	—	140 (d)	1735, 1600	—	525	—

[a] Molecular weight from mass spectral analysis = 735.16 [M$^+$ (based on ^{120}Sn isotope)-H].
[b] Could not be observed.

Table 2
^{1}H, ^{119}Sn NMR, AND ^{119m}Sn MÖSSBAUER DATA FOR ORGANOTIN STEROIDS

Compound	^{1}H NMR[a]						^{119}Sn NMR[c]	^{119m}Sn Mössbauer		Linewidths		QS/IS
	Ph$_3$Sn[b] or Me$_2$Sn	18-CH$_3$	19-CH$_3$	21-CH$_3$	26/27-CH$_3$			IS (mm · sec^{-1})	QS (mm · sec^{-1})	r$_1$	r$_2$	
Ph$_3$Sn(H$_3$chol) (I)	7.54 m	0.89	0.63 }[d] 0.69	1.03 }[d] 1.01 0.99 }[d] 0.97	—		−210.5[d]	—	—	—	—	—
(Ph$_3$Sn)$_2$(H$_2$chol) (II)	7.45 m	0.86	0.56 }[d] 0.66 J = 31.4 Hz	0.98 }[d] 0.96 J = 6.1 Hz 0.93 }[d] 0.91 J = 6.1 Hz	—		−168.9[d] −212.1	1.21(2)[e] 1.29(2)[e]	1.46(2)[e] 2.46(2)[e]	0.53 0.50	0.53 0.50	1.20 1.90
Ph$_3$Sn(cholest) (V)	7.30 m	0.60	0.93	0.83	0.75		−83.07[f]	1.12(3)[g]	1.61(2)[g]	0.91	0.92	1.43
Me$_2$Sn(H$_2$chol) (III)	0.86	0.84	0.66	0.98	—		−135.06[d]	—	—	—	—	—
(Me$_2$Sn)$_3$(Hchol)$_2$ (IV)	0.76	0.95	0.81	1.07	—		—	1.20(2)[e]	3.14(2)[e]	1.29	1.27	2.61

[a] δ Ppm relative to TMS; solvent: CDCl$_3$ (for IV: CD$_3$OD).
[b] Center of multiplet.
[c] δ Ppm relative to TMT.
[d] — Solvent: CD$_3$OD.
[e] Recorded at 4.2 K.
[f] — Solvent: CDCl$_3$.
[g] Recorded at 77 K.

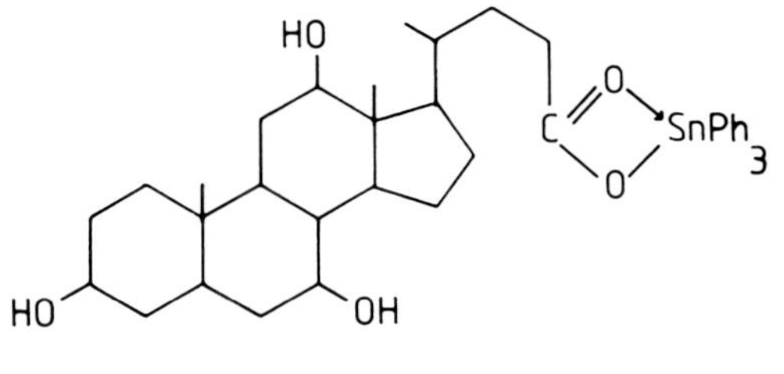

FORMULA 1

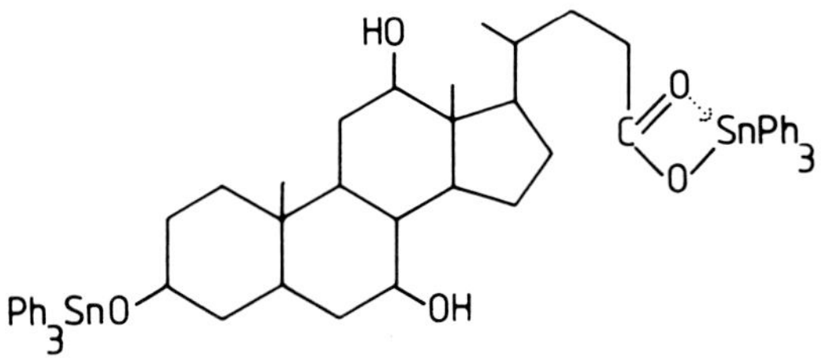

FORMULA 2

Solid state and data in methanolic solutions allow us to make the following tentative proposals for $(Ph_3Sn)_n(H_{4-n}chol)$ (n = 1,2) and for $Ph_3Sn(cholest)$ (Formula 1). In $Ph_3Sn(H_3chol)$ according to IR-data (Table 1) the carboxylate group is acting in a bidentate fashion rendering a five coordination at tin (Formula 1). The ^{119}Sn NMR data in methanolic solution (Table 2) indicate a coordination of at least five.[5] The molecular weight data in methanol suggest dissociation of the compound, which in term of solvolysis can be formulated as

$$Ph_3Sn(H_3chol) + n L \leftrightarrows (Ph_3SnL_n)^+ + H_3chol^-$$

(L = methanol; n may be, according to NMR, around 2)

The IR data for $(Ph_3Sn)_2(H_2chol)$ (Table 1) suggest a slightly different mode of coordination of the carboxylate group, a quasibidentate mode. The Mössbauer data indicate the presence of two tin sites (Table 2). One tin site is definitely four coordinate,[6] while the other value is slightly lower than five-coordinate tin would have given.[7] This observation, consistent with IR interpretation, gives a structure as shown in Formula 2. Substitution of H in OH at ^3C is indicated by ^{13}C NMR data and is consistent with the reactivities of hydroxyl groups in H_4chol.[8] The NMR data in methanolic solution (Table 2) again suggest the presence of two different tin centers; one value is approximately the same as obtained for $Ph_3Sn(H_3chol)$, and we assume that the species present is the same in the solutions of both compounds. The second NMR signal lies in the range of four and five coordination.[9] We postulate a dissociation mechanism based on molecular weight measurements (Table 1) and NMR data as

$$(Ph_3Sn)_2(H_2chol) + n L \leftrightarrows (Ph_3SnL_n)^+ + [Ph_3Sn(H_2chol)]^-$$
(A)

We assume the species A to be the residue left after dissociation of the Ph_3Sn group originally bonded to the carboxylate group. We made similar observations on analogous compounds.[10] Sn in A might be weakly coordinated by solvent molecules.

Preliminary results of Mössbauer measurements on $Ph_3Sn(cholest)$ (Table 2) suggest te-

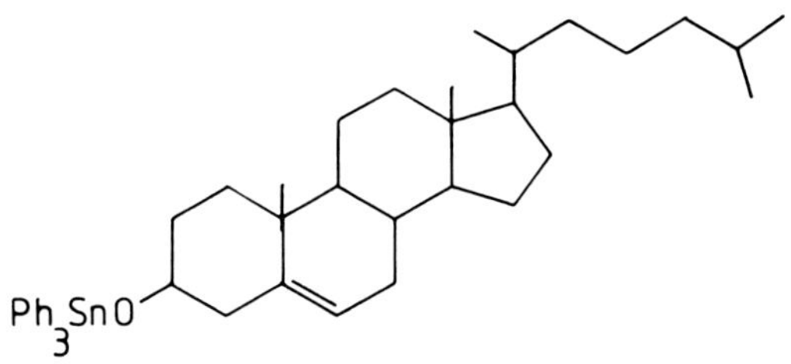

FORMULA 3

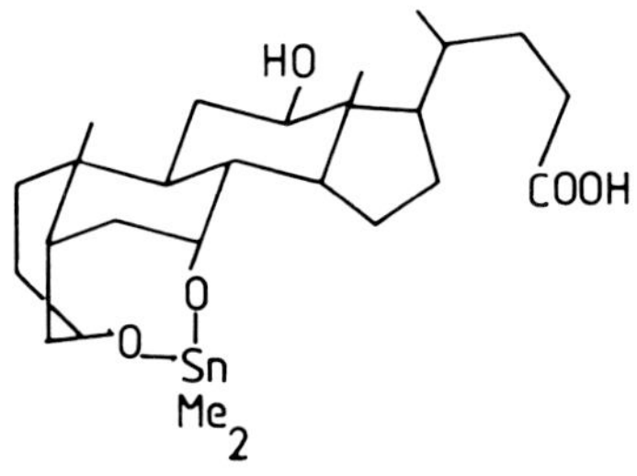

FORMULA 4

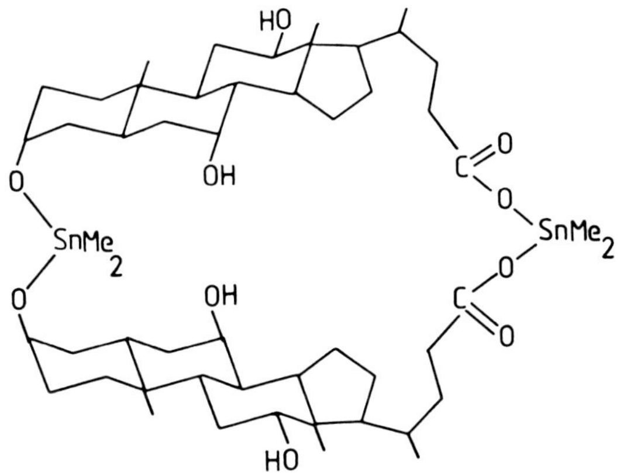

FORMULA 5

trahedral environment around tin in the solid state. We propose a tentative structure as shown in Formula 3.

Probable structures of $R_2Sn(H_2chol)$ (R = Me, Et, Ph) are shown in Formula 4. In Formula 4 the A ring of $R_2Sn(H_2chol)$ may have changed the conformation from chair to boat; thereby OH at ^{7}C is coming in proximity of OH at ^{3}C allowing normal O–Sn–O bonds. If ring A retains chair conformation, Formula 5 is assumed with two O–Sn–O bridges in sandwich structure. According to ^{119}Sn NMR and molecular weight data, Formula 4 seems to be preferred in methanolic solution. Mössbauer data of $(R_2Sn)_3(Hchol)_2$ (R = Me, Et, Ph) indicate only one tin site. We therefore have to assume that the skeleton of these compounds is different from those of $R_2Sn(H_2chol)$.

Studies are underway to draw a better picture of this and further types of compounds.

ACKNOWLEDGMENTS

For recording the ^{119}Sn Mössbauer spectra the authors thank Dr. J. Pebler, Fachbereich Chemie der Philipps-Universität Marburg, West Germany, (compounds II and $\overline{N}$) and Professor Dr. L. Pellerito, Istituto di Clinica Generale, Universitá di Palermo, Italy (compound V). Anil Saxena would like to thank Alexander von Humboldt Stiftung for the award of a Postdoctoral Research Fellowship.

REFERENCES

1. **Kanakkanatt, S. V.**, Synthesis of tin steroids and the relation between structure and anticancer activity, paper presented by Cardarelli, N. F., at 1st Int. Conf. Tin and Malignant Cell Growth, Scranton, Pa., May 1984.
2. **Hudec, J.**, cited in Spectroscopic properties of axially and equatorially substituted β-trimethylstannyl ketones and compounds with related chromophores, *J. Chem. Soc. Perkin Trans.*, 1, 1020, 1975.
3. **Pellerito, L., Cefalù, R., Girasolo, M. A., and Stocco, G. C.**, Synthesis and spectroscopic investigations of metallic and organometallic derivatives of biological molecules, 3rd Simp. Sulla Chimica dei Composti dei Metalli di Nontransizione, Parma, Italy, 1983, 83.
4. **Pellerito, L.**, personal communication, 1984.
5. **Smith, P. J. and Tupčianuskas, A. P.**, Chemical shifts of ^{119}Sn nuclei in organotin compounds, *Annu. Rev. NMR Spectrosc.*, 8, 291, 1978.
6. **Herber, R. H. and Leahy, M. F.**, Structure and bonding in organotins by gamma-resonance spectroscopy, Advances in Chemistry Ser. No. 157, American Chemical Society Washington, D.C., 1976, 155.
7. **Zuckerman, J. J.**, Applications of ^{119m}Sn Mössbauer spectroscopy to the study of organotin compounds, *Adv. Organomet. Chem.*, 9, 21, 1970; **Zuckerman, J. J.**, Organotin-119m Mössbauer spectroscopy: the first quarter century, in *Chemical Mössbauer Spectroscopy*, Herber, R. H., Ed., Plenum Press, New York, 1984, 267.
8. **Smith, W. B.**, Carbon-13 nmr spectroscopy of steroids, *Annu. Rev. NMR Spectrosc.*, 8, 199, 1978.
9. **Kennedy, J. D. and McFarlane, W.**, ^{119}Sn magnetic shielding in tin compounds, *Rev. Si, Ge, Tin Lead Compd.*, 1, 135, 1974.
10. **Saxena, A., Huber, F., and Pellerito, L.**, personal communication, 1985.

Chapter 6

TIN STEROIDS AS ANTICANCER AGENTS

Nate F. Cardarelli

TABLE OF CONTENTS

I.	Introduction	54
II.	Materials and Methods	54
III.	Results	55
IV.	Discussion	57
	Acknowledgments	57
	References	57

I. INTRODUCTION

Studies using COBS outbred mice (white albino strain, originally germfree, Charles River Laboratories, Wilmington, Mass.) showed that the thymus gland is a major accumulatory site for xenobiotic tin.[1,2] In a time-profile study using three mice strains administered ^{113}Sn, results indicated that tin is processed in the thymus of the noncancer-prone COBS strain while by-passing this organ in the AKR leukemia-prone subjects.[2] Tin circulation is through the lymphatic system in COBS, whereas the AKR subjects and the A/KI mammary adenocarcinoma strain contained appreciable tin concentrations in the blood.[3] Evidence indicates that the thymus of man, as well as rodent, processes tin in specific medullary cells.[3,4]

An organotin dietary supplement retarded transplanted tumor growth, but did not destroy the tumor.[5] Dermal application of the organotin, using dimethylsulfoxide (DMSO) as the carrier, over the tumor site was ineffective. It was noted that DMSO alone enhances tumor growth rate. Various researchers have shown that a number of organotin substances administered interperitonally to P-388-infected mice will extend life span.[6,7]

It is well recognized that the human and bovine thymus excrete various hormone-like substances.[8] At least three known thymic extracts are antiproliferative in vitro. Over 50 years ago Hanson noted that a specific bovine thymus extract administered daily to human patients caused a shrinkage in tumor size.[9,10] The most potent antiproliferative bovine thymus substance is an unknown material having a molecular weight of about 600 daltons with a steroid nucleus[8,11,12] termed the "S" fraction. It has never been fully characterized to our knowledge. It is recognized that the human thymus synthesizes cholesterol.[13] Although there is some small presumptive evidence available,[3] it was assumed that the "S" material is a tin-cholesterol derivative as a basic element in a tentative hypothesis linking thymus tin with cancer and the aging process. Isolation and analysis of the "S" fraction for tin content is in progress.

A series of tin cholesterol derivatives was prepared.[14,15] These included combinations of various organotin moieties with cholesterol and cholesterol derivatives. For comparison, tin combinations with other steroids were also synthesized. However, these materials have not been chemically characterized. The presence of isomers and some degree of contamination by starting materials are expected. This report presents a portion of the anticancer studies conducted with such materials.

II. MATERIALS AND METHODS

A/KI mice 6 to 9 weeks old were used as subjects. Rearing conditions have been reported in an earlier article of this series.[2] Adenocarcinoma tumor fragments of approximately 0.04 were subdermally inserted in subjects using a standard trochar (large hypodermic needle). Each test cohort contained mice of the same age ±2 days and about equal numbers of both sexes. A cohort consisted of no less than 10 mice and in some instances over 20 mice.

Mice were provided with the test chemical, either a tin steroid or one of the reaction products used in synthesizing the steroid, at 10 and 100 ppm in their drinking water. Presentment was initiated 15 days before transplant and continued for 30 days posttransplant. On the 31st day after transplantation, mice were sacrificed and the tumor, thymus, spleen, and liver completely excised and weighed. Test subjects were observed daily for signs of gross intoxication. Body weight was measured periodically. Upon necropsy, organs were examined for indication of lesions or other signs of intoxication.

Tin steroids were also sent to Dr. W. Lichter at The University of Miami School of Medicine for evaluation in cell tissue culture against human KB epidermoid tumor and P-388 mouse leukemia.

Table 1
ADENOCARCINOMA SUPPRESSION IN A/KI MICE USING TIN STEROIDS

Material[a]	Dosage (ppm)	C/T × 100	Subjects (no.)
Triphenyltin cholate	10	55	20
	100	354	20
Cholesteryl-*n*-butylstannate	10	86	16
Triphenyltin testosterone	10	255	10
	100	237	10
Tri *n* butyltin deoxycholate (I)	10	168	20
Triphenyltin cholesterol ether (I)	10	723 (3)[b]	10
	100	2350 (5)[b]	15
Tri-*n*-butyltin deoxycholate (II)	10	266 (2)[b]	10
	100	1352 (11)[b]	21
Triphenyltin cholesterol ether (II)	10	211 (2)[b]	10
	100	494 (1)[b]	10
Cholesteryl-tri-*n*-butyltin ether (I)	10	1707 (4)[b]	12
	100	2821 (6)[b]	10
Cholesteryl-tri-*n*-butyltin ether (II)	10	508 (3)[b]	10
	100	442 (5)[b]	10
Cholesteryl-tri-*n*-butyltin adipate (I)	10	Toxic	10
	100	Toxic	10
Cholesteryl-tri-*n*-butyltin adipate (II)	182	182	10
	100	2611 (2)[b]	10

[a] Not single species, since none shows sharp melting points. Preparations are found in Reference 15. The degree of contamination by starting materials is unknown, but believed to be less than 2%.

[b] The figure in parentheses refers to the number of mice wherein the tumor fragment could not be located, or when found was totally necrotic.

III. RESULTS

Table 1 depicts some of the tin steroids evaluated. The C/T × 100 index is used with the adenocarcinoma study and the ED_{50} inhibition index for the KB and P-388 evaluations. Table 3 presents the C/T × 100 values found for the reaction materials used in synthesis. In some instances, the tumor fragment could not be located after diligent search or when located was totally necrotic. Since all such instances were observed with specific tin steroids and no such results were found with the control animals, it is believed that effect of the the tin steroid was to destroy the fragment. All necrotic tumors lacked vascularization. Whether metastasis occurred in such circumstances is unknown. In cases where the fragment was missing or necrotic, no identifiable tumors were found in the GI tract, liver, spleen, or kidney. Fat and muscle tissue were not examined, however.

A total of 80 control mice were used, in 4 cohorts of 20 subjects each. In all cases, viable, large tumors were removed after sacrifice.

The ED_{50} values, where available, are also noted in Table 1. In several instances, the tin steroid was found to have more than one component upon purification by recrystallization. Components were separated and labeled as (I), (II), etc., to designate each fraction.[15] Qualitative test by the dithiol method indicated that each fraction contained tin. Table 2 designates the inhibition indices determined in cell culture studies.[16]

Table 2
INHIBITION INDICES FOR SEVERAL TIN STEROIDS[17]

	ED_{50} (mcg/mℓ)	
Compound[a]	Human KB tumor	Mouse P-388 leukemia
Triphenyltin cholate	0.22	0.18
Cholesteryl-*n*-butylstannate	29	25.5
Triphenyltin testosterone	0.2	0.004
Tri-*n*-butyltin deoxycholate (I)	0.25	0.26
Triphenyltin cholesterol ether II	0.1	0.2
Cholesteryl tri-*n*-butyltin ether (II)	0.3	5.0
Cholesteryl tri-*n*-butyltin adipate (II)	0.20	0.05
Triphenyltin cholesterol ether (I)	0.24	0.40
Tri-*n*-butyltin deoxycholate (II)	0.23	0.31
Tri-*n*-butyltin deoxycholate (III)	1.3	0.4
Testosteronyl-*n*-butylstannate	24.0	32.0
Estronyl-*n*-butylstannate	20	24

[a] Not single species, since none shows sharp melting points. Preparations are found in Reference 15. The degree of contamination by starting materials is unknown, but believed to be less than 2%.

Table 3
ADENOCARCINOMA SUPPRESSION IN A/KI MICE WITH SUBDERMAL TUMOR TRANSPLANTS IN THE MAMMARY REGION BY THE REACTANTS USED IN SYNTHESIZING TIN STEROIDS

Material	Dosage	Mice (no.)	C/T × 100
Triphenyltin hydroxide	10	10	109
	100	10	107
Triphenyltin chloride	10	13	101
	100	10	99
Cholic acid	10	10	102
	100	10	53
Testosterone	10	10	99
	100	10	119
Cholesterol	10	10	94
	100	10	108
Tri-*n*-butyltin adipate	10	10	128
	100	10	168
Tri-*n*-butyltin chloride	10	10	111
	100	10	217
Cholesterol chloride	10	10	53
	100	10	62
n-Butyltin hydroxide oxide	10	10	123
	100	10	117

IV. DISCUSSION

It is believed on the basis of the data reported in this paper that tin cholesterol derivatives are active against mouse adenocarcinoma, mouse P-388 leukemia, and human KB tumor.

Materials of higher activity have a tin-cholesterol linkage at ^{23}C (ether type) or ^{24}C (ester type) as determined by infrared spectroscopy. Oral presentment seems to be superior over i.p. administration. To date, National Cancer Institute (NCI) data using the 3PS31 protocol (five i.p. injections on five successive days) have only indicated reasonable activity with triphenyltin cholesterol either at 30- or 15-mg/kg dosages.

Anticarcinogenic activity appears to be dose dependent. The mechanism of action is unknown. Various tin compounds retard the growth rate of tumors and generally extend the lifetime of leukemic subjects.[6,7] However, the tin reactants used in the preparation of the products discussed herein show very little activity in the in vitro assays. Whether the action is somehow directed against the tumor cell or additional tin merely leads to a greater thymic anticancer hormone output has to be assessed. In preliminary studies there has been some indication that a tin supplement in the diet will retard the involution rate of the rodent thymus.[17] If it is assumed that the hormonal output of this gland decreases with involution, then slowing involution also slows the rate of decrease of thymic secretions. Changes in thymus hormone output as a function of age (i.e., involution) has yet to be evaluated.

ACKNOWLEDGMENTS

Tin steroids used in this study were prepared by S. V. Kanakkanatt at the Unique Technologies Inc. facilities in Mogadore, Ohio. The tissue culture studies were performed by W. Lichter of the University of Miami School of Medicine. This study was performed at Unique Technologies Inc. and was partially sponsored by the Griffin Corporation of Valdosta, Ga.

REFERENCES

1. **Cardarelli, N. F., Quitter, B. M., Allen, A., Dobbins, E., Hager, P., and Sherman, L.,** Organotin implications in anticarcinogenesis: background and thymus involvement, *Aust. J. Exp. Biol. Med. Sci.,* 62, 199, 1984.
2. **Cardarelli, N. F., Cardarelli, B., and Marioneaux, M.,** Tin as a vital trace nutrient, *J. Nutr. Growth Cancer,* 1, 181, 1985.
3. **Cardarelli, N. F., Ed.,** *Tin as a Vital Nutrient: Implications in Cancer Prophylaxis and Other Physiological Processes,* CRC Press, Boca Raton, Fla., 1985.
4. **Sherman, L. R., Bilgicer, K. I., and Cardarelli, N. F.,** Analysis of tin in mouse and human organs, *J. Nutr. Growth Cancer,* 2, 107, 1985.
5. **Cardarelli, N. F., Cardarelli, B. M., Libby, E. P., and Dobbins, E.,** Organotin implications in anticarcinogenesis: effect of several organotins on tumor growth rate in mice, *Aust. J. Exp. Biol. Med. Sci.,* 62, 209, 1984.
6. **Haiduc, I., Silvestru, C., and Gielen, M.,** Organotin compounds: new organometallic derivatives exhibiting antitumor activity, *Bull. Soc. Chem. Belg.,* 92, 187, 1983.
7. **Crowe, A. J., Smith, P. J., and Atassi, G.,** Investigations into the antitumor activity of organotin compounds. I. Diorganotin dihalide and di-pseudohalide complexes, *Chem. Biol. Interact.,* 32, 171, 1980.
8. **Luckey, T. D., Ed.,** *Thymic Hormones,* University Park Press, Baltimore, Md., 1973.
9. **Hanson, A. M.,** A report of four cases of inoperable carcinoma treated with intramuscular injections of karkinolysin, *Minn. Med.,* 13, 65, 1930.
10. **Hanson, A. M.,** Treatment of cancer with thymus extracts, *J.A.M.A.,* 94, 653, 1930.
11. **Potop, I., Sterescu, V., Boeru, V., Peloni, R., Petrescu, E., and Ghinea, E.,** Effect of an "S" purified thymus factor (isolated from IIB thymus fraction) on the *in vitro* proliferation of tumor cells, *Neoplasma,* 17, 655, 1970.

12. **Milcu, S. M., Potop, I., Holban-Petrescu, R., Boeru, V., Ghinea, E., and Tasca, C.,** Effect of some fractions isolated from the lipid thymus extract (extract IIB) on tumor cell proliferation *in vitro, Neoplasma,* 16, 473, 1969.
13. **Abraham, A.,** Evidence of steroid synthesis in the thymus of white rats using (1-^{14}C) acetate and (4-^{14}C) cholesterol as precursors, *Rev. Roum. Endocr.,* 8, 83, 1971.
14. **Kanakkanatt, S. V.,** Synthesis of tin steroids and the relation between structure and anticancer activity, in *Tin as a Vital Nutrient: Implications in Cancer Prophylaxis and Other Physiological Processes,* Cardarelli, N. F., Ed., CRC Press, Boca Raton, Fla., 1985.
15. **Cardarelli, N. F. and Kanakkanatt, S. V.,** Tin Steroids and Their Use as Antineoplastic Agents, U.S. Patent 4,541,956, 1985.
16. **Lichter, W.,** private communication, 1983 to 1985.
17. **Sherman, L. R., Masters, J. G., Peterson, R., and Levine, S.,** Tin concentration in the thymus glands of rats and mice and its relation to the involution of the gland, *J. Anal. Toxicol.,* 10, 6, 1986.

Chapter 7

CHEMISTRY AND BIOLOGY OF ORGANOTIN DERIVATIVES OF CARBOHYDRATES

Robert C. Poller

TABLE OF CONTENTS

I.	Introduction		60
II.	Synthetic Methods		60
	A.	Alkoxide Derivatives	60
		1. Trialkyltin Compounds	60
		2. Dialkyltin Compounds	64
	B.	Compounds Containing Tin-Carbon Bonds	67
	C.	Thiolate Derivatives	68
	D.	Indirect Methods of Linking Tin Atoms to Sugars	69

Acknowledgment ... 70

References ... 70

I. INTRODUCTION

Over the last decade interest in organotin derivatives of carbohydrates has been steadily increasing. It is opportune now to review developments in the subject which will be at least useful background material for the main purpose of this book, but could be of more central interest. There do not seem to be any reports of general evaluation of this class of compound for antitumor activities, though the writer is in the process of sending a number of compounds for evaluation.

Although there have been one or two incursions into polysaccharide chemistry, the work in this field has generally been with sugars, almost entirely mono- and disaccharides and compounds derived from them. The major interest and motivation in this area is chemical, and the bulk of the paper is therefore concerned with chemistry. Nevertheless, a minority of compounds have been submitted to some kind of biological evaluation, and these results are also discussed.

II. SYNTHETIC METHODS

Carbohydrates are polyhydroxy compounds and, when methods of attaching organotin groups are contemplated, utilization of these hydroxyl groups (which may be primary alcoholic, secondary alcoholic or glycosidic) is the obvious approach. Further examination of the problem, however, suggests four distinct methods of linking organotin groups to sugars which are summarized in Figure 1.

The first and most widely used method in which the sugar is converted to an organotin alkoxide has already been referred to. In method 2 the organotin group is directly attached to a sugar carbon atom. The third approach is to use some bifunctional species X to link the organotin and sugar moieties. Finally, method 4 involves conversion of a hydroxyl to a thiol group and, hence, formation of an organotin thiolate. Although most of the compounds discussed in this paper were made by the first method, derivatives made by methods 2 through 4 will also be considered.

A. Alkoxide Derivatives

1. Trialkyltin Compounds

Conversion of an alcohol to a trialkyltin alkoxide increases electron density at the oxygen atom and thereby activates the alcohol to electrophilic attack. This is illustrated in Scheme 1 where the cationic benzoyl group is the electrophile. This ability of organotin groups to activate alcohols has been exploited commercially in the use of organotin catalysts for the production of polyurethanes. Here, the essential reaction is between an alcohol and an isocyanate; the catalytic cycle is shown in Scheme 2.

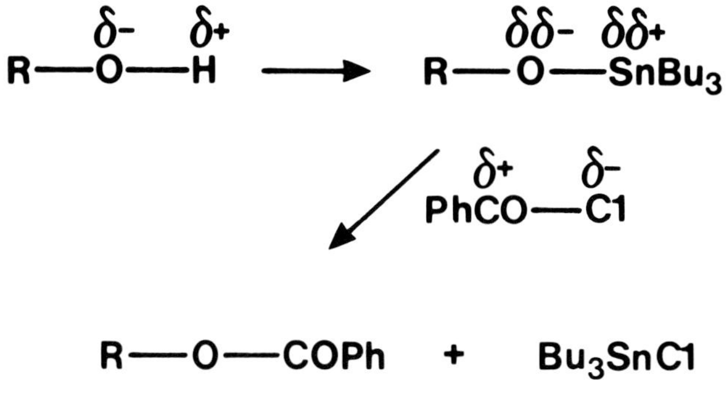

$$R\overset{\delta-}{-}O\overset{\delta+}{-}H \longrightarrow R\overset{\delta\delta-}{-}O\overset{\delta\delta+}{-}SnBu_3$$

$$\overset{\delta+}{PhCO}\overset{\delta-}{-}Cl \diagdown$$

$$R-O-COPh \;+\; Bu_3SnCl$$

SCHEME 1

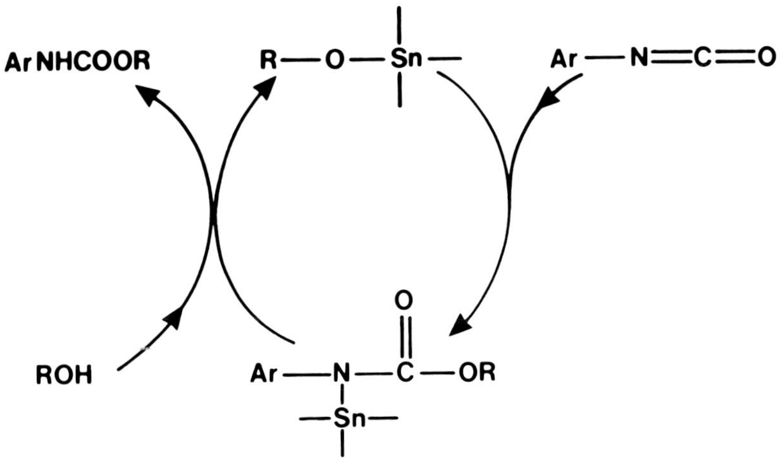

SCHEME 2

Much research in carbohydrate chemistry is concerned with the need for selective reaction at one or more predetermined hydroxylic sites, while the remainder of the molecule is unaffected. Since stannylation occurs regioselectively, it can be used for selective activation. Ogawa and Matsui[1] suggested that stannylation of a particular hydroxyl group would be favored if the coordination number at tin was increased from four to five by donation of a lone pair from an appropriately positioned oxygen atom. Thus, of the two primary hydroxyls in hexan-1,2,6-triol shown in Scheme 3, that on C-1 is stannylated as stabilization by coordination from the C-2 hydroxyl occurs. This is followed by benzoylation which occurs exclusively at the stannylated-hydroxyl group.

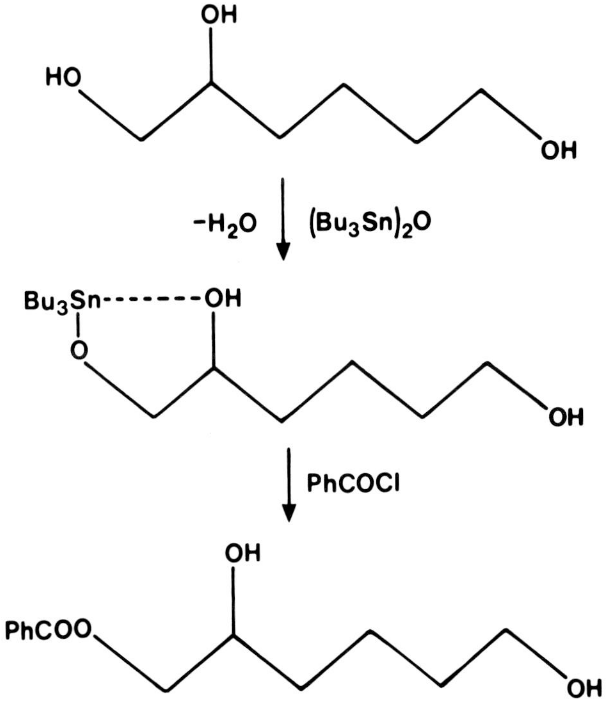

SCHEME 3

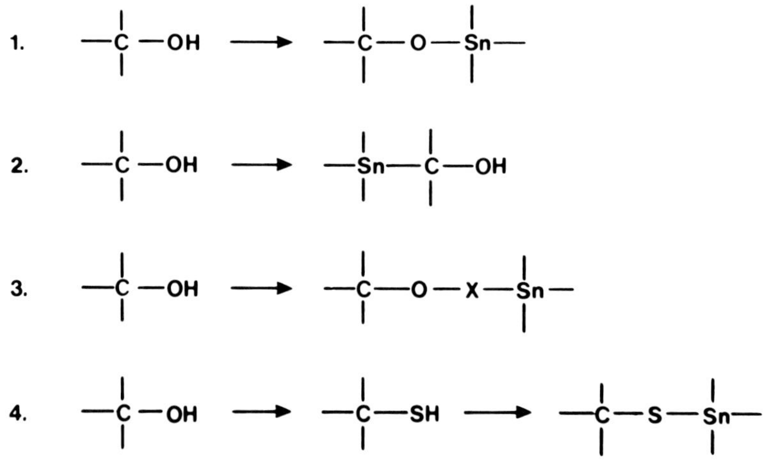

FIGURE 1. Methods of joining organotin groups to sugars.

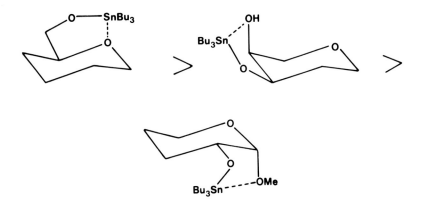

FIGURE 2. Stability order for stannylated sugar derivatives.

Applying these ideas to the aldopyranose sugars, it has been shown that on treatment with one equivalent of bis(tri-*n*-butyltin) oxide in benzene with azeotropic removal of water, the order of reactivity is as follows. Most favored is the primary hydroxyl, the stannoxide being stabilized by donation from the ring-oxygen atom; next is a vicinal pair of *cis*-hydroxyls in which the equatorial hydroxyl is stannylated with coordination from the axial group; and finally, in α-glycosides, an equatorial hydroxyl on C-2 is attacked, stabilization occurring by coordination from the glycosidic oxygen (Figure 2).[2] The 5-coordination shown must be weak since it is not detected by ^{119}Sn NMR measurement[3] but, nevertheless, this concept allows successful prediction of the site of stannylation.

In the following brief survey of stannylations with bis(tri-*n*-butyltin) oxide we begin with diols in which the other hydroxyl groups are masked and then progress to sugar derivatives with increasing numbers of free hydroxyls. In Scheme 4 the *N*-phthaloylglucosamine derivative is regioselectively stannylated at the primary hydroxyl and the tin group subsequently displaced with benzyl[4] (N.B. throughout this paper Bz = benzyl). A compound with a vicinal *cis*-diol pair is illustrated by the mannose derivative in Scheme 5 where the equatorial hydroxyl is stannylated; when the product was benzylated, the 3-benzyl compound was obtained in 73% yield.[5] Specific stannylation at the O-2 position in an α-glycoside is exemplified by the glucose derivative in Scheme 6.[6]

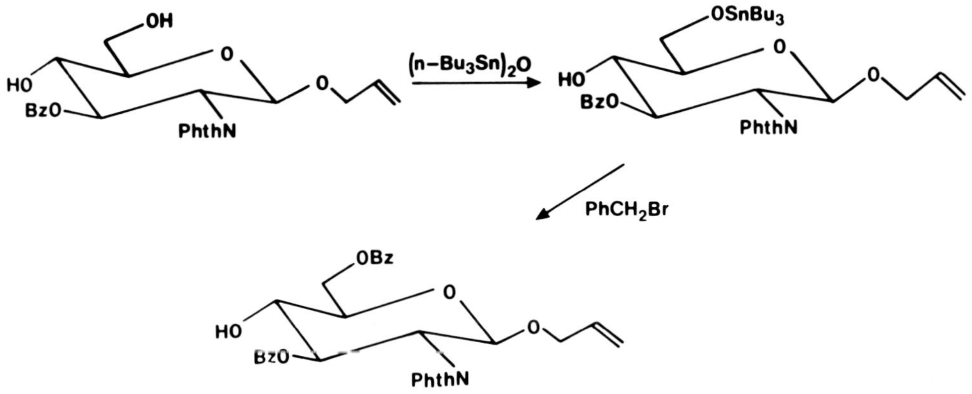

SCHEME 4

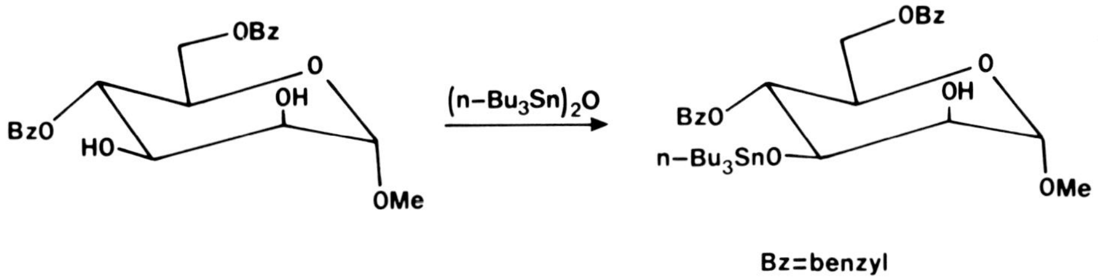

SCHEME 5

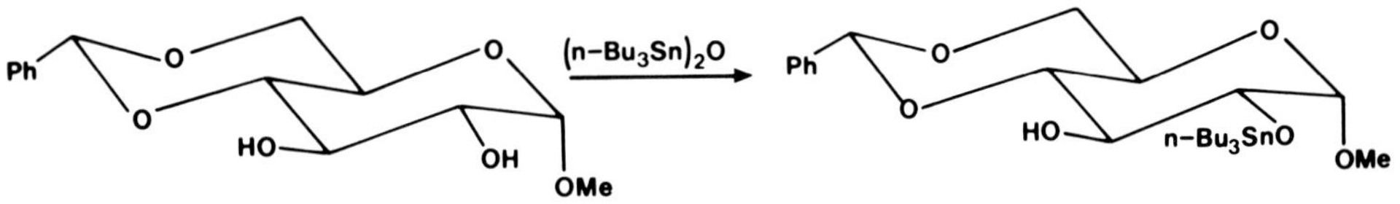

SCHEME 6

The mannose derivative shown in Scheme 7 has three free hydroxyl groups on adjacent carbon atoms, but only the hydroxyls on C-2 and C-3 have the required *cis* relationship and, accordingly, it is the equatorial group on C-3 which is stannylated.[7] A number of other sugar triols have been shown to react similarly.

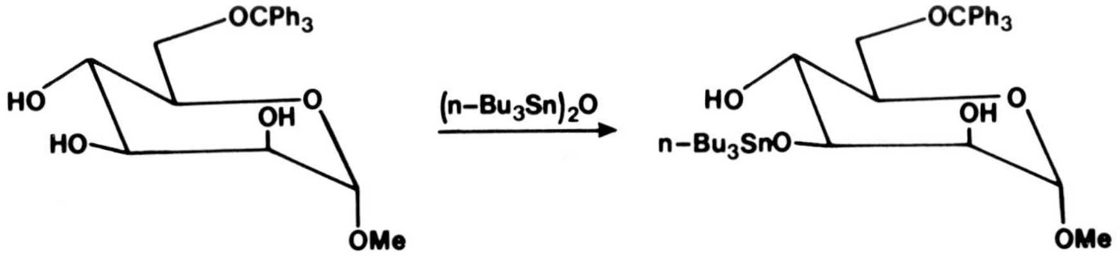

SCHEME 7

When methyl α-D-glucopyranoside is treated with three equivalents of bis(tri-*n*-butyltin) oxide we predict that only the C-6 and C-2 hydroxyls should be stannylated. Scheme 8 represents what was observed.[1]

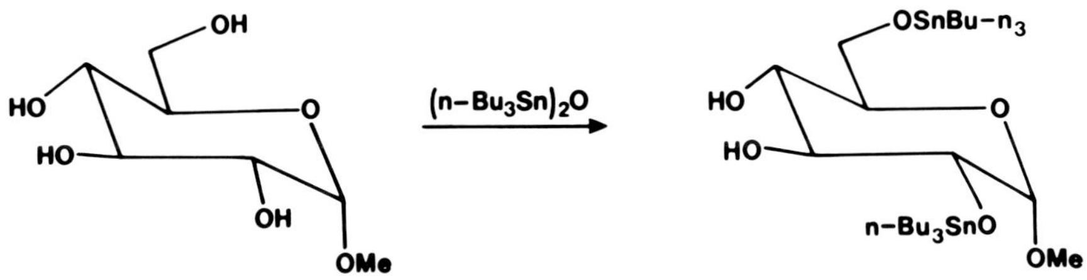

SCHEME 8

Two general points should be noted about selective tri-*n*-butylstannylation. The first is that in almost all cases the structures have been inferred from those of the products of further substitution. Second, although hydroxyl groups are activated by stannylation, the relative order of reactivity is not affected, for example, the primary hydroxyl group remains the most reactive. It will be seen later that stannylation with dibutyltin groups can profoundly alter relative reactivities.[2]

Recently a technique for perstannylation has been reported[8] in which the hydroxylic hydrogens are first replaced with diethylboron groups and subsequently with tri-*n*-butyltin residues by treatment with tri-*n*-butyltin acetylacetonate (Scheme 9). Using this technique octastannylsucrose and perstannylated oligosaccharides were prepared.

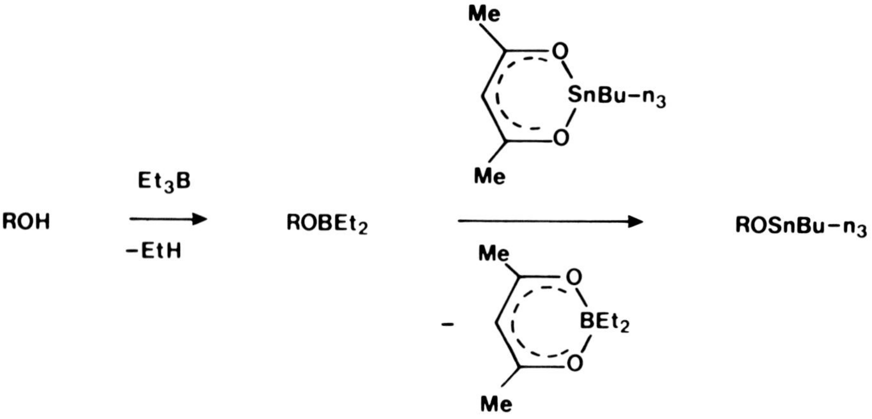

SCHEME 9

2. Dialkyltin Compounds

Vicinal diol units, *cis* or *trans*, react with di-*n*-butyltin oxide in methanol (where the effective reagent is *n*-Bu$_2$Sn[OMe]$_2$) or in benzene under conditions for azeotropic dehydration to give the cyclic di-*n*-butylstannylene derivatives (Scheme 10). This reaction was first applied to nucleoside chemistry by Moffat and co-workers[9] who isolated a series of crystalline di-*n*-butylstannylene derivatives of ribonucleosides in which the O-2 and O-3 atoms were bridged by tin (Scheme 11). Acylation of the stannylene derivatives led to substitution at these oxygens and not at the primary O-5 or the NH positions in the bases (i.e., a change in relative reactivities).

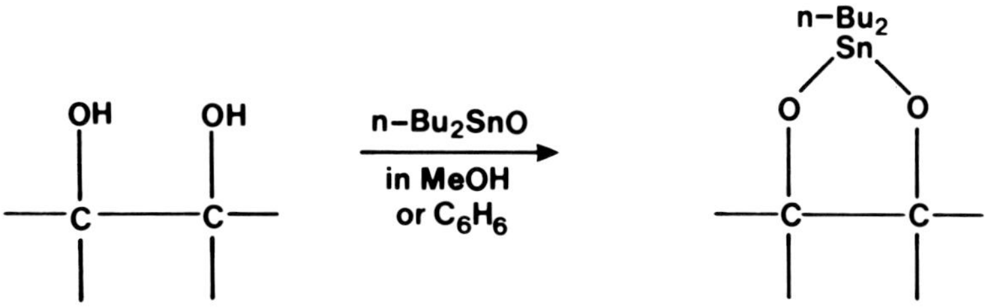

SCHEME 10

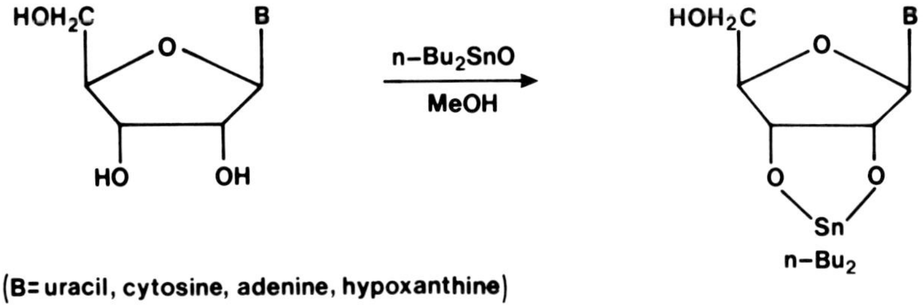

SCHEME 11

(B = uracil, cytosine, adenine, hypoxanthine)

Turning from ribonucleosides to consider di-*n*-butylstannyl derivatives of sugars more generally, our interpretation of the chemistry is aided by the existence of two X-ray crystal structure determinations. The essential structure of the dimeric dibutylstannyl derivative of methyl 4,6-di-*O*-benzylidine-α-D-glucopyranoside[10] (omitting conformation) is shown in Scheme 12.

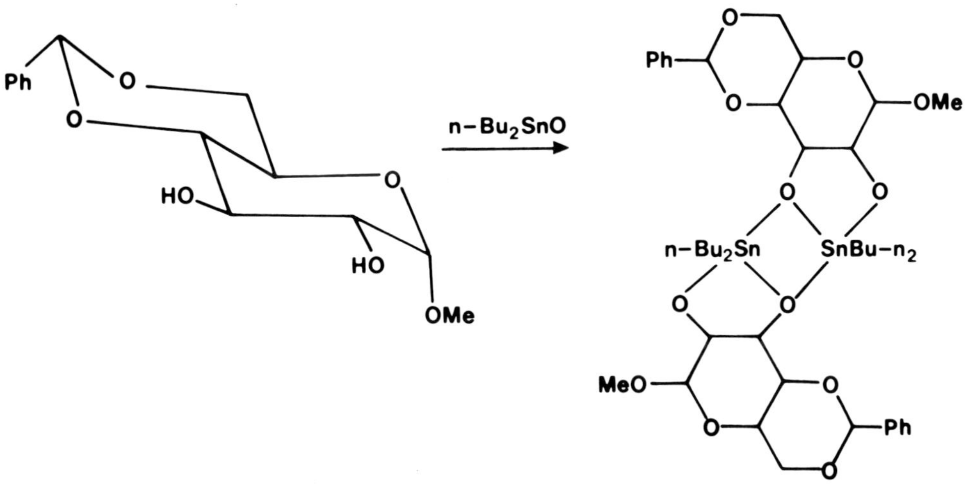

SCHEME 12

The two molecules are held together by coordination from O-3 to tin. The dimeric structure persists in noncoordinating solvents such as toluene, but in donor solvents the molecules exist as solvated monomers. Hence, in noncoordinating solvents only O-2 is activated to electrophilic substitution, but in donor solvents O-3 is also activated. Accordingly, we find that benzoylation of this stannylene derivative in benzene gave exclusively[10] or mainly[6] the

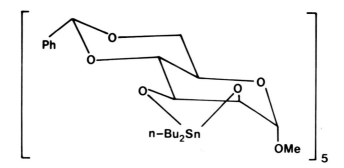

FIGURE 3. X-ray crystal structure shows pentamer; molecules joined by coordination from O-2 and O-3 to tin.[11]

2-O-benzoate, whereas methyl iodide in 1,2-dimethylformamide (DMF) gave a 2:1 mixture of the 2-O- and 3-O-methyl ethers.[10]

The crystal structure of the dibutylstannyiene derivative of the corresponding mannose compound, in which the two hydroxyls bridged by tin are *cis* instead of *trans*, revealed a pentameric unit in the solid state[11] (Figure 3). The molecules are joined via coordination from O-2 and O-3 to tin and in noncoordinating solvents O-2 is preferentially attacked. In donor solvents, or on addition of a basic species, it appears that solvated monomers are formed and now regioselective substitution occurs at the equatorial O-3.

Where more than one pair of vicinal hydroxyls are free, di-*n*-butyltin oxide will react preferentially at a *cis* (equatorial/axial) rather than a *trans* (equatorial/equatorial, usually) grouping. Subsequent electrophilic substitution then occurs predominantly at the equatorial oxygen in donor solvents and at the axial oxygen in noncoordinating media. These generalizations are illustrated by the chlorosugar shown in Scheme 13 where stannylene formation occurs at the *cis*-hydroxyls. Further reaction in donor solvents leads to electrophilic substitution at O-3.[6]

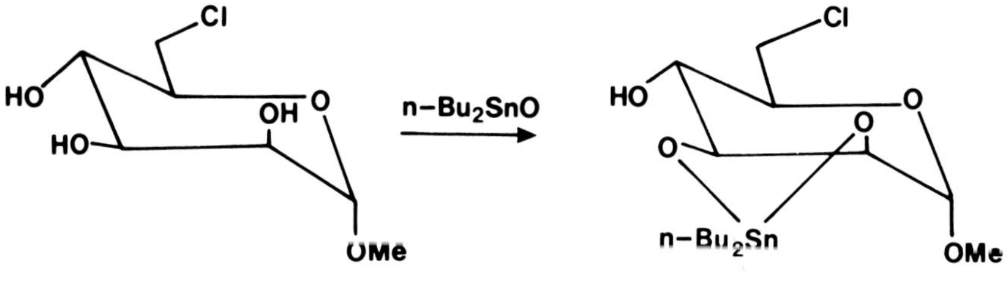

SCHEME 13

Even when a primary hydroxyl group is free, as in benzyl 2-*O*-benzyl-β-D-galactopyranoside, stannylation still occurs at the *cis*-diol grouping at C-3 and C-4[12] (Scheme 14).

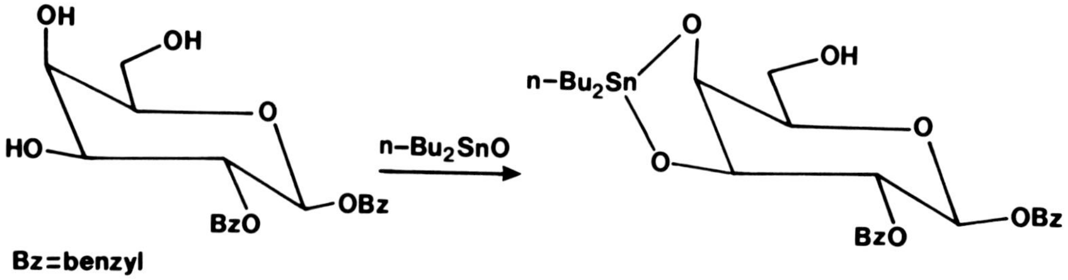

Bz=benzyl

SCHEME 14

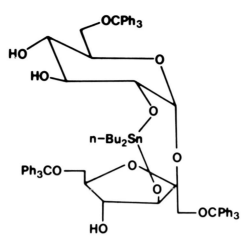

FIGURE 4. Proposed structure of di-*n*-butylstannylene derivative of 6,1',6'-tri-*O*-tritylsucrose.[11]

There is reasonable evidence that, where no vicinal *cis*-diol unit is present, tin will bridge oxygen atoms which are more widely separated. A particularly striking example is 6,1',6'-tri-*O*-tritylsucrose in which the hydroxyl groups attached to C-2 and C-3' are activated leading to the proposed structure shown in Figure 4 in which the dibutyltin group acts as a second bridge between the glucose and fructose residues.[13]

B. Compounds Containing Tin-Carbon Bonds

This class contains only a very few compounds which were prepared for a number of reasons. The first two, both triphenylstannyl derivatives, were prepared primarily as NMR reference compounds. Thus, treatment of the glucofuranose derivative shown in Scheme 15 with triphenyltin lithium caused nucleophilic displacement of the tosyloxy group on C-6 by the triphenylstannyl moiety.[14] Using the same reagent an epoxy sugar reacted to give the triphenylstannyl substituent on a secondary carbon atom[14] (Scheme 16). Although biological properties of organotin sugar derivatives are mentioned in a general way in this paper no biological tests on the products are reported and apparently no attempts were made to remove the protecting groups.

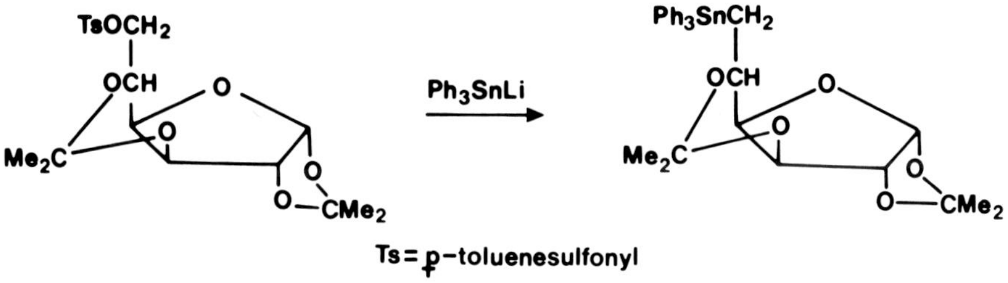

SCHEME 15

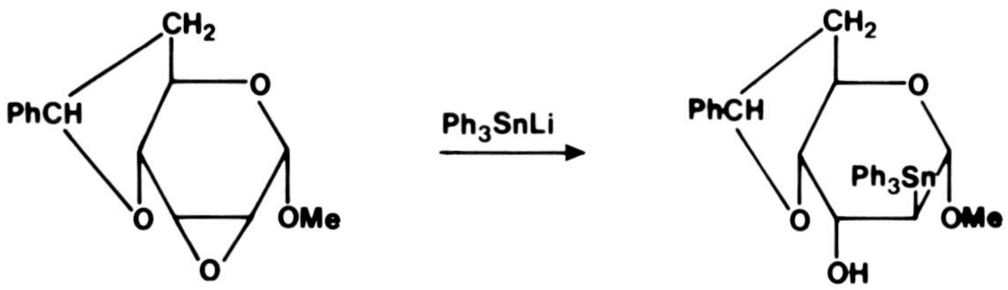

SCHEME 16

More recently, a stannylated sugar alkene was prepared by the addition of tri-*n*-butyltin hydride to an acetylenic sugar[15] (Scheme 17). In this case the product was a synthetic intermediate, and the tin moiety was replaced by bromine to give a compound of potential pharmaceutical interest.

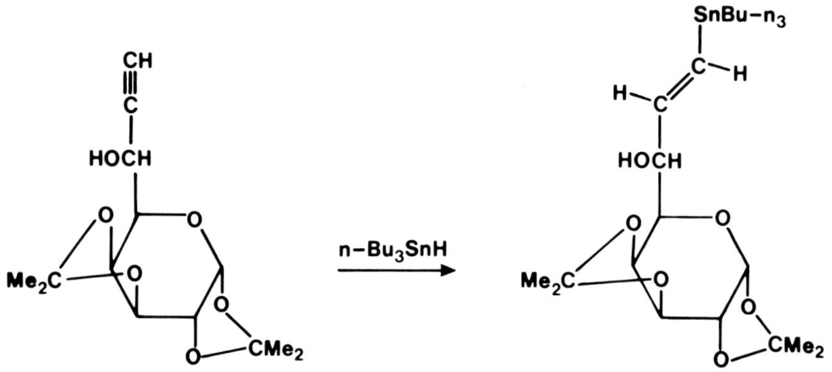

SCHEME 17

C. Thiolate Derivatives

Stable organotin derivatives of glucose were prepared either by treatment of 2,3,4,6-tetra-*O*-acetyl-1-thio-β-D-glucopyranose with organotin oxides and hydroxides or by reaction between 2,3,4,6-tetra-*O*-acetyl-α-D-glucopyranosyl bromide and organotin lithium sulfides[16] (Scheme 18). Careful treatment of the products shown in Scheme 18 with catalytic amounts of sodium methoxide allowed the isolation of the tri-*n*-butyl- and triphenyl-tin derivatives of free glucose. The triphenyltin compound was given preliminary screening for biological activity (see Tables 1 and 2), and as it appeared to be less active than other compounds which interested us at the time, the biological tests of this type of compound were not pursued.

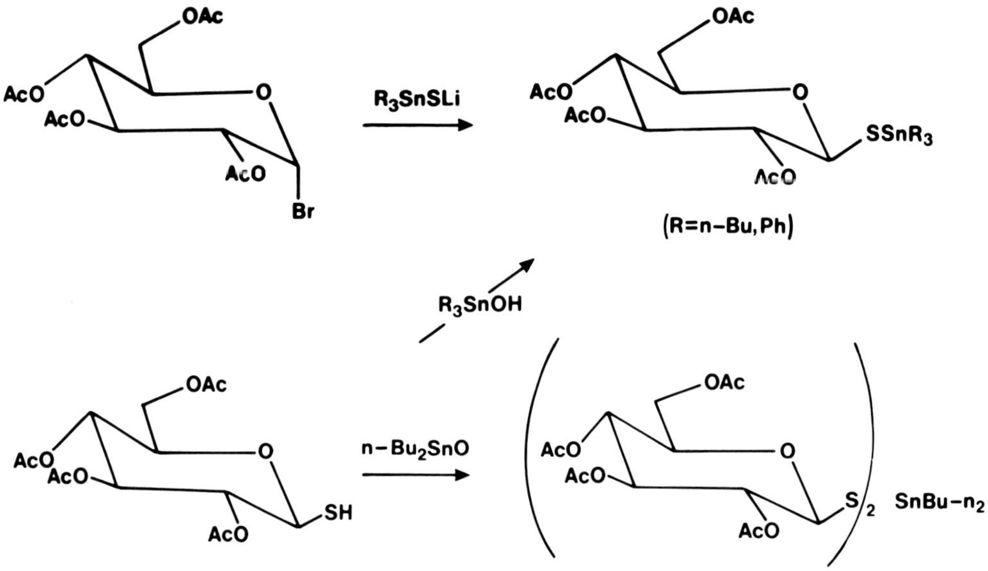

SCHEME 18

Table 1
FUNGICIDAL TESTS

Compound	No. of fungi showing inhibition of spore germination (max 16)		
	100 ppm	10 ppm	1 ppm
n-Bu$_3$SnOCOC$_6$H$_4$COOsucrose	16	16	6
Ph$_3$SnOCOC$_6$H$_4$COOsucrose	16	14	4
(C$_6$H$_{11}$)$_3$OCOC$_6$H$_4$COOsucrose	3	0	0
n-Bu$_3$SnOCOCH$_2$CH$_2$COOsucrose	16	16	10
Ph$_3$SnOCOCH$_2$CH$_2$COOsucrose	16	15	9
SucroseOCOC$_6$H$_4$COO(CH$_2$)$_3$SnPh$_2$Br	16	7	0
Ph$_3$SnSglucose	14	14	6
(n-Bu$_3$Sn)$_2$O	13	13	12

Table 2
ALGICIDAL TESTS

Compounds Tested against *Enteromorpha* in Sea Water Modified with Algal Nutrients

Compound	Concentration	
	1 ppm	0.1 ppm
n-Bu$_3$SnOCOC$_6$H$_4$COOsucrose	+	+
Ph$_3$SnOCOC$_6$H$_4$COOsucrose	+	+
(C$_6$H$_{11}$)$_3$SnOCOC$_6$H$_4$COOsucrose	−	−
n-Bu$_3$SnOCOCH$_2$CH$_2$COOsucrose	+	+
Ph$_3$SnOCOCH$_2$CH$_2$COOsucrose	+	+
SucroseOCOC$_6$H$_4$COO(CH$_2$)$_3$SnPh$_2$Br	+	+
Ph$_3$SnSglucose	+	−

Note: + = effective; − = not effective; minimum concentration at which (n-Bu$_3$Sn)$_2$O is effective = 0.3 ppm.

D. Indirect Methods of Linking Tin Atoms to Sugars

Some years ago we were interested in preparing organotin derivatives of sucrose and assessing their potential as commercial biocides. After surveying a number of possible methods, we decided to treat sucrose with cyclic anhydrides and thereby prepare monosucrose esters of dibasic acids, the free carboxyl group subsequently being used for attachment to tin. By this means organotin sucrose phthalates and succinates were prepared, but the corresponding maleates proved to be more difficult to prepare, and initial experiments were not pursued[17] (Scheme 19). Because we were seeking products for commercial exploitation, we used unprotected sucrose and had to accept that we were dealing with mixtures; a typical sample of "sucrose phthalate" contained 36% sucrose, 37% monoester, 26% diester, and 1% higher esters.[17] Maximum biological activity is found in compounds containing three carbon-tin bonds, i.e., of the R$_3$SnX type, and the sucrose compounds discussed so far all had the sugar residue incorporated into the X group. The sequence shown in Scheme 20 was used to prepare a compound containing the sucrose residue in the R group to determine whether this affected biological activity.[18]

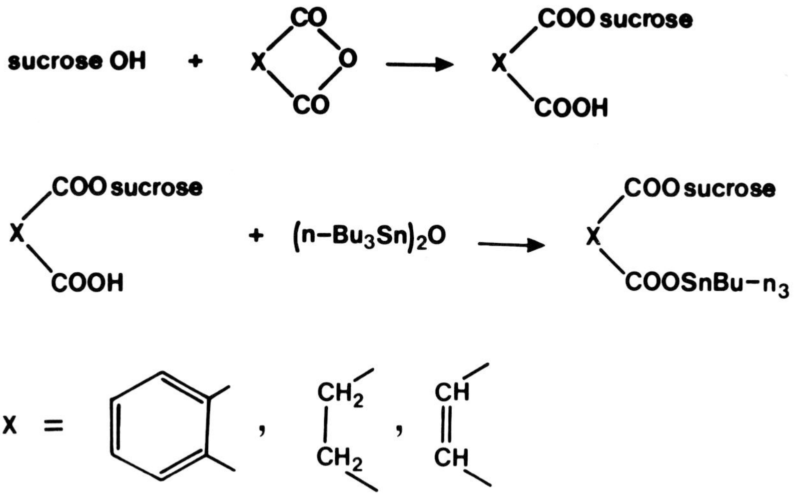

$$\text{sucrose OH} + X\begin{matrix}\diagup\text{CO}\\ \diagdown\text{CO}\end{matrix}\!\!\!\diagdown\!\!\text{O} \longrightarrow X\begin{matrix}\diagup\text{COO sucrose}\\ \diagdown\text{COOH}\end{matrix}$$

$$X\begin{matrix}\diagup\text{COO sucrose}\\ \diagdown\text{COOH}\end{matrix} + (n\text{-Bu}_3\text{Sn})_2\text{O} \longrightarrow X\begin{matrix}\diagup\text{COO sucrose}\\ \diagdown\text{COOSnBu-}n_3\end{matrix}$$

X = *ortho*-phenylene, –CH$_2$–CH$_2$–, –CH=CH–

SCHEME 19

$$\text{NaOCOC}_6\text{H}_4\text{COOsucrose} + \text{Ph}_3\text{SnCH}_2\text{CH}_2\text{CH}_2\text{Br}$$
$$\downarrow$$
$$\text{Ph}_3\text{SnCH}_2\text{CH}_2\text{CH}_2\text{OCOC}_6\text{H}_4\text{COOsucrose} + \text{NaBr}$$
$$\downarrow \text{Br}_2$$
$$\text{BrPh}_2\text{SnCH}_2\text{CH}_2\text{CH}_2\text{OCOC}_6\text{H}_4\text{COOsucrose} + \text{PhBr}$$

SCHEME 20

The compounds were tested for their ability to inhibit spore germination using 16 species of fungi which attack paint films.[18] The results are summarized in Table 1. If the tri-*n*-butyltin compounds are compared at the 10-ppm level when they will all be in solution, the sucrose residues appear to alter the biological specificity so that the two fungal species not attacked by bis(tri-*n*-butyltin) oxide became susceptible. The thioglucose derivative is included for comparison.

Since an important use of organotin compounds is in antifouling paints it was important to test the compounds against the marine alga *Enteromorpha;* the results are shown in Table 2. It is striking that the sucrose compounds are generally more effective than bis(tri-*n*-butyltin) oxide even though their tin content is much reduced.

Because the introduction of a sucrose residue increased both the range and degree of biological activity, it seemed unlikely that this is due simply to solubility effects. It was decided to extend the sucrose work to include other sugars. We were particularly attracted to trehalose because of its role in the metabolism of fungi and other microorganisms as well as of some insects, but we included many other sugars. Apart from some improvements in technique, the same method of reaction between the cyclic anhydride was adopted, and a number of the mixed sugar esters have been fully separated and characterized.[19] Biological testing of these compounds is incomplete, but herbicidal evaluation has been carried out (Table 3). From these results we note that, in contrast to the previous tests, the sugar derivatives are less active than the standard organotin compounds (*n*-Bu$_3$Sn)$_2$O and Ph$_3$SnOH.

Table 3
HERBICIDAL TESTS[a]

Compound		Score[b]	EF[c]
Trehalose			
Succinate	n-Bu[d]	17	1.6
	Ph[e]	11	1.7
Phthalate	n-Bu	15	1.5
	Ph	15	2.5
Cl$_4$phthalate	n-Bu	18	2.1
Lactose			
Succinate	n-Bu	17	1.6
	Ph	12	1.8
Phthalate	n-Bu	17	1.7
	Ph	12	2.0
Cl$_4$phthalate	n-Bu	16	1.9
	Ph	12	2.3
Maltose			
Succinate	n-Bu	18	1.7
	Ph	17	2.6
Phthalate	n-Bu	17	1.7
	Ph	11	1.8
Sucrose			
Succinate	n-Bu	17	1.7
	Ph	12	1.8
Phthalate	n-Bu	14	1.4
	Ph	16	2.7
Raffinose			
Succinate	n-Bu	22	2.2
	Ph	9	1.5
Phthalate	Ph	12	2.0
(n-Bu$_3$Sn)$_2$O		26	
Ph$_3$SnOH		14	

- [a] Plants: beet, maize, mustard, peas, rye, and linseed. Treated with 1% solution of compound in aqueous acetone.
- [b] For each plant, compound given a score of 5 (rapid kill) to 0 (no effect); maximum score = 30.
- [c] Enhancement factor (EF) = actual score/score expected by comparison of tin content with that of (Bu$_3$Sn)$_2$O (for tributyltin compounds) or Ph$_3$SnOH (for triphenyltin compounds).
- [d] n-Bu = tri-n-butylstannyl.
- [e] Ph = triphenylstannyl.
- [f] Cl$_4$phthalate = tetrachlorophthalate.

However, in terms of tin content, their biological activities are enhanced, but not strikingly and with no great variation from one sugar to another. The generalization that alkyltin compounds are more phytotoxic than the aryltins holds in most cases.

The results of some tests against bacteria and fungi are shown in Table 4. Although the enhancement factors are somewhat larger, there are, again, no large differences between the various sugars, with the highest single value of a three-fold enhancement for tri-n-butyltin sucrose phthalate.

To summarize, large numbers of organotin derivatives of sugars have been prepared, though few have been assessed for biological activity. The introduction of sugar residues can have profound effects on the biological properties in ways which are difficult to explain

Table 4
BACTERIAL AND FUNGICIDAL TESTS[a,b]

Compound		Bactericidal				Fungicidal			
		1 ppm		0.1 ppm		1 ppm		0.1 ppm	
		Score[c]	EF[d]	Score	EF	Score	EF	Score	EF
Trehalose	succinate n-Bu	25	2.5	22	2.7	25	2.0	13	2.5
Lactose	succinate n-Bu	25	2.5	22	2.7	26	2.1	13	2.5
Maltose	succinate n-Bu	25	2.5	17	2.1	26	2.1	13	2.5
Sucrose	succinate n-Bu	23	2.6	22	3.0	28	2.3	12	2.4

[a] Bacteria: *C. michiganense, P. syringae, S. aureus, P. auruginosa,* and *K. aerogenes*. Fungi: *R. oligosporus, A. niger, C. globulosum, P. irregulare,* and *B. fabae*. Yeasts: *S. cerevisae, C. utilis,* and *T. verstilis*.
[b] Bacteria: five species examined, maximum score 25. Fungi and yeasts: eight species examined, maximum score 40.
[c] Score: maximum activity = 5, no activity = 0 for each microorganism.
[d] Enhancement factor (EF) = actual score/score expected by comparison of the tin content with that of $(Bu_3Sn)_2O$. The score for $(Bu_3Sn)_2O$ was the one obtained for the particular specimens of mocroorganisms used for assessing the test compounds.

in terms of solubility alone. More work is needed, and we are hopeful that further tests on compounds we have already prepared will help our understanding of this phenomenon.

ACKNOWLEDGMENT

The work carried out jointly by Patel and Poller was supported by the Science and Engineering Research Council and by Tate and Lyle, Ltd.

REFERENCES

1. **Ogawa, T. and Matsui, M.,** *Tetrahedron*, 37, 2363, 1981.
2. **Tsuda, Y., Haque, M. E., and Yoshimoto, K.,** *Chem. Pharm. Bull.*, 31, 1612, 1983.
3. **Blunden, S., Smith, P. J., Benyon, P. J., and Gillies, D. G.,** *Carbohydr. Res.*, 88, 9, 1981.
4. **Ogawa, T., Kitajima, T., and Nukada, T.,** *Carbohydr. Res.*, 123, C5, 1983.
5. **Handa, V. K., Barlow, J. J., and Matta, K. L.,** *Carbohydr. Res.*, 76, C1, 1979.
6. **Holzapfel, C. W., Koekemoer, J. M., and Marais, C. F.,** *S. Afr. J. Chem.*, 37, 19, 1984.
7. **Alais, J. and Veyrières, A.,** *J. Chem. Soc. Perkin Trans. 1*, p. 377, 1981.
8. **Taba, K. M., Koester, R., and Dahlhoff, W. V.,** *Synthesis*, p. 399, 1984.
9. **Wagner, D., Verheyden, J. P. H., and Moffatt, J. G.,** *Org. Chem.*, 39, 24, 1974.
10. **David, S., Pascard, C., and Cesario, M.,** *Nouv. J. Chim.*, 3, 63, 1979.
11. **Holzapfel, C. W., Koekemoer, J. M., Marais, C. F., Kruger, G. J., and Pretorius, J. A.,** *S. Afr. J. Chem.*, 35, 80, 1982.
12. **David, S., Thiefry, A., and Veyrières, A.,** *J. Chem. Soc. Perkin Trans. 1*, p. 1796, 1981.
13. **Holzapfel, C. W., Koekemoer, J. M., and Marais, C. F.,** *S. Afr. J. Chem.*, 37, 57, 1984.
14. **Hall, L. D., Steiner, P. R., and Miller, D. C.,** *Can. J. Chem.*, 57, 38, 1979.
15. **Neeser, J. R., Hall, L. D., and Balatoni, J. A.,** *Helv. Chim. Acta*, 66, 1018, 1983.
16. **Husain, A. F. and Poller, R. C.,** *J. Organomet. Chem.*, 118, C11, 1976.
17. **Parkin, A. and Poller, R. C.,** *Carbohydr. Res.*, 62, 83, 1978.
18. **Parkin, A. and Poller, R. C.,** *Int. Pest Control*, 19, 5, 1977.
19. **Patel, A. and Poller, R. C.,** Main group, *Metal Chem.*, 10, 287, 1987; *Rec. Trav. Chim.*, 1988, in press. **Patel, A., Poller, R. C., and Rathbone, E. B.,** *Appl. Organometallic Chem.*, 1, 325, 1987.

Chapter 8

APPLICATION OF SOLID STATE NMR TO PROBLEMS IN STRUCTURAL ORGANOTIN CHEMISTRY

Thomas P. Lockhart

TABLE OF CONTENTS

I.	Introduction	74
II.	Results	74
III.	Discussion	75
	A. General Features of CPMAS NMR Spectra of Organotin Compounds	75
	B. Dependence of $\|J\|$ on Me–Sn–Me Angle	78
	C. Analysis of Medium Effects on Molecular Structure	79
	D. Structural Analysis of Amorphous Methyltin(IV) Polymers	79
IV.	Conclusions on the Use of Solid State NMR for the Structural Analysis of Organotin Anticancer Agents	80
	Acknowledgments	81
	References	81

I. INTRODUCTION

NMR is an important tool for investigating the structure of organotin compounds in solution. However, because medium effects obscure the relationship of solid state molecular structure to the structure present in solution, only qualitative relationships between molecular structure and NMR parameters such as chemical shift[1] and spin coupling to tin[2] have been developed. With solid state NMR one can obtain spectral data on compounds in the state of matter where their structure is accurately known (from X-ray), and thus this technique offers a chance to investigate rigorously the relationship of NMR and structural parameters. Even in the absence of X-ray data, solid state and solution NMR can be used to deduce the changes in molecular structure on changing phase.

I will describe some results of our studies of methyltin(IV)s by magic-angle spinning (MAS), cross-polarized (CP) solid state ^{13}C-NMR (CPMAS ^{13}C-NMR). As we will be concerned primarily with tin-carbon spin coupling it should be noted that there are two spin-$1/2$ isotopes of Sn, ^{117}Sn and ^{119}Sn, of useful natural abundance (7.6 and 8.6%, respectively). In CPMAS as in solution ^{13}C-NMR experiments, ^{117}Sn and ^{119}Sn satellites are symmetrically displaced about the uncoupled, central resonance[3] (recall that 84% of all molecules will contain no NMR-active Sn isotope) and can be observed for many organotin solids.

Studying structurally characterized methyltin(IV) solids, we have discovered[4] a simple relationship of the magnitude of tin-carbon spin coupling, $|^1J(^{119}\text{Sn-}^{13}\text{C})|$ (hereafter referred to by $|J|$), to the C–Sn–C angle. Several examples will serve to illustrate the use of the new relationship in elucidating the structure of methyltin(IV)s in both the solid-state and solution. CPMAS NMR structural analysis of insoluble, amorphous methyltin(IV) polymers not amenable to study by X-ray will also be described. At the end of the report I will discuss contributions that such studies can make toward understanding the structure of organotin anticancer agents and their interactions with biological molecules.

II. RESULTS

CPMAS ^{13}C-NMR spectra were obtained at 15.08 MHz with high-power proton decoupling (the spectroscopic method has been published elsewhere[5]). All methyltin(IV)s were prepared by published procedures and, when details were given, were crystallized under the conditions used in the X-ray studies.

A list of tin-carbon coupling constants, $|J|$, of structurally characterized polycrystalline methyltin(IV) solids measured by CPMAS ^{13}C-NMR, is given in Table 1. A plot of $|J|$ vs. the Me–Sn–Me angle reveals a simple, linear relationship between these two parameters for all but two of the points (Figure 1). The equation of the line relating $|J|$ and the Me–Sn–Me angle, Θ, is

$$|J| \text{ (Hz)} = 11.6(\Theta) - 899$$

($r = 0.992$, $n = 14$ points). In Table 2 Me–Sn–Me angles of two dimethyltin(IV) bis(dithiocarbamates) predicted from CPMAS ^{13}C-NMR are compared with those subsequently determined by single crystal X-ray diffraction studies.

The influence of medium (solid state, solution) on the NMR data and structure of several methyltin(IV)s is shown in Table 3. The ^{117}Sn, ^{119}Sn satellites have also been observed in the spectra of amorphous methyltin(IV) polymers (Figure 2); CPMAS NMR data for two are given in Table 4.

Table 1
CPMAS ^{13}C NMR OF METHYLTIN(IV) SOLIDS $|^1J(^{119}Sn,^{13}C)|$ vs. Me-Sn-Me ANGLE

No.	Compound[a]	Sn coordinate no.	Me-Sn-Me angle (°)	Ref.	$|^1J(^{119}Sn-^{13}C)|$[b] Hz
1	Me$_4$Sn	4	109.5	c	336[c]
2	Me$_2$SnPh$_2$ · 2Cr(CO)$_3$	4	115.5	d	380
3	[Me$_2$SnS]$_3$	4	118	e	430
4	Me$_3$SnCl	5	117.2	f	470
5	Me$_3$SnOAc	5	120	g	540
6	Me$_2$PhSnOAc	5	128.1	h	610
7	Me$_2$Sn[ON(H)CH(CH$_3$)O]$_2$	6	109.1	i	600
8	Me$_2$Sn(oxinate)$_2$	6	110.7	j	630
9	[Me$_2$SnCl$_2$(salicylaldehyde)]$_2$	6	131.4	k	675
10	Me$_2$Sn(S$_2$CNEt$_2$)$_2$	6	135.6	11	680
11	Me$_2$Sn(S$_2$CNMe$_2$)$_2$	6	136	l	670
12	Me$_2$Sn(NO$_3$)(OH)	5[m]	139.9	m	730
13	[Me$_2$SnCl$_2$ · lut-N-O)$_2$	6	145.3	n	810
14	Me$_2$SnCl$_2$ · 2DMF	6	165.0	o	990
15	Me$_2$SnCl$_2$ · 2DMSO	6	170.4	p	1060
16	Me$_2$Sn(acac)$_2$	6	180.0	6	1175[q]

[a] Abbreviations: OAc = acetate; oxinate = anion of 8-hydroxyquinoline; lut-N-O = lutidine-N-oxide; DMF = N,N-dimethylformamide; DMSO = dimethylsulfoxide; acac = acetylacetonate.

[b] Calculated from distance (Hz) separating pairs of fused ^{117}Sn, ^{119}Sn satellites × 1.023.

[c] Petrosyan, V. S., Permin, A. B., Reutov, O. A., and Roberts, J. D., Av. solution value, *J. Magn. Res.*, 40, 511, 1980.

[d] Schubert, U., Willeford, B. R., and Zuckerman, J. J., *J. Organomet. Chem.*, 215, 367, 1981.

[e] Menzebach, P. and Bleckmann, P., Tetragonal modification, *J. Organomet. Chem.*, 91, 291, 1975.

[f] Lefferts, J. L., Molloy, K. C., Hossain, M. B., van der Helm, D., and Zuckerman, J. J., *J. Organomet. Chem.*, 240, 349, 1982.

[g] Chih, H. and Penfold, B. R., *J. Cryst. Mol. Struct.*, 3, 285, 1973.

[h] Amini, M. M., Heeg, M. J., and Zuckerman, J. J., unpublished results.

[i] Harrison, P. G., King, T. J., and Phillips, R. C., *J. Chem. Soc. Dalton Trans.*, 2317, 1976.

[j] Schlemper, E. O., *Inorg. Chem.*, 11, 2012, 1967.

[k] Ng, S.-W. and Zuckerman, J. J., *J. Chem. Soc. Chem. Commun.*, 475, 1982.

[l] Kimura, T., Yasuoka, N., Kasai, N., and Kakudo, M., *Bull. Chem. Soc. Jpn.*, 45, 1649, 1972.

[m] Domingos, A. M. and Sheldrick, G. M., *J. Chem. Soc. Dalton Trans.*, 475, 1975. Although they assigned Sn a coordination number of five, an additional, short intramolecular Sn-O distance (2.92 Å) implies hexacoordination.

[n] Ng, S.-W., Barnes, C. L., van der Helm, D., and Zuckerman, J. J., *Organometallics*, 2, 600, 1983.

[o] Aslanov, L. A., Ionov, V. M., Attiya, V. M., Permin, A. B., and Petrosyan, V. S., *J. Struct. Chem.*, 91, 1978.

[p] Isaacs, N. W. and Kennard, C. H. L., *J. Chem. Soc.*, 1257, 1970; Aslanov, L. A., Ionov, V. M., Attiya, W. M., Permin, A. B., and Petrosyan, V. S., *J. Organomet. Chem.*, 144, 39, 1978.

[q] $|^1J(^{119}Sn,^{13}C)|$ observed directly for this compound.

III. DISCUSSION

A. General Features of CPMAS NMR Spectra of Organotin Compounds

The solid state NMR spectrum of Me$_2$Sn(acac)$_2$ (acac = acetylacetonate), Figure 3, gives an idea of the resolution attainable in CPMAS NMR spectra of polycrystalline organotin compounds. The ^{119}Sn and ^{117}Sn satellites are fully resolved, and the ratio of the coupling constants, $|^1J(^{119}Sn,^{13}C)|/|^1J(^{117}Sn^{13}C)|$, 1.05, is equal to the ratio of the gyromagnetic ratios of ^{119}Sn and ^{117}Sn (1.046). The narrow line widths, 5 Hz at half-height, reveal an unexpected multiplicity of the acac-carbonyl carbons (191.4, 192.2 ppm) and the acac-methyl carbons

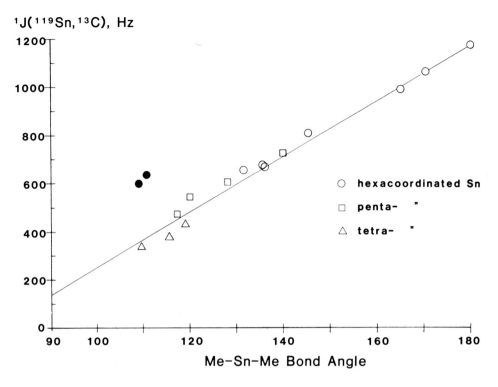

FIGURE 1. Plot of $|^1J(^{119}Sn\text{-}^{13}C)|$ (from CPMAS ^{13}C NMR) vs. Me–Sn–Me bond angle, Θ. Compound numbers defined in Table 1. Filled circles omitted from linear regression (see text).

Table 2
COMPARISON OF CPMAS ^{13}C NMR AND X-RAY STRUCTURES OF TWO DIMETHYLTIN(IV) BIS(DITHIOCARBAMATES)

Compound	CPMAS NMR		X-ray Me-Sn-Me angle (°)	Ref.
	$\|^1J(^{119}Sn-^{13}C)\|$, Hz	Estimated Me-Sn-Me angle (°)		
Me$_2$Sn(S$_2$CNEt$_2$)$_2$ (orthorhombic modification)	675	136	135.6(6)	11
Me$_2$Sn[S$_2$CN(CH$_2$)$_4$]$_2$	705	138	137.4	12

(29.2, 29.5 ppm), both of which appear as partially resolved doublets. Reference to the published X-ray structure[6] shows that this feature arises from asymmetry of the acac ligands, in which there is considerable localization of double and single bond character.

Line widths of 4 to 8 Hz are generally observed for polycrystalline organotin(IV)s.[3] However, the presence of abundant NMR-active nuclei, including quadrupolar nuclei such as ^{14}N and ^{35,37}Cl, can produce severe line broadening and may obscure the Sn satellites.[5] Structural inhomogeneity of noncrystalline methyltin(IV)s (in which the methyls bonded to tin reside in a variety of magnetic environments owing to the random distribution of molecular orientations) also produces line broadening.[7] Line widths of the amorphous polymers in Figure 2 are five to ten times greater than for crystalline compounds.

Table 3
INFLUENCE OF MEDIUM ON STRUCTURE OF METHYLTIN(IV)S

	$|^1J(^{119}Sn-^{13}C)|$, Hz[a]	
Compound	Solid state	Solution
Me_3SnOAc	540	401 ($CDCl_3$)
Me_3SnOH	600	388 ($CDCl_3$)
Me_3SnCl	470	380 (CCl_4)[b]
Me_3SnF	550	369 (CCl_4)[b]
Me_3SnNO_3	500	395 ($CDCl_3$)
		497 (acetone-d_6)
$Me_2Sn(acac)_2$	1175	966 ($CDCl_3$)
		929 (C_6H_6)

[a] $|^1J(^{119}Sn-^{13}C)|$ for solid-state (CPMAS) NMR data calculated as in Table 1; observed directly in solution NMR experiments.

[b] Data from footnote c, Table 1.

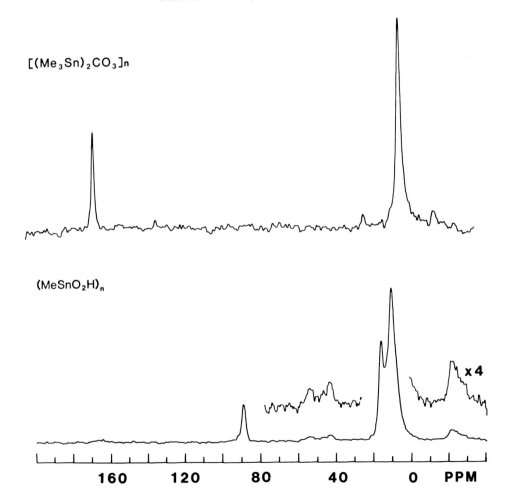

FIGURE 2. CPMAS ^{13}C NMR spectra of amorphous bis(trimethyltin) carbonate and methylstannonic acid polymers. Internal reference, delrin, appears at 89.1 ppm.

Table 4
CPMAS ^{13}C-NMR SPECTRA OF AMORPHOUS METHYLTIN(IV) POLYMERS

Compound	^{13}CH$_3$-Sn chemical shift (ppm)	Line width at half-height (Hz)	$\|^1J(^{119}\text{Sn-}^{13}\text{C})\|$ (Hz)
(MeSnOOH)$_n$	16.2, 10.0	70	1160, 1030
[(Me$_3$Sn)$_2$CO$_3$]	0.4	45	590

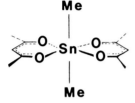

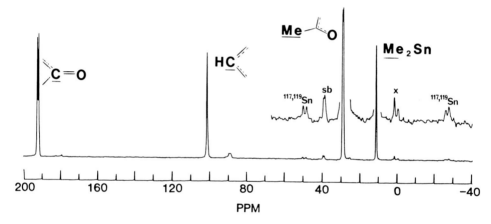

FIGURE 3. CPMAS ^{13}C NMR spectrum of Me$_2$Sn(acac)$_2$. X-ray structure of molecule represented at top left. ^{117,119}Sn indicates Sn satellites; sb = spinning side band; x = unidentified impurity (< ca. 5×).

B. Dependence of |J| on the Me-Sn-Me Angle

As stated in the introduction, it was our goal to examine the structural dependence of tin-carbon spin coupling by taking advantage of the ability of CPMAS NMR to provide data on compounds in the solid state where their molecular structure is accurately known. We have worked with methyltin(IV)s because of their relatively simple NMR spectra and the large body of X-ray structure data available for them.[8] This approach has revealed[4] (Figure 1) that |J| is linearly related to the Me-Sn-Me angle, Θ, for a wide structural variety of methyltin(IV)s: tetramethyltin and tetra-, penta-, and hexacoordinated di- and trimethyltin(IV)s.

The methyltin(IV)s lie within 5° of the line, and most within 2 to 3°, with the exception of Me$_2$Sn(oxinate)$_2$ and Me$_2$Sn[ON(H)CH(CH$_3$)O]$_2$ which are structurally unique[8] hexacoordinated *cis*-dimethyltin(IV)s. The deviation of these two points is theoretically intriguing, but they are frustrating exceptions to an otherwise simple relationship. At this time it is best to exercize caution when estimating the Me-Sn-Me angle of compounds for which |J| is less than about 640 Hz and for which hexacoordination of Sn is possible.

Although the results described here relate specifically to methyltin(IV)s, the relationship of |J| to the C-Sn-C angle likely takes a similar form for other organotin(IV)s. The large number of hexacoordinated *cis*-diphenyltin(IV)s known[8] may provide a means of exploring the deviation from linearity of hexacoordinated *cis*-diorganotin(IV)s.

The power of the |J|/angle correlation in the structural characterization of methyltin(IV)s is illustrated by the case of the two dimethyltin(IV) bis-(dithiocarbamates) in Table 2. Incompatibility of the CPMAS NMR |J| values of these compounds with the published X-ray data[9,10] led us to redetermine their X-ray structures. One, $Me_2Sn(S_2CNEt_2)_2$, proved to be a new crystalline modification,[11] and the Me–Sn–Me angle assigned by NMR was shown to be correct. Our X-ray analysis[12] of $Me_2[S_2CN(CH_2)_4]_2$ showed the earlier structure[10] to be in error: the Me-Sn-Me angle originally reported was 130(2)° vs. 137.4° in the redetermined structure (NMR estimate, 138°).

C. Analysis of Medium Effects on Molecular Structure

It is worth emphasizing explicitly that J couplings observed by CPMAS and solution NMR are the same parameter. Therefore, the |J|/angle correlation can be used to determine the structure of methyltin(IV)s in either medium and provides a powerful tool for examining the influence of medium on the molecular structure of a given compound.

The change in association (e.g., depolymerization) of numerous polymeric trimethyltin(IV) solids,[13] Me_3SnX (X = acetate, halide, hydroxide, etc.), on dissolution can be clearly documented by comparison of CPMAS and solution NMR |J| values (Table 3): solution values of |J| are 90 Hz, or more, smaller than the values measured for the polymeric Me_3SnX solids, corresponding to a change in the tin conformation from approximately trigonal bipyramidal ($\Theta = 120°$) in the polymer to tetrahedral ($\Theta = 109.5°$) in solution. Interestingly, when the good 2-electron donor, acetone-d_6, was used as NMR solvent, |J| of Me_3SnNO_3 increased from the value in $CDCl_3$ (395 Hz) to 497 Hz, the value observed in the penta-coordinated polymer.

The Me-Sn-Me angle calculated for the trimethyltin(IV)s (Table 3) in solution (109 to 112°) are credible, but there is some difficulty with the angles calculated from the CPMAS NMR data: though the largest possible average Me-Sn-Me angle for an Me_3Sn group is just 120°, the CPMAS NMR data for Me_3SnOH, Me_3SnF, and Me_3SnOAc indicate angles of 129, 125, and 124°, respectively. This suggests that a sizable substituent effect is operating for these molecules. The poor quality of the X-ray data for these three compounds[8] precludes a search for a possible structural basis of the NMR result.

Changes in molecular conformation in different media can also be detected by a comparison of solid state and solution NMR data, as shown by the NMR spectra of $Me_2Sn(acac)_2$ (Table 3). The conformation of $Me_2Sn(acac)_2$ in solution has been the subject of some debate, arguments in support of both a *trans-* and *cis-* dimethyltin structure having been presented.[14] The |J| in the CPMAS spectrum of crystalline $Me_2Sn(acac)_2$, where the Me-Sn-Me angle is known to be 180.0°,[6] is 1175 Hz, the largest we have observed. In solution, |J| drops more than 200 Hz indicating Me-Sn-Me angles of only 161° in $CDCl_3$ and 158° in benzene (Table 3). Thus, our data confirm dipole moment[15] and IR[16] studies which implicated a nonlinear Me–Sn–Me group, but they further allow an estimate of the angle adopted in different solvents to be made. NMR data for $Me_2Sn(acac)_2$ in solution have been used in earlier attempts to explore the relationship between $|^1J(^{119}Sn-^{13}C)|$ and $|^2J(^{119}Sn-^1H)|$ and Θ;[2,9,17] the unexpected, large decrease in the Me–Sn–Me angle in solution revealed by our data illustrates the vulnerability of such studies to unpredictable medium effects.

D. Structural Analysis of Amorphous Methyltin(IV) Polymers

Amorphous and microcrystalline compounds are unsuited for X-ray analysis and are a major frustration for the structural chemist. We have obtained CPMAS NMR data for methyltin(IV) polymers not amenable to crystallographic study (Table 4, Figure 2).[5] ^{119}Sn Mössbauer spectroscopy has given little insight into the structure of these compounds, and our CPMAS NMR studies lead to new structural proposals.

It has been suggested[18] that bis (trialkyltin) carbonates are associated linear polymers with

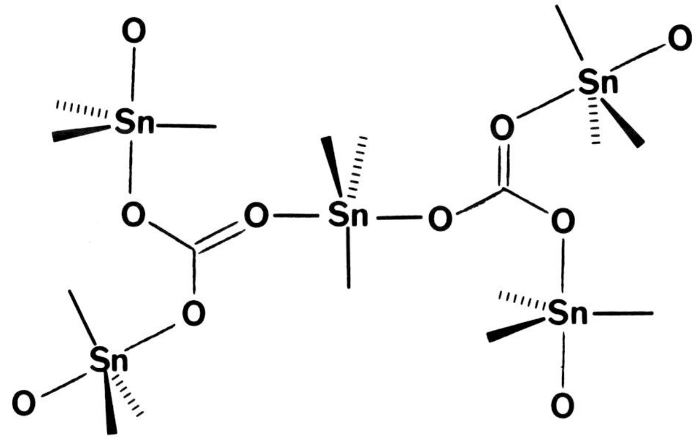

FIGURE 4. Structure proposed for amorphous $(Me_3Sn)_2CO_3$ polymer based on CPMAS ^{13}C NMR.

one Sn of each unit pentacoordinated, forming the backbone of thepolymer, and the second, tetracoordinated Sn pendant to the chain. The CPMAS NMR spectrum of bis(trimethyltin) carbonate, however, is inconsistent with such a picture: only one methyl ^{13}C resonance and one pair of Sn satellites ($|J| = 590$ Hz) are observed. Thus, there appears to be only a single structural type of Me_3Sn unit in the molecule, and Sn is pentacoordinated (cf. $|J|$ values of the Me_3SnX polymers in Table 3). The polymer structure suggested is shown in Figure 4.

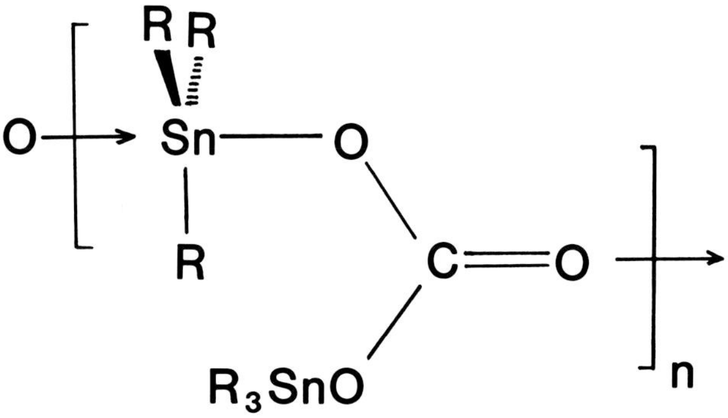

Mössbauer data for methylstannonic acid has been interpreted[19] in terms of a linear polymer with tetracoordinated Sn. The large values of $|J|$, 1160 and 1030 Hz, of the solid are inconsistent with such a picture and instead strongly implicate a higher Sn coordination number. We believe that the polymer is densely cross-linked and that most or all Sn atoms are hexacoordinated.

IV. CONCLUSIONS ON THE USE OF SOLID STATE NMR FOR THE STRUCTURAL ANALYSIS OF ORGANOTIN ANTICANCER AGENTS

Organotin structural analysis and the understanding of medium effects on molecular structure are major preoccupations of chemists in their quest to design more effective organotin anticancer agents. The results I have described can facilitate such studies in several ways. described can facilitate such studies in several ways.

First, with the $|J|$/angle correlation I have described, it is possible to perform structural analyses of unprecedented accuracy on methyltin(IV) compounds in solution using routine solution NMR spectrometers. Such work complements X-ray structural analysis in a very important way in that it can provide insight into the effect of various environments, e.g., aqueous, nonpolar, and crystal lattice on organotin structure. The $|J|$ values for other alkyltin(IV)s are also likely to be linearly related to the C–Sn–C bond angle, so differences in $|J|$ for compounds with the same organic substituent (or changes in $|J|$ for one compound in various solvents) may be attributed to changes in molecular geometry.

The application of solid state NMR by organotin chemists, at least in the immediate future, will be constrained by the limited availability of spectrometers capable of recording such data and their access to them. I have already given several examples of the kinds of contributions that CPMAS ^{13}C-NMR can make to structural organotin chemistry. Let me point out further that CPMAS NMR measurements of organotin solids may serve to focus and extend limited resources for X-ray structural analysis by indicating structural relationships between classes of uncharacterized compounds and by identifying members likely to have unique structural features.

Perhaps the most direct contribution that solid-state NMR could make to an understanding of the biological activity of organotin compounds would come from investigations of organotin-biomolecule complex structures. However, under such conditions the organotin moiety would be present in minor amounts, and the prospects for detecting the signals of interest are poor even for ^{13}C-labeled organotins. The possibility of observing spin-coupling constants is even lower.

The greatest potential, therefore, seems to lie in the use of CPMAS ^{119}Sn NMR, although only one report of the technique has appeared.[20] The higher sensitivity of ^{119}Sn than ^{13}C,[21] and the fact that the ^{119}Sn signals will arise only from species of interest should produce simple spectra. Considerable information about coordination environment may be obtained from the ^{119}Sn chemical shift.[1] The use of ^{13}C-labeled organotins offers the possibility of detecting $|^1J(^{119}\text{Sn}-^{13}\text{C})|$ even at relatively low levels (perhaps as low as 0.1% Sn by weight). The use of ^{117}Sn or ^{119}Sn-labeled compounds would lower the detection limit much further and raises the possibility that organotin species in biological media might be detected and characterized.

ACKNOWLEDGMENTS

The contributions of my collaborator, William F. Manders (NBS), are gratefully acknowledged. I would also like to thank Professor J. J. Zuckerman (University of Oklahoma) for helpful discussions and F. E. Brinckman (NBS) for his continuing support.

REFERENCES

1. **Smith, P. J. and Tupciauskas, A. P.**, Chemical shifts of ^{119}Sn nuclei in organotin compounds, *Annu. Rep. NMR Spectrosc.*, 8, 292, 1978; **Nadvornik, M., Holecek, H., Handlir, K., and Lycko, A.**, The ^{13}C and ^{119}Sn NMR spectra of some four- and five-coordinate tri-*n*- butyltin (IV) compounds, *J. Organomet. Chem.*, 275, 43, 1984.
2. **Mitchell, T. M.**, Carbon-13 NMR investigations on organotin compounds, *J. Organomet. Chem.*, 59, 189, 1973.
3. **Manders, W. F. and Lockhart, T. P.**, High resolution CPMAS ^{13}C NMR of organometallic solids. Observation of J coupling to tin, *J. Organomet. Chem.*, 143, 297, 1985.
4. **Lockhart, T. P., Manders, W. F., and Zuckerman, J. J.**, Structural investigation by solid-state ^{13}C NMR. Dependence of $|^1J(^{119}\text{Sn}, ^{13}\text{C})|$ on Me-Sn-Me angle in methyltin(IV)s, *J. Am. Chem. Soc.*, 107, 4546, 1985.
5. **Lockhart, T. P. and Manders, W. F.**, Structural analysis of methyltin(IV) polymers by solid-state ^{13}C NMR Spectroscopy, *J. Am. Chem. Soc.*, 107, 5863, 1985.
6. **Miller, G. A. and Schlemper, E. O.**, Crystal and molecular structure of bis(2,4-pentanedionato)dimethyltin(IV), *Inorg. Chem.*, 12, 677, 1973.

7. **Balimann, G. E., Groombridge, C. J., Harris, R. K., Packer, K. J., Say, G. J., and Tanner, S. F.**, Chemical applications of high-resolution ^{13}C NMR spectra for solids, *Philos. Trans. R. Soc. London, Ser. A*, 229, 654, 1981.
8. **Smith, P. J.**, A bibliography of X-ray crystal structures of organotin compounds, *J. Organomet. Chem. Libr.*, 12, 97, 1981; **Zubieta, J. A. and Zuckerman, J. J.**, Structural tin chemistry, *Prog. Inorg. Chem.*, 24, 251, 1978.
9. **Morris, J. S. and Schlemper, E. O.**, Crystal and molecular structure of tin(IV) dithiocarbamates. IV. Monoclinic and triclinic bis(N,N-diethyldithiocarbamato)dimethyltin(IV), unusual six coordination, *J. Cryst. Mol. Struct.*, 9, 13, 1979.
10. **Malik, K. M. A., Lindley, P. F., and Jeffery, J. W.**, Crystal and molecular structure of dimethyltin bis(1-pyrrolidinylcarbodithiato-S,S)stannane, *J. Bangaladesh Acad. Sci.*, 5, 53, 1981.
11. **Lockhart, T. P., Manders, W. F., and Schlemper, E. O.**, Elucidation of medium effects on molecular structure by solid-state and solution ^{13}C NMR. Identification and x-ray structure of the orthorhombic modification of dimethyltin(IV) bis(N,N-diethyldithiocarbamate), *J. Am. Chem. Soc.*, 108, 4074, 1986.
12. **Lockhart, T. P., Manders, W. F., and Schlemper, E. O.**, Solid-state ^{13}C NMR determination of methyltin(IV) structure. Crystal and molecular structure of dimethylitn bis(1-pyrrolidinecarbodithiate), *J. Am. Chem. Soc.*, 107, 7451, 1985.
13. **Smith, P. J. and Tupciauskas, A. P.**, Chemical shifts of ^{119}Sn nuclei in organotin compounds, *Annu. Rep. NMR Spectrosc.*, 8, 303, 1978.
14. **Serpone, N. and Hersh, K. A.**, Kinetic analysis of the configurational rearrangements in and the stereochemistry of some organotin(IV) β-ketonenolate complexes, *Inorg. Chem.*, 13, 2901, 1974.
15. **Moore, C. Z. and Nelson, W. H.**, A dipole moment study of six-coordinate organotin chelate compounds, *Inorg. Chem.*, 8, 138, 1969; **Hayes, J. W., Nelson, W. J., and Radford, D. V.**, Atomic polarization in metal chelates. II. Dielectric loss measurements on some diketone chelates of tin(IV), *Aust. J. Chem.*, 26, 871, 1973.
16. **LeBlanc, R. B. and Nelson, W. H.**, Evidence for *cis*-bis (2,4-pentanedionato)dimethyltin(IV) in solution: a spectroscopic study, *J. Organomet. Chem.*, 113, 257, 1976.
17. **Otera, J., Hinoishi, T., Kawabe, Y., and Okawara, R.**, ^{119}Sn, ^{13}C, and ^{1}H NMR studies on six-coordinate dimethyltin bis (chelate) compounds, *Chem. Lett.*, 273, 1981.
18. **Blunden, S. J., Hill, R., and Ruddick, J. N. R.**, The structure of bis(trialkyltin)carbonates: evidence for two non-equivalent tin sites, *J. Organomet. Chem.*, 267, C5, 1984.
19. **Davies, A. G., Smith, L., and Smith, P. J.**, The structure and reactions of some mono-organotin(IV) compounds, *J. Organomet. Chem.*, 39, 279, 1972.
20. **Lippmaa, E. T., Alla, M. A., Pehk, T. J., and Engelhardt, G.**, Solid-state high resolution NMR spectroscopy of spin 1/2 nuclei (^{13}C, ^{29}Si, ^{119}Sn) in organic compounds, *J. Am. Chem. Soc.*, 100, 1929, 1978.
21. **Harris, R. K. and Mann, B. E.**, *NMR and the Periodic Table*, Academic Press, New York, 1978, 5.

Chapter 9

SUPPRESSION OF CELL PROLIFERATION BY CERTAIN ORGANOTIN COMPOUNDS

Yasuaki Arakawa and Osamu Wada

TABLE OF CONTENTS

I.	Introduction	84
II.	Experimental	84
	A. Materials and Appliances	84
	B. In Vivo Studies	85
	C. In Vitro Studies	85
III.	Results	87
	A. Effect of Organotin Compound on the Proliferation of Malignant Cells	87
	B. The Direct Cytotoxic Effects of Organotin Compounds on Thymocytes	88
	C. Effect of Organotin Compounds on the Biochemical Events in the Early Stage of Lymphocyte Transformation	92
IV.	Discussion	98
References		104

I. INTRODUCTION

Di-substituted organotin compounds were reported to inhibit α-keto acid oxidation, probably by their combination with coenzymes or enzymes possessing vicinal dithiol groups, e.g., lipoyl dehydrogenase.[1]

Recently, Seinen et al.[2,3] described that di-n-alkyltin compounds such as di-n-butyltin and di-n-octyltin produced selective atrophy of thymus and thymus-dependent lymphoid tissue in rats and affected the immune system by selective inhibition of T-lymphocyte activity, and further they suggested that these compounds may hold potential as anti-T-cell tumor agents.

More recently, Crowe et al.[4] have reported some diorganotin complexes possessing antitumor activity in the P-388 lymphoid leukemia system.

We also found that dialkytin compounds particularly di-n-butylin, exhibited antitumor activity in vivo towards the Ehrlich-ascites tumor, IMC-carcinoma, P-388 lymphocytic leukemia, and sarcoma 180 in descending order of activity in mice, and also the compounds dramatically inhibited the proliferation of thymic lymphosarcoma cells and HeLa cells in cell cultures in vitro.

Therefore, in order to investigate the biochemical mechanism for the inhibitory effects of organotin compounds on the proliferation system of cancer cells, the transformation of lymphocytes by various mitogens was selected as a convenient cellular model system in which a resting cell is stimulated to enlarge and divide. The transformation of lymphocytes by various mitogens is a consequence of the binding of the mitogen to specific receptors on the cell surface.[5] The receptors rapidly form clusters ("patches") which may aggregate into polar "caps" at higher mitogen concentration. These events initiate a series of membrane-related biochemical changes: increased glucose, amino acid, and nucleoside transport,[6,7] potassium[8] and Ca^{2+} influx,[9-11] membrane fluidity,[12] cyclic GMP level,[13,14] phospholipid methylation,[15] phosphatidyl inositol (PI) turnover,[16-19] arachidonate release,[20,21] RNA synthesis,[22,23] histone acetylation,[24] and increased nonhistone protein phosphorylation,[25-27] which culminate in DNA synthesis and mitosis 48 to 72 hr later. Although the sequence, relative importance, and control of these events is not yet fully defined, the following two hypotheses are proposed for a main pathway leading to DNA synthesis and ultimate mitotic division on the basis of relative dependency studies among events. (1) The stimulation of DNA synthesis may be triggered by in-turn transient stimulation of phospholipid methylation, increase of Ca^{2+} influx, transient changes of membrane fluidity, and activation of phospholipase A_2. (2) The activation of phospholipase C may be the first event in a sequence of reactions leading to arachidonate release, and it may initiate PI turnover on one hand; on the other hand, the resulting unsaturated diacylglycerol may serve as a messenger which in turn activates protein kinase C in the presence of Ca^{2+} and phospholipid such as PI and phosphatidyl serine (PS).[28] (3) RNA synthesis and protein synthesis are related to phospholipase activation and arachidonate release.

In this chapter, the effects of various organotin compounds on these essential biochemical events at the early stage of lymphocyte transformation were examined with rat thymocytes.

II. EXPERIMENTAL

A. Materials and Appliances

The following organotin compounds were used in this study: monomethyltin trichloride ($MeSnCl_3$), mono-n-butyltin trichloride (n-$BuSnCl_3$), dimethyltin dichloride (Me_2SnCl_2), di-n-propyltin dichloride (n-Pr_2SnCl_2), and di-n-butyltin dichloride (Bu_2SnCl_2) were purchased from K & K Laboratories (Plainview, N.Y.); di-n-octyltin dichloride (n-Oct_2SnCl_2), tri-methyltin chloride (Me_3SnCl), triethyltin chloride (Et_3SnCl), tri-n-butyltin chloride (n-

Bu$_3$SnCl), triphenyltin chloride (Ph$_3$SnCl), tetramethyltin (Me$_4$Sn), tetraethyltin (Et$_4$Sn), and tetra-n-butyltin (n-Bu$_4$Sn) were obtained from the Aldrich Chemical Co., Inc. (Milwaukee, Wis.). The purity of these compounds was not less than 98%. All of radiolabeled compounds were purchased from the Japan Isotope Center. The RPMI medium 1640 (with L-glutamine), fetal bovine serum (heat inactivated), and penicillin-streptomycin solution (5000 U/mℓ to 5000 μg/mℓ) were purchased from Gibco Laboratories (New York). Phytohemagglutinin P (PHA) and bacto-concanavalin A (Con A) were purchased from Difco Laboratories (Detroit, Mich.).

Ionophore A 23187 (Antibiotic A 23187, calcium ionophore-free acid) was obtained from the Calbiochem-Behring Corp. (La Jolla, Calif.). Standard phospholipids such as PI, PS, phosphatidyl ethanolamine (PE), phosphatidyl choline (PC), phosphatidic acid (PA), 1,2-diacylglycerol (DAG), and arachidonic acid (AA) were purchased from Sigma Chemical Company (St. Louis, Mo.). Dimilume-30 and Soluene-350 were obtained from Packard. Other reagents included special-grade organic solvents such as chloroform, methanol, ethanol, and acetone (each provided by Wako Pure Chemicals Co., [Tokyo, Japan]). Further, culture tubes (12 × 75-mm style, clear with cap from Falcon Co., [Oxnard, Calif.]), Acrodisc (disposable filter assembly, pore size: 1.2 μm, diameter: 25 mm, from Gelman Science, Inc. [Michigan]) and liquid scintillation vials from Wheaton Scientific (Millville, N.J.) were used as the experimental appliances.

B. In Vivo Studies

The antitumor activity of organotin compounds in vivo was examined towards the sarcoma 180, IMC-carcinoma, P-388 lymphocytic leukemia, and Ehrlich ascites tumor in male mice. The mice were inoculated in the peritoneal cavity with an ascitic tumor at a level of $5 \cdot 10^6$ cells. Organotin compounds were suspended in a Tween-80/distilled water/alcohol mixture (1:97:2). One day after inoculation, the mice were injected intraperitoneally with the suspensions of the compounds. A total of one to five injections were given at daily intervals in one experiment. The dose per injection was kept in the range of 10 to 0.1 mg/kg body weight. The results of the screening were evaluated by computing the T/C, which is the mean survival time of the treated group divided by that of the control group, and the increase in life span of treated animals as compared to the controls, since the increase in life span = (T/C)% − 100. A T/C value of 100 means that the drug has no effect of either increasing or decreasing the tumor, while a T/C value >115 means significant activity.

C. In Vitro Studies

Thymocytes were obtained by mincing rat thymus gland with scissors in cold RPMI 1640 medium and by gently passing the mince through a stainless steel sieve (220 μm diameter) with the same cold medium.

The viability of the cells (1 to 3 × 10^6 cells in 1 mℓ) was determined in hemocytometers with a 0.04% erislosin solution in saline after the incubation with 10^{-4} to 10^{-8} M individual organotin compounds in RPMI 1640 medium containing 10% fetal calf serum, penicillin (100 units/mℓ), and streptomycin (100 μg/mℓ) at 37°C in a humidified atmosphere of 5% CO_2 in air for 24 hr.

The individual organotin compound was dissolved in ethanol, and 5 μℓ of it was added to 1 mℓ of the cell suspension. The final concentration of ethanol in the medium should be less than 0.5%, the concentration that did not affect cell survival.

The synthesis of DNA and RNA was determined by measuring the incorporation of [6-^{3}H]thymidine into DNA and of [5-^{3}H]uridine into RNA. Thymocytes (1 to 3 × 10^6 cells) were suspended in 1 mℓ of RPMI 1640 medium containing 10% fetal calf serum, penicillin (100 units/mℓ), and streptomycin (100 μg/mℓ) and preincubated in the absence or presence of 10^{-6} to 10^{-7} M organotin compounds (5 μℓ in EtOH solution) at 37°C for 1 to 2 hr. For the evaluation of DNA synthesis, the cells were radiolabeled with 1.0 μCi of [6-^{3}H]thymidine (5.0 Ci/m mol, RCC [Amersham, England]) per culture during the final 4 hr of a 24-hr culture. For the evaluation of RNA synthesis, the cells were radiolabeled with 2.0 μCi of [5-^{3}H]uridine (25 to 30 Ci/mmol RCC [Amersham, England]) per culture for variable intervals. When the synthesis of DNA and of RNA in the mitogen-stimulated cells was to be determined, the cells were first stimulated by the addition of concanavalin A (Con A, 5 μg/mℓ) after the 1- to 2-hr preincubation with organotin compound. This concentration of Con A gave a maximal stimulation of [6-^{3}H]thymidine incorporation into DNA after 24 hr incubation. After the incubation, the cultures were cooled in ice and the cells were harvested by aspiration through an Acrodisc Filter Assembly (pore size: 1.2 μm; diameter: 25 mm) from the culture tubes. The cells collected on the filter discs were washed by aspirating 3 to 4 mℓ of cold 5% trichloroacetic acid (TCA) aqueous solution for DNA assay and of 10% TCA for RNA assay into the syringe. The TCA-insoluble fractions on the filter discs were transferred to glass scintillation vials (Falcon) by pressure elution with 0.6 mℓ of Soluene-350 (Packard) prefilled in the syringe, homogenized with 5 mℓ of Dimilume-30 (Packard), and then counted in a Packard Tri-Carb 3255 liquid scintillation spectrometer.

The total RNA polymerase activity was assayed by the incorporation of labeled nucleotides into RNA, with a modification of the method described by Pogo.[29,30] Thymocytes (1×10^7 cells) were preincubated in 1 mℓ of 0.01 M Tris-HCl buffer, pH 8.0, containing 0.3 M sucrose, 4 mM MgCl$_2$ or 1.8 mM MnCl$_2$, 0.06 M NaCl, 30 mM 2-mercaptoethanol, and 0.4 μmol each of four unlabeled nucleotide adenosine triphosphate (ATP), cytidine triphosphate (CTP), gluanosine triphosphate (GTP), and uridine triphosphate (UTP) in the absence or presence of 10^{-6} to 10^{-7} M organotin compounds at 37°C for 2 hr. After the preincubation, the thymocyte stimulation was started by the addition of Con A (5 μg/mℓ). At the same time 1 μCi of [5-^{3}H]UTP (10 to 30 Ci/mmol, RCC [Amersham, England]) was added to all cultures and the incubations were continued at 37°C for variable intervals. The cultures were then harvested by aspiration through an Acrodisc Filter Assembly, as described above, and washed with 3 to 4 mℓ of 10% cold TCA containing 0.05 M sodium pyrophosphate. The precipitates on the filter discs were transferred to glass scintillation vials by pressure elution with 0.6 mℓ of Soluene-350 as described above, and the radioactivity was determined.

Influx of ^{45}Ca^{2+} (10 to 40 mCi/mg Ca, [Amersham, England]) was assayed in a modified Hanks balanced solution (phosphate-free). A cell suspension of thymocytes (10^6 cells per millimeter) was incubated with 10 μCi of ^{45}Ca^{2+} per 1 mℓ in the absence and presence of 10^{-9} to 10^{-4} M organotin compounds at 37°C for variable intervals. At specified times, the cultures were harvested by aspiration through an Acrodisc Filter Assembly, as described above. The cell pellets on the filter was dissolved in 0.6 mℓ of Soluene-350 solubilizer and mixed with 3 mℓ of Dimilume scintillator, and the radioactivity was determined.

Phospholipid synthesis was measured by the incorporation of carrier-free ^{32}P-phosphoric acid (100 mCi/mℓ, [Japan Isotope Center]) into the lipid fraction of the cultured cells. Thymocytes (1 to 4×10^7 cells in 1 mℓ) were incubated in RPMI 1640 medium containing 10% fetal calf serum with 1 to 10 μCi of ^{32}P-phosphoric acid in the absence and presence of 10^{-6} to 10^{-7} M n-Bu$_2$SnCl$_2$ at 37°C for variable intervals. The stimulation of cells was performed by the addition of Con A (5 μg/mℓ) 2 hr after the incubation with organotin compound, and the reaction was terminated by the addition of 1 mℓ of ice-cold 10-mM phosphate-buffered saline, pH 7.4. After the incubation, the cells were washed twice with iced phosphate-buffered saline. The packed cells were then extracted with 3 mℓ of chloroform-methanol-water (1:2:0.8, v/v) for 30 min with occasional shaking. After centrifugation at 3000 rpm for 10 min, the supernatant was carefully aspirated and diluted with 1 mℓ of chloroform and 1 mℓ of water. Further centrifugation at 3000 rpm for 10 min resolved the emulsion into two phases. The lower phase (1 mℓ) was removed, and the radioactivity of total lipid extracts was determined by a Model 3255 Packard liquid scintillation spectrometer.

When the incorporation of radioactive label into the individual phosphatides was to be determined, the phospholipid components in the lower phase (1 mℓ) were first separated by means of the two dimensional thin layer chromatography (TLC) on a commercially precoated, silica gel plate (20 cm × 20 cm, Art. 5721, Merk, [Darmstadt]) using solvent systems of chloroform-methanol-28% ammonia (65:25:5, v/v; the first dimension) and chloroform-acetone-methanol-acetic acid-water (50:20:10:10:5, v/v; the second dimension).[17] The separated phosphatides were detected and identified by comparing their localization with that of standard phospholipids. In order to measure the radioactivity incorporated into the separated phospholipid components from ^{32}P phosphoric acid, the thin layer plates were exposed to Kodak Safety X-ray film for 4 days. The films were developed and again placed over the plates. The areas on the plates which corresponded to the darkened areas on the film were scraped and extracted. The extracts were then counted for radioactivity.

When total cellular incorporation of ^{32}P was determined, the ^{32}P-labeled cells were washed twice with iced phosphate-buffered saline, and the packed cells were dissolved with 0.6 mℓ of Soluene-350 and homogenized with 5 mℓ of Dimilume-30 for determinations of radioactivity.

Phospholipase activity was measured by the release of [^{14}C] AA from the cellular lipids, mainly phospholipids with a modification of the method described by Hirata.[15,20] Thymocytes (1 × 10^7 cells per milliliter) were preincubated in a total volume of 20 mℓ of RPMI 1640 medium containing 1% fetal calf serum with 20 μCi of [1-^{14}C] AA (55.5 mCi/mmol, DuPont-New England Nuclear [NEN] Products [Billerica, Mass.]) at 37°C in a humidified atmosphere of 5% CO_2/95% air for 1 hr. The cells were washed twice with fresh media containing 0.5% fatty acid-free albumin in order to remove the excess radioactive AA and resuspended in 20 mℓ of the same media and divided as to contain 1 mℓ of cell suspension (1 × 10^7 cells) per culture tube. The prelabeled cells of each tube were further incubated in the absence and presence of 10^{-5} to 10^{-8} M organotin compound for variable intervals at 37°C. The thymocytes stimulation was performed by adding Con A (5 μg/mℓ) or fMet-Leu-Phe (1 · 10^{-8} M) after the organotin treatment. The reaction was terminated by adding 1 mℓ of ice cold 10-mM phosphate-buffered saline, pH 7.4. After centrifugation at 600 × g for 5 min, an aliquot (1 mℓ) of the supernatant was transferred into a counting vial. To the counting vial was added 8 mℓ of an aqueous counting scintillant, ACS II (Amersham), and the counts per minute (cpm) of each sample were determined with a Packard Tri-Carb 3255 liquid scintillation spectrometer.

III. RESULTS

A. Effect of Organotin Compound on the Proliferation of Malignant Cells

The antitumor activity of organotin compounds in vivo towards various tumor systems was investigated (Table 1). As a result, n-Bu$_2$SnCl$_2$ was found to exhibit reproducible activity in vivo towards Ehrlich-ascites tumor, IMC-carcinoma, P-388 lymphocytic leukemia, and sarcoma 180 systems in descending order of activity. Particularly, the compound showed the highest activity against the Ehrlich-ascites tumor system and gave T/C value in the range of 98 to 186 with dosage ranging from 0.1 to 3.0 mg/kg, the maximum activity being observed at a single dose of 3 mg/kg in the present case. Generally, a total of one to two injections of high dose levels (2 to 3 mg/kg), at which the compound do not show any toxicity, were more effective against any tumor than five injections of low dose levels (0.1 to 0.3 mg/kg).

Further, thymic lymphosarcoma cells (BW5147) and HeLa cells were selected as malignant culture cells, and the effects of organotin compounds on the proliferation of these cells in vitro were examined being compared with those of thymocytes in which DNA synthesis is more active than in other normal tissue cells (Figure 1). The result was that DNA syntheses of thymic lymphosarcoma cells and HeLa cells were more dramatically (and also in dose-

Table 1
SCREENING DATA FOR ANTITUMOR ACTIVITY OF DI-n-BUTYLTIN COMPOUND

	Dose[a]		Life span	
Tumor	mg/kg i.p.	Injection time	Survival time (days)	T/C%[b]
Sarcoma 180	0	5	15.1	100
	0.1	5	17.6	117
	0.3	5	17.8	118
	1.0	5	15.8	105
	2.0	2	15.0	100
	2.0	4	15.0	100
	3.0	1	13.2	87
	3.0	2	13.0	86
IMC-Carcinoma	0	5	16.5	100
	0.1	5	18.6	113
	0.3	5	19.1	116
	1.0	5	19.8	120
	2.0	2	20.8	126
	2.0	4	21.3	129
	3.0	1	21.0	127
	3.0	2	22.0	133
Lymphocyte leukemia P-388	0	5	10.4	100
	0.1	5	10.6	102
	0.3	5	12.1	116
	1.0	5	11.8	114
	2.0	2	12.3	118
	2.0	4	12.2	117
	3.0	1	12.1	116
	3.0	2	12.5	120
Ehrlich ascites tumor	0	5	21.1	100
	0.1	5	20.7	98
	0.3	5	21.8	104
	1.0	5	22.7	108
	2.0	2	29.1	138
	2.0	4	28.1	133
	3.0	1	39.3	186
	3.0	2	37.6	178

[a] A total of one to five injections were given at daily intervals in one experiment.
[b] The increase in survival of treated animals over control is expressed as T/C (%). The values are the means of ten animals per group.

related fashion) inhibited by $n\text{-Bu}_2\text{SnCl}_2$ of more than 10^{-7} M as compared with those of mitogen and nonstimulated thymocytes. By the way, at the concentration of range from 10^{-7} to 10^{-6} M, $n\text{-Bu}_2\text{SnCl}_2$ affected little cell viability of thymocytes, much less that of other tissue cells. These results, taken together, suggest that $n\text{-Bu}_2\text{SnCl}_2$ may inhibit the further growth of malignant cell population by preventing the mitotic division of the cells and that the compound may be available as an anticancer agent.

B. The Direct Cytotoxic Effects of Organotin Compounds on Thymocytes

To investigate the sensitivity of thymocytes to various organotin compounds, cell viability and DNA synthesis of rat thymocytes were determined after 24 hr of incubation with individual organotin compounds. As a result, it was found that both cell viability and DNA

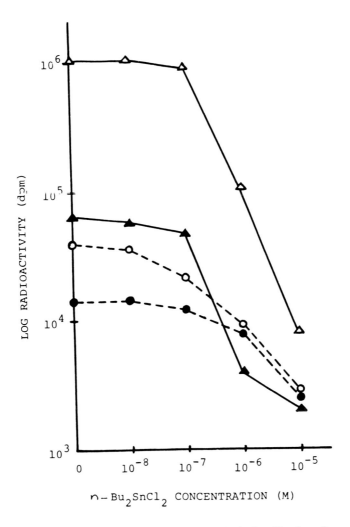

FIGURE 1. Effect of n-Bu_2SnCl_2 on DNA synthesis of proliferating cells. Cells (each, 1×10^6 cells per milliliter) were cultured with varying amounts of n-Bu_2SnCl_2 in octuple during 24 hr, and [^{3}H]thymidine was present during the last 4 hr of the culture period. Con A-stimulated thymocytes (○), nonstimulated thymocytes (●), thymic lymphosarcoma cells (△), HeLa cells (▲).

synthesis were significantly suppressed by n-Bu_2SnCl_2 and, to a lesser degree, Me_2SnCl_2, n-Pr_2SnCl_2, n-Oct_2SnCl_2, Et_3SnCl, n-Bu_3SnCl, and Ph_3SnCl, whereas almost no significant effect was noted with $MeSnCl_3$, Me_4Sn, and n-Bu_4Sn (Tables 2 and 4). Moreover, these organotin-induced suppressions of both cell viability and DNA synthesis were dose dependent and their dose-response curves were parallel to each other (Figure 2). Particularly, DNA synthesis of thymocytes was significantly inhibited by n-Bu_2SnCl_2 even at the concentration of 10^{-7} M at which cell viability was not yet impaired. These results seem to suggest that organotin compounds may primarily induce an inhibition of cell proliferation and secondarily cause cell death.

On the basis of these results, n-Bu_2SnCl_2, Ph_3SnCl, and $MeSnCl_3$ were selected and employed in the subsequent in vitro studies as a representative compound for the assessment of cytotoxic effects on the biochemical events leading to DNA synthesis of thymocytes.

In analogy with the inhibition of DNA synthesis, RNA synthesis was also significantly inhibited at 3 hr after the addition of $1 \cdot 10^{-6}$ M n-Bu_2SnCl_2, and this inhibitory effect

Table 2
CELL VIABILITY AND DNA SYNTHESIS OF RAT THYMOCYTES INCUBATED FOR 24 HR WITH 10^{-4} M OF INDIVIDUAL ORGANOTIN COMPOUNDS

Organotin compound	Cell viability[a] (% of control)	DNA synthesis[a] (% of control)
$MeSnCl_3$	82.8 ± 3.5	80.5 ± 5.6
Me_2SnCl_2	54.8 ± 3.2	48.2 ± 4.3
Me_3SnCl	49.4 ± 2.8	42.2 ± 4.5
Me_4Sn	93.6 ± 6.8	93.4 ± 7.5
Et_3SnCl	40.5 ± 3.4	41.4 ± 2.6
Et_4Sn	64.2 ± 5.1	68.8 ± 4.2
$n\text{-}Pr_2SnCl_2$	44.9 ± 5.6	42.8 ± 2.8
$n\text{-}BuSnCl_3$	63.8 ± 7.8	63.4 ± 3.0
$n\text{-}Bu_2SnCl_2$	34.2 ± 2.8	22.8 ± 4.0
$n\text{-}Bu_3SnCl$	39.5 ± 3.0	32.9 ± 3.6
$n\text{-}Bu_4Sn$	80.4 ± 5.5	76.7 ± 5.8
$n\text{-}Oct_2SnCl_2$	47.2 ± 3.6	41.4 ± 2.5
Ph_3SnCl	43.8 ± 5.3	35.6 ± 2.3

[a] The mean value determined in the control cultures (without organotin compound) was taken as 100% and compared to the mean value determined in the organotin-treated cultures.

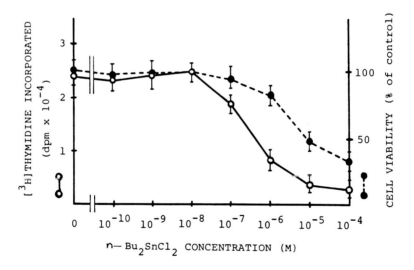

FIGURE 2. Effect of $n\text{-}Bu_2SnCl_2$ concentrations on DNA synthesis (○) and viability (●) of rat thymocytes. Cells (10^6 cells per milliliter) were cultured in triplicate during 24 hr, and [^{3}H]thymidine was present during the last 4 hr of the culture period.

continued throughout the 8-hr time period of the experiment (Figure 3). Similarly, total RNA polymerase activity was markedly reduced at 3 hr after the addition of $1 \cdot 10^{-6}$ M $n\text{-}Bu_2SnCl_2$ (Figure 4). The increases in intracellular concentration of cAMP, AMP, ADP, ATP (Figure 5), and the decreases in P, Fe, and Zn concentrations (Figure 6) were also observed after 3 hr exposure of thymocytes to $n\text{-}Bu_2SnCl_2$. However, each of these phe-

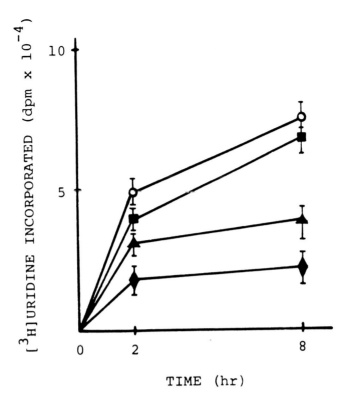

FIGURE 3. Effect of organotin compounds on RNA synthesis. Incorporation of [^{3}H]uridine into RNA of nonstimulated thymocytes (10^6 cells per milliliter) was measured in the absence (○) and presence of 10^{-6} M n-Bu$_2$SnCl$_2$ (▲), 10^{-6} M Ph$_3$SnCl (♦), or 10^{-6} M MeSnCl$_3$ (■). Vertical bars indicate the standard error (SE) of the mean for five determinations.

nomena did not exhibit a sharp dose-dependency. Probably, these phenomena arose from secondary effects.

The total incorporation of ^{32}P into the thymocytes was strongly inhibited only when the cells had been preincubated in the presence of n-Bu$_2$SnCl$_2$ for 24 hr (Figure 7). When the cells were exposed to n-Bu$_2$SnCl$_2$ at the time of addition of isotope (0 time), there was only a slight effect on the uptake of the ^{32}P.

An inhibition of ^{32}PO$_4$ incorporation into the lipid fraction could not be observed during the first 3 to 5 hr of incubation of thymocytes with $1 \cdot 10^{-6}$ M n-Bu$_2$SnCl$_2$ (Figure 8). However, a 50% inhibition of incorporation of the label was observed during the subsequent 5-hr period. These results could indicate an inhibition of phospholipid turnover, or they could reflect the inhibition of total phosphorus uptake. Therefore, in order to determine if the n-Bu$_2$SnCl$_2$-induced inhibition of phospholipid synthesis was restricted to certain phosphatides, the labeled phospholipids were separated by TLC.

Table 3 shows the relative distribution of the ^{32}P label among the separated phosphatides. An increase in ^{32}PO$_4$ incorporation into PI and a decrease in ^{32}PO$_4$ incorporation into PC, PE, and PS were observed during 3 to 6 hr after the addition of $1 \cdot 10^{-6}$ M n-Bu$_2$SnCl$_2$. In the incubation with $1 \cdot 10^{-7}$ M n-Bu$_2$SnCl$_2$, however, there were no major differences in the distribution of the label. These results suggested that the n-Bu$_2$SnCl$_2$-induced alteration of phospholipid metabolism might be due to the inhibition of PI turnover or the blockage of the phospholipase activation system.

From these points of view, the effect of organotin compounds on the degradation of phospholipids was further investigated by measuring the release of AA and its metabolites

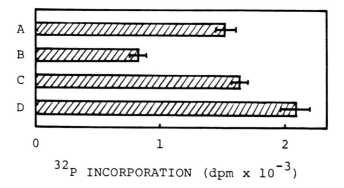

FIGURE 7. Effect of organotin compounds on total ^{32}P incorporation into thymocytes. Thymocytes (2×10^6 cells per milliliter) were incubated during 24 hr in the absence (A) and presence of 10^{-6} M n-Bu$_2$SnCl$_2$ (B), 10^{-6} M MeSnCl$_3$ (C) or 10^{-6} M Ph$_3$SnCl (D), and ^{32}P phosphoric acid (1 μCi/mℓ) was present during the last 1 to 2 hr of the culture period. Vertical bars indicate SE of the mean for five determinations.

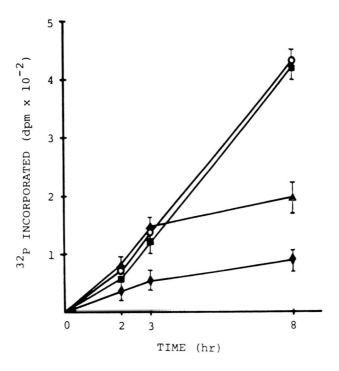

FIGURE 8. Effect of organotin compounds on phospholipid synthesis. Phospholipid synthesis was measured by the incorporation of ^{32}P into the lipid fraction of nonstimulated thymocytes (3×10^6 cells per milliliter) in the absence (○) and presence of 10^{-6} M n-Bu$_2$SnCl$_2$ (▲), 10^{-6} M Ph$_3$SnCl (♦), or 10^{-6} M MeSnCl$_3$ (■). Vertical bars indicate the SE of the mean for five determinations.

lymphocyte transformation were examined by the stimulation of organotin-preincubated thymocytes with various mitogens such as PHA, Con A, Ca^{2+}, Ca^{2+} ionophore A23187,[32] and ATP.[33]

Although PHA and Con A stimulate mainly mature T cells, whereas ATP activates immature T cells, the acceleration of DNA synthesis was inhibited in a dose-related fashion by the concentration of more than $1 \cdot 10^{-7}$ M of n-Bu$_2$SnCl$_2$ in all mitogen-stimulated

Table 3
EFFECT OF ORGANOTIN COMPOUNDS ON PHOSPHOLIPID METABOLISM OF RAT THYMOCYTES[a]

Phospholipid isolated	Control	Organotin compound (1×10^{-6} M)	
		n-Bu$_2$SnCl$_2$	Ph$_3$SnCl
Phosphatidyl inositol	21.7 ± 0.92	41.0 ± 0.51	25.9 ± 0.85
Phosphatidyl choline	54.8 ± 0.75	33.0 ± 0.26	43.5 ± 0.52
Phosphatidyl ethanolamine	5.5 ± 0.15	2.2 ± 0.10	3.9 ± 0.03
Phosphatidyl serine	2.6 ± 0.10	1.3 ± 0.06	1.5 ± 0.02
Phosphatidic acid	4.0 ± 0.19	6.0 ± 0.29	6.8 ± 0.13

[a] The total recovered radioactivity from one sample was taken as 100%, and the relative distribution of ^{32}P in the separated phospholipid components was determined from this value. Each result is the mean ± standard error (SE) of four determinations.

Table 4
DNA SYNTHESIS OF RAT THYMOCYTES INCUBATED FOR 24 HR WITH OR WITHOUT ORGANOTIN COMPOUNDS[a]

Organotin compound	Thymidine incorporation (dpm)	
	Without Con A[b]	With Con A[c]
None	10224 ± 518	46008 ± 4187
n-Bu$_2$SnCl$_2$	3312 ± 833	6548 ± 576
MeSnCl$_3$	8633 ± 1119	34600 ± 2906
Ph$_3$SnCl	4958 ± 732	17854 ± 760

[a] [^{3}H] Thymidine was present during the last 4 hr of the culture period.
[b] Thymocyte suspension (1 × 10^6 cells per milliliter) was incubated with $1 \cdot 10^{-6}$ M of organotin compounds.
[c] Thymocyte suspension (1 × 10^6 cells per milliliter) was incubated with $1 \cdot 10^{-7}$ M of organotin compounds.

thymocytes as well as in nonstimulated thymocytes (Figure 12 and Table 4). The acceleration of RNA synthesis in mitogen-stimulated thymocytes was also significantly inhibited by the presence of $1 \cdot 10^{-7}$ M n-Bu$_2$SnCl$_2$ as well as in nonstimulated thymocytes (Figure 13). Also, Ph$_3$SnCl inhibited the acceleration of DNA synthesis and of RNA synthesis at 10^{-7} M, although to a lesser extent (Figure 13 and Table 4). In addition, MeSnCl$_3$ (10^{-7} M) has almost no inhibitory effect on DNA synthesis and RNA synthesis (Figure 13 and Table 4).

An increase of ^{45}Ca^{2+} influx within 30 to 60 min after the addition of mitogens except ATP was not inhibited by the presence of organotin compounds tested at all, although the maximal Ca^{2+} uptake responses occurred at the optimal concentration of each mitogen for stimulation of DNA synthesis (Figures 14 and 15). However, an increase in ^{45}Ca^{2+} uptake in ATP-stimulated thymocytes was suppressed in a dose-related fashion in the presence of n-Bu$_2$SnCl$_2$ (Figure 15), although it was not sharp.

On the contrary, an acceleration of ^{32}PO$_4$ incorporation into the lipid fraction during the 5 min after the addition of Con A was significantly inhibited by the presence of $1 \cdot 10^{-7}$ M n-Bu$_2$SnCl$_2$ and $1 \cdot 10^{-7}$ M Ph$_3$SnCl (Figure 16). However, MeSnCl$_3$ had no significant

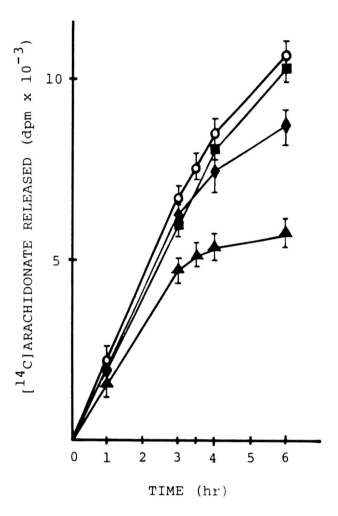

FIGURE 9. Effect of organotin compounds on arachidonate release from cellular lipids of nonstimulated thymocytes. Thymocytes (1.5×10^6 cells per milliliter) prelabeled with [1-^{14}C]arachidonic acid (1 μCi/mℓ) were incubated in the absence (○) and presence of 10^{-6} M n-Bu$_2$SnCl$_2$ (▲), 10^{-6} M Ph$_3$SnCl (◆), or 10^{-6} M MeSnCl$_3$ (■) for the indicated times. The released radioactivity into the media, expressed as [^{14}C]arachidonic acid released, included free arachidonic acid and its metabolites. Vertical bars denote SE of the mean for five determinations.

inhibitory effect on phospholipid synthesis. Further, since Con A has been reported to produce a remarkable stimulation in ^{32}PO$_4$ incorporation into PI and PA at the earliest stage of lymphocyte transformation,[16,19] the effect of n-Bu$_2$SnCl$_2$ on the ^{32}PO$_4$ incorporation into various phospholipids during the first 5 to 30 min of the thymocyte stimulation was examined in order to clarify whether the n-Bu$_2$SnCl$_2$-induced inhibition of phospholipid synthesis was restricted to certain phosphatides. As shown in Figure 17, the remarkable acceleration of ^{32}PO$_4$ incorporation into PI during the 5 min after the addition of Con A was significantly and transiently inhibited by the presence of $1 \cdot 10^{-7}$ M n-Bu$_2$SnCl$_2$. A transient increase in ^{32}PO$_4$ incorporation into PA during the 5 min after the addition of the mitogen was also inhibited by the presence of $1 \cdot 10^{-7}$ M n-Bu$_2$SnCl$_2$. Since in vivo the generated DAG which is produced from PI is immediately and efficiently phosphorylated to PA by a diacylglycerol-kinase,[18,34] these results indicate that n-Bu$_2$SnCl$_2$ inhibits transiently the acceleration of PI turnover. Further, although ^{32}PO$_4$ incorporation into PC and, to a lesser degree, PE and PS

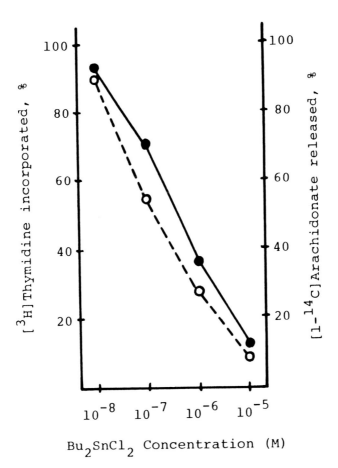

FIGURE 10. Inhibition of DNA synthesis (○) and [1-^{14}C]arachidonate release (●) by n-Bu$_2$SnCl$_2$.

were reduced to below the control levels incorporated without Con A during the first 1 hr of treatment of lymphocyte with the mitogen, and at least 3 hr exposure was required for the detectable increase of ^{32}PO$_4$ incorporation into these phospholipids, the presence of 1 · 10^{-7} M n-Bu$_2$SnCl$_2$ produced a transient increase of ^{32}PO$_4$ incorporation into PC only during the first 5 min of the lymphocyte stimulation. Also, n-Bu$_2$SnCl$_2$ had little or no effect on ^{32}PO$_4$ incorporation into PE and PS during this period. These results suggest that n-Bu$_2$SnCl$_2$ may inhibit transiently the activation of phospholipase A$_2$, an enzyme that removes an unsaturated fatty acid from phospholipids.

Therefore, the effects of organotin compounds on the stimulation of arachidonate release from phospholipids were examined by the use of mitogens such as Con A and synthetic chemoattractant N-formyl-methionyl-leucyl-phenylalanine. As for the results, the stimulation of arachidonate release during the first 5 to 30 min of treatment of thymocytes with mitogen was also significantly inhibited by the presence of 10^{-6} to 10^{-7} M n-Bu$_2$SnCl$_2$ (Figure 18). Also, this inhibition was dose dependent, and a parallelism was found between dose-dependent inhibition of acceleration of arachidonate release and that of DNA synthesis by n-Bu$_2$SnCl$_2$ as well as in nonstimulated thymocytes. By contrast, MeSnCl$_3$ had no inhibitory effect on the release of AA.

In analogy with the results of the studies with nonstimulated thymocytes, these results indicated that n-Bu$_2$SnCl$_2$ produced a significant inhibitory effect on the PI turnover and the

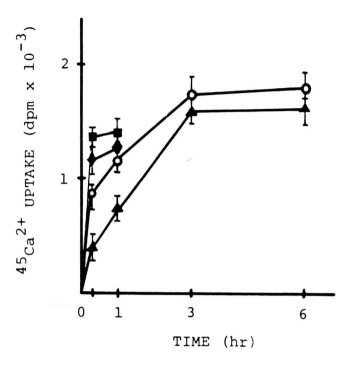

FIGURE 11. Effect of organotin compounds on calcium uptake by non-stimulated thymocytes. Thymocytes (10^6 cells per milliliter) were incubated with 10 μCi of $^{45}CaCl_2$ in the absence (○) and presence of 10^{-6} M n-Bu$_2$SnCl$_2$ (▲), 10^{-6} M Ph$_3$SnCl (◆), or 10^{-6} M MeSnCl$_3$ (■) for the indicated times. Vertical bars indicate SE of the mean for five determinations.

phospholipase-activation system which might play an important role in the induction of lymphocyte transformation.

IV. DISCUSSION

The lymphocyte is a convenient cellular model for studying the initiation of proliferation in eukaryotic organisms. However, the lymphocyte population in the thymus gland consists of two distinct subpopulations. The larger part (80 to 90%) of the population is made up of small, nonproliferating lymphocytes,[35-37] and the remaining 10 to 20% of the population consists of mitotically active, large, and medium-sized lymphoblasts which give rise to the small lymphocytes during a series of rapid cell divisions.[35] Moreover, about 20% of the total cell population appears to be initially either in the DNA-synthetic phase or near the threshold of this phase, and that the progression of thymocytes into mitosis is stimulated by promoting the initiation of DNA synthesis.

On the other hand, the T-lymphocyte population within the thymus divides into cortisone-sensitive cells (immunologically incompetent or immature T cells) and cortisone-resistant cells (immunocompetent or mature T cells). Cortisone-resistant thymocytes show a much greater response to all mitogens than unselected thymocytes.[38] However, Con A activates a considerable response in the latter population. By the way, PHA scarcely stimulates unselected thymocytes, although PHA and Con A stimulate mature T but not B cells.

Therefore, the effects of organotin compounds on thymic lymphocytes should be examined with due regard to the property of these lymphocyte populations and selectivity of mitogens for T cells.

Our present results demonstrate that n-Bu$_2$SnCl$_2$ inhibits selectively PI turnover, arachi-

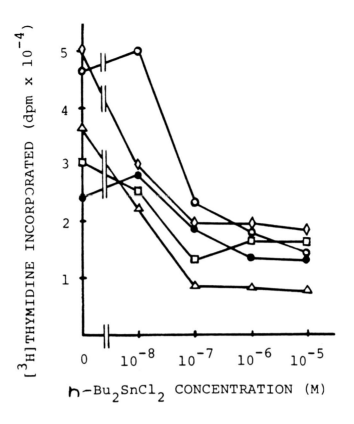

FIGURE 12. Effect of n-Bu$_2$SnCl$_2$ on the stimulation of DNA synthesis with various mitogens. Incorporation of [^{3}H]thymidine into DNA of thymocytes (10^6 cells per milliliter) 24 hr after stimulation with Con A (○), Ca^{2+} (△), ATP (◇), and Ca^{2+} ionophore (□), or that of nonstimulated thymocytes (●) was measured in the presence of various concentration of n-Bu$_2$SnCl$_2$. The optimal concentration of each mitogen for stimulation of DNA synthesis was 5 μg/mℓ for Con A, 5 mM for Ca^{2+}, 4 mM for ATP, and 0.05 μg/mℓ for Ca^{2+} ionophore.

donate release, and DNA synthesis of not only nonstimulated thymocytes, but also mitogen-stimulated thymocytes, and that each of these inhibitions is dose dependent and their dose-response curves are parallel to each other. An increase of Ca^{2+} influx within 30 to 60 min after the addition of mitogens except ATP, which has been also reported as one of the main events in the early stage of lymphocyte transformation, was not inhibited by the presence of organotin compounds at all.

These findings suggest that the organotin-induced inhibition of DNA synthesis may be due to the early effects of organotin compounds on the phospholipid metabolism of the cell membrane, in particular, on the activation system of phospholipases such as phospholipase A$_2$ and endogenous phospholipase C which might provoke arachidonate release and PI turnover and might play an important role in the induction of lymphocyte transformation.

Recently, we found that organotin compounds such as n-Bu$_2$SnCl$_2$ and Ph$_3$SnCl inhibited selectively the release of arachidonate and β-glucuronidase in rabbit neutrophils,[39,40] chemotactic response of neutrophils to stimulation by the synthetic chemoattractant fMet-Leu-Phe,[41] and carrageenan-induced inflammation,[42] and that there was a close association among the dose-dependent inhibitions of arachidonate release, β-glucuronidase release, and chemotaxis by organotin compounds.[41] Furthermore, we demonstrated that these compounds inhibited the phosphorylation of lipomodulin, a phospholipase inhibitory protein, in che-

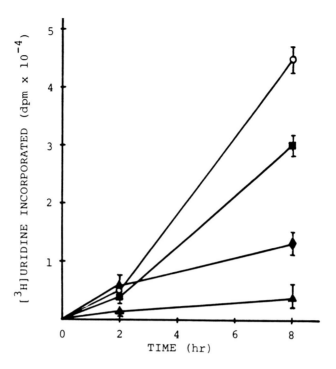

FIGURE 13. Effect of organotin compounds on RNA synthesis. Incorporation of [^{3}H]uridine into RNA of thymocytes (10^6 cells per milliliter) after stimulation with Con A (5 μg/mℓ) was measured in the absence (○) and presence of 10^{-7} M n-Bu$_2$SnCl$_2$ (▲), 10^{-7} M Ph$_3$SnCl (◆), or 10^{-7} M MeSnCl$_3$ (■). Each point is corrected for radioactivity incorporated without Con A at each incubation time. Vertical bars denote the SE of the mean for five determinations.

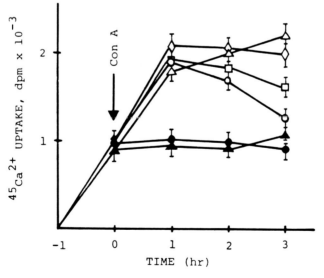

FIGURE 14. Effect of organotin compounds on calcium uptake. Incorporation of ^{45}Ca^{2+} into thymocytes (10^6 cells per milliliter) after stimulation with Con A (5 μg/mℓ) was measured in the absence (○) and presence of 10^{-7} M n-Bu$_2$SnCl$_2$ (△), 10^{-7} M Ph$_3$SnCl (◇), or 10^{-7} M MeSnCl$_3$ (□), and ^{45}Ca^{2+} uptake by nonstimulated thymocytes was measured in the absence (●) and presence (▲) of 10^{-7} M n-Bu$_2$SnCl$_2$. Vertical bars denote the SE of the mean for five determinations.

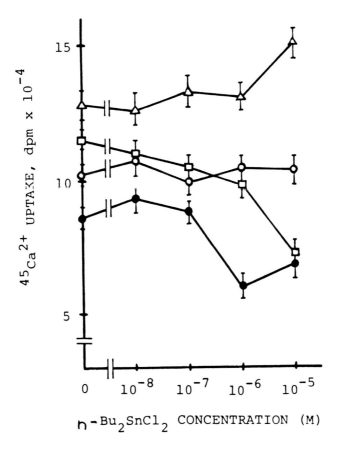

FIGURE 15. Effect of n-Bu$_2$SnCl$_2$ on the stimulation of calcium uptake with various mitogens. Incorporation of ^{45}Ca^{2+} into thymocytes (2×10^6 cells per milliliter) after stimulation with the optimal concentration of Con A (○), Ca^{2+} (△), and ATP (□), or that of nonstimulated thymocytes (●) was measured in the presence of various concentration of n-Bu$_2$SnCl$_2$. Vertical bars indicate the SE of the mean for five determinations.

moattractant-stimulated neutrophils of rabbits, without affecting directly phospholipase A$_2$ and C, although the phosphorylation of lipomodulin took place within 30 sec after stimulation with 10^{-8} M fMet-Leu-Phe and reached a maximal level at 1 min and subsequently gradually decreased to the control level by 3 min.[43]

These results of the studies with rabbit neutrophils are compatible with those observed with rat thymocytes, and all of these observations strongly suggest that organotin compounds such as n-Bu$_2$SnCl$_2$ and Ph$_3$SnCl have a selective inhibitory effect on the activation system of phospholipase activity. Probably, this inhibition of phospholipase activation may reflect the inhibition of phosphorylation of lipomodulin.

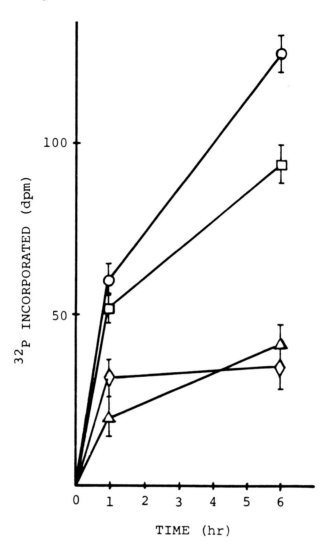

FIGURE 16. Effect of organotin compounds on phospholipid synthesis of rat thymocytes. Phospholipid synthesis was measured by the incorporation of ^{32}P into the lipid fraction of the cultured cells (1.5×10^6 cells per milliliter) after stimulation with Con A (5 μg/mℓ) in the absence (○) and presence of 10^{-7} M n-Bu$_2$SnCl$_2$ (△), 10^{-7} M MeSnCl$_3$ (□), or 10^{-7} M Ph$_3$SnCl (◇). Each point is corrected for radioactivity incorporated without Con A at each incubation time. Vertical bars denote the SE of the mean for five determinations.

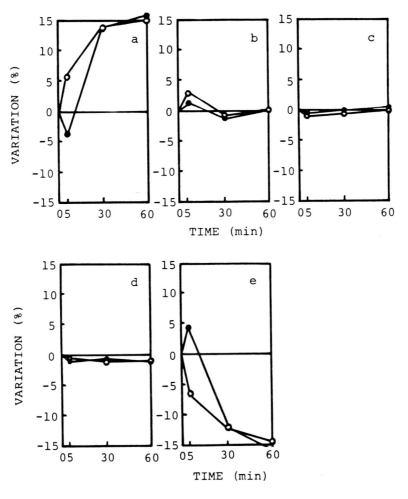

FIGURE 17. The variation of relative distribution ratio of ^{32}P in the major phospholipid classes after the stimulation of thymocytes (10^7 cells per milliliter) with Con A (5 μg/mℓ) in the absence (○) and presence (●) of 10^{-7} M n-Bu$_2$SnCl$_2$. The total recovered radioactivity from one sample was taken as 100%, and the relative distribution was determined from this value, and further the mitogen-induced variation of the distribution ratio was corrected for the distribution ratio taken without Con A at each incubation time. Represented are a, Phosphatidyl inositol; b, phosphatidic acid; c, phosphatidyl serine; d, phosphatidyl ethanolamine; and e, phosphatidyl choline.

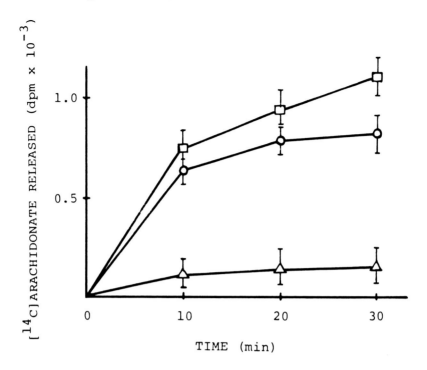

FIGURE 18. Time course of release of arachidonic acid. [1-^{14}C]Arachidonate release was measured after stimulation with 5 μg of Con A in the absence (○) and presence of 10^{-6} M n-Bu$_2$SnCl$_2$ (△) or 10^{-6} M MeSnCl$_3$ (□). Each point is corrected for radioactivity released without Con A at each incubation time. Vertical bars denote the SE of the mean for five determinations.

REFERENCES

1. **Aldridge, W. N. and Cremer, J. E.**, The biochemistry of organotin compounds, *Biochem. J.*, 61, 406, 1955.
2. **Seinen, W. and Willems, M. I.**, Toxicity of organotin compounds. I. Atrophy of thymus and thymus-dependent lymphoid tissue in rats fed di-n-octyltindichloride, *Toxicol. Appl. Pharmacol.*, 35, 63, 1976.
3. **Seinen, W., Vos, J. G., Van Spanje, I., Snoek, M., Brands, R., and Hooykaas, H.**, Toxicity of organotin compounds. II. Comparative in vivo and in vitro studies with various organotin and organolead compounds in different animal species with special emphasis on lymphocyte cytotoxicity, *Toxicol. Appl. Pharmacol.*, 42, 197, 1977.
4. **Crowe, A. J., Smith, P. J., and Atassi, G.**, Investigations into the antitumor activity of organotin compounds. I. Diorganotin dihalide and di-pseudohalide complexes, *Chem. Biol. Interact.*, 32, 171, 1980.
5. **Greaves, M. F., Bauminger, S., and Janossy, G.**, Lymphocyte activation. III. Binding sites for phytomitogens on lymphocyte subpopulations, *Clin. Exp. Immunol.*, 10, 537, 1972.
6. **Peters, J. H. and Hausen, P.**, Effect of phytohemagglutinin on lymphocyte membrane transport. II. Stimulation of "Facilitated Diffusion" of 3-O-methyl-glucose, *Eur. J. Biochem.*, 19, 502, 1971.
7. **Hadden, J. W., Hadden, E. M., Haddox, M. K., and Goldberg, N. D.**, Guanosine 3′,5′-cyclic monophosphate: a possible intracellular mediator of mitogenic influences in lymphocytes, *Proc. Natl. Acad. Sci. U.S.A.*, 69, 3024, 1972.
8. **Quastel, M. R. and Kaplan, J. G.**, Early stimulation of potassium uptake in lymphocytes treated with PHA, *Exp. Cell Res.*, 63, 230, 1970.
9. **Whitney, R. B. and Sutherland, R. M.**, Characteristics of calcium accumulation by lymphocytes and alterations in the process induced by phytohemagglutinin, *J. Cell Physiol.*, 82, 9, 1973.

10. **Whitfield, J. F., Perris, A. D., and Youdale, T.**, The calcium-mediated promotion of mitotic activity in rat thymocyte populations by growth hormone, neurohormones, parathyroid hormone and prolactin, *J. Cell Physiol.*, 73, 203, 1969.
11. **Maino, V. C., Green, N. M., and Crumpton, M. J.**, The role of calcium ions in initiating transformation of lymphocytes, *Nature*, 251, 324, 1974.
12. **Barnett, R. E., Scott, R. E., Furcht, L. T., and Kersey, J. H.**, Evidence that mitogenic lectins induce changes in lymphocyte membrane fluidity, *Nature*, 249, 465, 1974.
13. **Peters, J. H. and Hausen, P.**, Effect of phytohemagglutinin on lymphocyte membrane transport. I. Stimulation of uridine uptake, *Eur. J. Biochem.*, 19, 502, 1971.
14. **Katagiri, T., Terao, T., and Osawa, T.**, Activation of mouse splenic lymphocyte guanylate cyclase by calcium ion, *J. Biochem.*, 79, 849, 1976.
15. **Hirata, F., Toyoshima, S., Axelrod, J., and Waxdal, M.**, Phospholipid methylation: a biochemical signal modulating lymphocyte mitogenesis, *Proc. Natl. Acad. Sci. U.S.A.*, 77, 862, 1980.
16. **Fischer, D. B. and Mueller, G. G.**, An early alteration in the phospholipid metabolism of lymphocytes by phytohemagglutinin, *Proc. Natl. Acad. Sci. U.S.A.*, 60, 1396, 1968.
17. **Masuzawa, Y., Osawa, T., Inoue, K., and Nojima, S.**, Effects of various mitogens on the phospholipid metabolism of human peripheral lymphocytes, *Biochim. Biophys. Acta*, 326, 339, 1973.
18. **Billah, M. M., Lapetina, E. G., and Cuatrecasas, P.**, Phosphatidylinositol-specific phospholipase-C of platelets: association with 1,2-diacylglycerolkinase and inhibition by cyclic-AMP, *Biochem. Biophys. Res. Commun.*, 90, 92, 1979.
19. **Kennerly, D. A., Sullivan, T. J., Sylwester, P., and Parker, C. W.**, Diacylglycerol metabolism in mast cells: a potential role in membrane fusion and arachidonic acid release, *J. Exp. Med.*, 150, 1039, 1979.
20. **Hirata, F., Corcoran, B. A., Venkatasubramanian, K., Schiffmann, E., and Axelrod, J.**, Chemoattractants stimulate degradation of methylated phospholipids and release of arachidonic acid in rabbit leukocytes, *Proc. Natl. Acad. Sci. U.S.A.*, 76, 2640, 1979.
21. **Bell, R. L., Kennerly, D. A., Stanford, N., and Majerus, P. W.**, Diglyceride lipase: a pathway for arachidonate release from human platelets, *Proc. Natl. Acad. Sci. U.S.A.*, 76, 3238, 1979.
22. **Cooper, H. L. and Rubin, A. D.**, RNA metabolism in lymphocytes stimulated by phytohemagglutinin: initial responses to phytohemagglutinin, *Blood*, 25, 1014, 1965.
23. **Ono, T., Terayama, H., Takaku, F., and Nakao, K.**, Inhibitory effects of hydrocortisone upon the phytohemagglutinin-induced RNA-synthesis in human lymphocytes, *Biochim. Biophys. Acta*, 161, 361, 1968.
24. **Pogo, B. G. T., Allfrey, V. G., and Mirsky, A. E.**, RNA synthesis and histone acetylation during the course of gene activation in lymphocytes, *Proc. Natl. Acad. Sci. U.S.A.*, 55, 805, 1966.
25. **Kleinsmith, L. J., Allfrey, V. G., and Mirsky, A. E.**, Phosphorylation of nuclear protein early in the course of gene activation in lymphocyte, *Science*, 154, 780, 1966.
26. **Johnson, E. M., Karn, J., and Allfrey, V. G.**, Early nuclear events in the induction of lymphocyte proliferation by mitogens: effects of concanavalin A on the phosphorylation and distribution of non-histone chromatin proteins, *J. Biol. Chem.*, 249, 4990, 1974.
27. **Levy, R., Levy, S., Rosenberg, S. A., and Simpson, R. T.**, Selective stimulation of nonhistone chromatin protein synthesis in lymphoid cells by phytohemagglutinin, *Biochemistry*, 12, 224, 1973.
28. **Takai, Y., Kishimoto, A., Kikkawa, U., Mori, T., and Nishizuka, Y.**, Unsaturated diacylglycerol as a possible messenger for the activation of calcium-activated, phospholipid-dependent protein kinase system, *Biochem. Biophys. Res. Commun.*, 91, 1218, 1979.
29. **Pogo, B. G. T.**, Early events in lymphocyte transformation by phytohemagglutinin. I. DNA-dependent RNA polymerase activities in isolated lymphocyte nuclei, *J. Cell Biol.*, 53, 635, 1972.
30. **Johnson, L. D. and Hadden, J. W.**, Cyclic GMP and lymphocyte proliferation: Effects on DNA-dependent RNA polymerase I and II activities, *Biochem. Biophys. Res. Commun.*, 66, 1498, 1975.
31. **Honma, M., Satoh, T., Takezawa, J., and Ui, M.**, An ultrasensitive method for the simultaneous determination of cyclic AMP and cyclic GMP in small-volume samples from blood and tissue, *Biochem. Med.*, 18, 257, 1977.
32. **Hovi, T., Allison, A. C., and Williams, S. C.**, Proliferation of human peripheral blood lymphocytes induced by A23187, A streptomyces antibiotic., *Exp. Cell Res.*, 96, 92, 1976.
33. **Gregory, S. H. and Kern, M.**, Mitogenic response of T-cell subclasses to agarose-linked and to free ribonucleotides, *Immunology*, 42, 451, 1981.
34. **Kennerly, D. A., Parker, C. W., and Sullivan, T. J.**, Use of diacylglycerol kinase to quantitate picomole levels of 1,2-diacylglycerol, *Anal. Biochem.*, 98, 123, 1979.
35. **Metcalf, D.**, *The Thymus. Recent Results in Cancer Research*, Springer-Verlag, New York, 1966.
36. **Miller, J. A. F. P. and Osoba, D.**, Current concepts of the immunological function of the thymus, *Physiol. Rev.*, 47, 437, 1967.
37. **Rixon, R. H.**, The effect of radiation on the survival in vitro by rat thymocytes of different size, *Radiat. Res.*, 32, 42, 1967.

38. **Janossy, G. and Greaves, M. F.,** Lymphocyte activation. II. Discriminating stimulation of lymphocyte subpopulations by phytomitogens and heterologous antilymphocyte sera, *Clin. Exp. Immunol.*, 10, 525, 1972.
39. **Arakawa, Y. and Wada, O.,** Immunotoxicity of organotin compounds, Proc. 1st Symp. Immunotoxic Metals, Tokyo, October 13, 1984.
40. **Arakawa, Y.,** Organotin compounds and lymphocytes, Proc. 1st Symp. Roles Metals Biol. React. Biol. Med., Tokyo, June 21, 1982, 100 1983; *J. Pharm. Dyn.*, 6, s-23, 1983.
41. **Arakawa, Y. and Wada, O.,** Inhibition of neutrophil chemotaxis by organotin compounds, *Biochem. Biophys. Res. Commun.*, 123, 543, 1984.
42. **Arakawa, Y. and Wada, O.,** Inhibition of carrageenan edema formation by organotin compounds, *Biochem. Biophys. Res. Commun.*, 125, 59, 1984.
43. **Hirata, F.,** The regulation of lipomodulin, a phospholipase inhibitory protein, in rabbit neutrophils by phosphorylation, *J. Biol. Chem.*, 256, 7730, 1981.

Chapter 10

INTERACTION OF TRIETHYLTIN BROMIDE WITH CAT HEMOGLOBIN

F. Taketa, K. R. Siebenlist, and A. G. Mauk

TABLE OF CONTENTS

I.	Introduction		108
II.	The Triethyltin-Binding Sites		108
	A.	Nature of Bonding	108
	B.	The Donor Amino Acid Residues	108
		1. Thiol Group of Cysteine 13α	108
		2. Imidazole Group of Histidine 113α	111
III.	Effects of Triethyltin Binding		111
	A.	Oxygen Affinity	111
		1. Change in P_{50}	111
		2. Preferential Binding to Liganded Hemoglobin	113
	B.	Oxidation and Reduction of the Hemes	114
	C.	Changes in Heme Spectra	114
IV.	Discussion		114
Acknowledgments			115
References			115

I. INTRODUCTION

The trialkyltin species, trimethyltin (Me_3Sn^+) and triethyltin (Et_3Sn^+), are potent neurotoxicants[1,2] that demonstrate selectivity in their interactions with proteins.[3] In efforts to understand the structural basis for this selectivity, Aldridge and colleagues examined the binding of Et_3Sn^+ to a variety of well-characterized proteins and found that cat and rat hemoglobins were among the few that bound these organometals.[4-6] Two molecules of Et_3Sn^+, for example, were bound to each of these hemoglobins with an affinity constant of about $5 \times 10^5 M^{-1}$. Since Et_3Sn^+ did not bind to other animal hemoglobins, or to denatured cat or rat hemoglobin, a specific three-dimensional arrangement of donor ligands at the Et_3Sn^+ binding site was indicated. As the interaction of the trialkyltin with cat hemoglobin can be regarded as a prototype for the interaction of such compounds with other proteins, subsequent work has focused upon efforts to characterize the structure of the binding site in cat hemoglobin and to ascertain the nature of functional alterations that are induced in the protein.

II. THE TRIETHYLTIN-BINDING SITES

A. Nature of Bonding

Participation of thiol groups of cysteine and imidazole groups of histidine residues in Et_3Sn^+ binding was initially suggested by the observation that binding was abolished or diminished when such groups in cat or rat hemoglobins were modified by chemical or physical methods.[5-7] That two donor ligands are involved in the formation of 5-coordinated trialkyltin to hemoglobin complex at each Et_3Sn^+-binding site was indicated by the lack of binding of internally 5-coordinated triorganotin compounds whose tin atom is capable of only a single additional coordination with a ligand. The tin-119m Mössbauer spectrum of the trialkyltin/hemoglobin complex also indicated that the organotin is 5-coordinated and that a single class of binding site is involved in which the two protein donor ligands are at 90° to each other.[7] Thus, the participation of a cysteine and a histidine residue at each of the two Et_3Sn^+ binding sites was suggested.

B. The Donor Amino Acid Residues
1. Thiol Group of Cysteine 13α

That cysteines in cat hemoglobin participate in Et_3Sn^+ binding was suggested by the observation that two of the eight "reactive" thiol groups in the protein become unavailable for reaction with the reagents *N*-ethylmaleimide (NEM) and 4,4'-dipyridyldisulfide (PDS) in the presence of the organotin.[8] They become unmasked and available for reaction when the protein is denatured and the Et_3Sn^+ released. Evidently, they are directly involved in triethyltin binding and are thereby protected from reaction with the thiol reagents. The eight "reactive" thiol groups in the cat hemoglobin tetramer ($\alpha_2\beta_2$) are distributed three to each α and one to each β subunit.[9] There is, in addition, a thiol group in each α and β subunit that is "buried" and, therefore, unreactive in the native protein.[10-12] Thus, there is a total of four cysteines in each α subunit and two in each β subunit, or six per αβ dimer and 12 in the $\alpha_2\beta_2$ tetramer. The position of each of the cysteines in the sequences of the α and β chains deduced from amino-acid compositions and sequence homology, as well as partial sequence analyses,[10-12] is indicated in Tables 1A and B. Comparison of each sequence with the corresponding sequences of rat, human, and other animal hemoglobins[13] indicates that the differences in number and positions of cysteines in the α chain distinguishes cat hemoglobin from the others, the number and positions of the β chain cysteines being identical in all animal hemoglobins. Cys 104α occurs in all animal α chains and Cys 111α is found in a few, including that of the rat. Cys 13α, however, is found only in cat and rat α chains,

Table 1A
THE ALPHA CHAIN SEQUENCES OF HUMAN AND CAT HEMOGLOBINS

```
                        5                  10                 15                 20                 25
human β     val-his-leu-thr-pro-glu-lys-ser-ala-val-thr-ala-leu-trp-gly-lys-val-asn-val-asp-glu-val-gly-gly-glu-ala-leu-
cat βᴬ      gly-phe-leu-ser-ala-glu-glu-lys-asn-leu-val-gly-leu-trp-gly-lys-val-asn-val-asp-glu-val-gly-gly-glu-ala-leu-
cat βᴮ      X-ser-

                        30                 35                 40                 45                 50                 55
human β     gly-arg-leu-leu-val-val-tyr-pro-trp-thr-gln-arg-phe-phe-glu-ser-phe-gly-asp-leu-ser-thr-pro-asp-ala-val-met-gly-
cat βᴬ      gly-arg-leu-leu-val-val-tyr-pro-trp-thr-gln-arg-phe-phe-glu-ser-phe-gly-asp-leu-ser-ser-asx-asp-ala-ile-met-ser-
cat βᴮ

                        60                 65                 70                 75                 80
human β     asn-pro-lys-val-lys-ala-his-gly-lys-lys-val-leu-gly-ala-phe-ser-asp-gly-leu-ala-his-leu-asp-asn-leu-lys-gly-thr-
cat βᴬ      asn-ala-lys-val-lys-ala-his-gly-lys-lys-val-leu-asn-ser-phe-ser-asp-gly-leu-lys-asn-leu-asp-asp-ile-lys-gly-ala-
cat βᴮ

                        85                 90                 95                 100                105                110
human β     phe-ala-thr-leu-ser-glu-leu-his-cys-asp-lys-leu-his-val-asp-pro-glu-asn-phe-arg-leu-leu-gly-asn-val-leu-val-cys-
cat βᴬ      phe-ala-lys-leu-ser-gly-leu-his-cys-asp-lys-leu-his-val-asp-pro-glu-asn-phe-arg-leu-leu-gly-asn-val-leu-val-cys-
cat βᴮ

                        115                120                125                130                135                140
human β     val-leu-ala-his-his-phe-gly-lys-glu-phe-thr-pro-pro-val-gln-ala-ala-tyr-gln-lys-val-val-ala-gly-val-ala-asn-ala-
cat βᴬ      val-leu-ala-his-his-phe-gly-asn-glu-phe-asn-pro-his-val-gln-ala-ala-phe-gln-lys-val-val-ala-gly-val-ala-asn-ala-
cat βᴮ                                                                                                                  -ser-

                        145
human β     leu-ala-his-lys-tyr-his-
cat βᴬ      leu-ala-his-lys-tyr-his-
cat βᴮ          -arg-
```

Table 1B
THE BETA CHAIN SEQUENCES OF HUMAN AND CAT HEMOGLOBINS

```
                       10                                    20
human α  val-leu-ser-pro-ala-asp-lys-thr-asn-val-lys-ala-ala-trp-gly-lys-val-gly-ala-his-ala-gly-glu-tyr-gly-ala-glu-ala-
cat   α  val-leu-ser-ala-ala-asp-lys-ser-asp-val-lys-ala-cys-trp-gly-lys-ile-gly-ser-his-ala-gly-tyr-gly-ala-glu-ala-
                                                  .....
                  30                                    40                                    50
human α  leu-glu-arg-met-phe-leu-ser-phe-pro-thr-thr-lys-thr-tyr-phe-pro-his-phe-asp-leu-ser-his-gly-ser-ala-gln-val-lys-
cat   α  leu-glu-arg-thr-phe-cys-ser-phe-pro-thr-thr-lys-thr-tyr-phe-pro-his-phe-asp-leu-ser-his-gly-ser-ala-glu-val-lys-
                             ---
              60                                    70                                    80
human α  gly-his-gly-lys-lys-val-ala-asp-ala-leu-thr-asn-ala-val-ala-his-val-asp-asp-met-pro-asn-ala-leu-ser-ala-leu-ser-
cat   α  ala-his-gly-gln-lys-val-ala-asp-ala-leu-thr-gln-ala-val-ala-his-met-asp-asp-leu-pro-thr-ala-met-ser-ala-leu-ser-
                       90                                   100                                   110
human α  asp-leu-his-ala-his-lys-leu-arg-val-asp-pro-val-asn-phe-lys-leu-leu-ser-his-cys-leu-leu-val-thr-leu-ala-ala-his-
cat   α  asp-leu-his-ala-tyr-lys-leu-arg-val-asp-pro-val-asn-phe-lys-leu-leu-ser-his-cys-leu-leu-val-thr-leu-ala-cys-his-
                                                                                                                ---
                 120                                   130                                   140
human α  leu-pro-ala-glu-phe-thr-pro-ala-val-his-ala-ser-leu-asp-lys-phe-leu-ala-ser-val-ser-thr-val-leu-thr-ser-lys-tyr-
cat   α  his-pro-ala-glu-phe-thr-pro-ala-val-his-ala-ser-leu-asp-lys-phe-leu-ala-ser-val-ser-thr-val-leu-thr-ser-lys-tyr-
         .....

human α  arg
```

and cys 34α in the cat α chain alone. The thiol groups of residues 13α, 34α, and 111α are all "reactive", but among them, the group on 111α is less reactive than the other two.[14] Direct analysis of the effects of Et_3Sn^+ on the reactivity of thiol groups in the isolated α and β subunits of cat hemoglobin was not possible because the separated chains proved to be highly unstable.[14] As an alternative, the stable cat-human hybrid hemoglobins, $α_2^{Cat} β_2^{Human}$ and $α_2^{Human} β_2^{Cat}$, were prepared and their interactions with Et_3Sn^+ assessed by determining the effects of the organotin on the kinetics and stoichiometry of the reaction of their thiol groups with PDS. The results of this analysis indicated that Et_3Sn^+ "masks" the availability of two of the eight "reactive" thiol groups in $α_2^{Cat} β_2^{Human}$ and in cat hemoglobin, but has no influence on the reactivity of the thiol groups in $α_2^{Human} β_2^{Cat}$ or human hemoglobin. Two thiol groups associated with the α subunits of the cat hemoglobin tetramer were thus implicated in Et_3Sn^+ binding.[8] This meant that a single cysteine in each of the two α subunits within the hemoglobin tetramer was involved. Cys 13α appeared to be the likely residue as it occurs uniquely in cat and rat hemoglobins, the only hemoglobins known to bind Et_3Sn^+. Its involvement was indicated by the finding[8] that its thiol group is selectively protected from reaction with NEM in the presence of Et_3Sn^+. Analysis of the peptide maps of the tryptic digests of cat hemoglobin that were reacted with ^{14}C-NEM in the presence and absence of Et_3Sn^+ showed that the radiolabeling of peptide αT-3 containing Cys 13α was markedly reduced in the presence of organotin. That the two Cys 13α residues of the hemoglobin tetramer are involved at separate Et_3Sn^+ binding sites is suggested by the fact that they are far removed from one another in the three-dimensional structure of the protein.[15] Assignment of each to two independent Et_3Sn^+ binding sites is in agreement with earlier findings that a single class of binding site is involved in binding of two molecules of the organotin to the protein.

2. Imidazole Group of Histidine 113α

Previously, His 20α had been proposed as a possible second donor ligand in the formation of a 5-coordinated Et_3Sn^+ to hemoglobin complex. This was based on its proximity in the protein sequence to Cys 13α.[8] However, recent examination of a simulated three dimensional structure of cat hemoglobin, based on the known high-resolution structures of human hemoglobin, rules out involvement of this residue since it is separated from the sulfur atom of Cys 13α by the adjacent peptide backbone of the A helix.[16,17] Instead, it appears that the imidazole group of His 113α is the second donor ligand as this is the only functional group that is in close juxtaposition with the -SH group of Cys 13α. A search of the coordinate file in the computer-generated structure for other sulfur-imidazole separations indicated that none are similarly juxtaposed. The assignment of Cys 13α and His 113α to the Et_3Sn^+ binding site is also in accord with the fact that this pair of residues occurs uniquely in the sequences of cat and rat α globins.[12,13] Other hemoglobins that fail to bind the triethyltin lack one or both residues (Table 2) and are thus evidently unable to form stable 5-coordinated complexes with triethyltin. Interestingly, most hemoglobins, like those of humans, contain the nonpolar residues at positions 13α and 113α, respectively. These residues are clearly incapable of coordination with the tin atom. A diagram of each of the two proposed Et_3Sn^+ binding sites in cat and rat hemoglobins is depicted in Figure 1. Its validation awaits the results of X-ray crystallographic analysis of the triethyltin to cat hemoglobin complex.

III. EFFECTS OF TRIETHYLTIN BINDING

A. Oxygen Affinity
1. Change in P_{50}

The oxygen affinity of cat hemoglobin is increased as a result of Et_3Sn^+ binding (Table 3). Human hemoglobin, by contrast, shows no response to the effects of the organotin. In

Table 2
AMINO ACID RESIDUES AT POSITIONS 13 AND 113 IN THE SEQUENCES OF VARIOUS ALPHA GLOBIN CHAINS

Species	Residues	
	13α	113α
Human	ALA	LEU
Horse	ALA	LEU
Bovine	ALA	LEU
Pig	ALA	LEU
Dog	SER	HIS
Rabbit	ALA	VAL
Cat	CYS	HIS
Rat	CYS	HIS
Mouse	ALA	HIS
Chicken	ILE	LEU
Carp	ALA	LEU

Table 3
EFFECT OF TRIETHYLTIN ON THE OXYGEN EQUILIBRIA OF HUMAN AND CAT HEMOGLOBINS[a]

HbA sample	Triethyltin (mM)	P_{50}[b]
Human	0.0	14 ± 1
	0.5	14 ± 1
Cat	0.0	33 ± 2
	0.1	32 ± 1
	0.2	30 ± 1
	0.4	25 ± 1
	0.5	24 ± 1
	0.8	24 ± 1
	1.0	24 ± 1

[a] The concentration of hemoglobin was 0.1 mM in 0.15 M phosphate buffer, pH 7.4. Oxygen saturation curves were generated in an Aminco Hem-O-Scan at 37°C.
[b] Partial pressure of oxygen at 50% saturation.

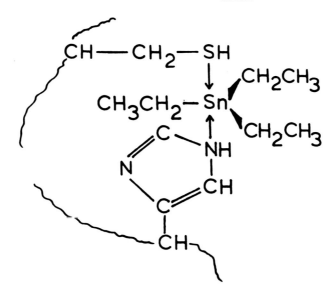

FIGURE 1. Suggested mode of Et_3Sn^+ binding to the alpha subunit of cat hemoglobin.

the presence of saturating amounts of the compound, the P_{50} value (O_2 pressure at 50% saturation) of cat hemoglobin is decreased by about 7 to 10 mm, an effect that is similar to that which is found when two of the thiol groups in the protein are derivatized with NEM.[9] Since factors that enhance stabilization of the R quaternary conformation of hemoglobin invariably produce an increase in the oxygen affinity of the protein,[17] preferential binding of Et_3Sn^+ to the R form and stabilization of this form of the protein over the T quaternary form with which it is in equilibrium[18] was indicated.

Table 4
BINDING OF TRIETHYLTIN TO VARIOUS FORMS OF CAT HEMOGLOBIN

Hemoglobin	$K_a(M^{-1})$[a]	Stoichiometry (mol Et_3Sn^+/mol Hb)
Oxy-Hb	9.5×10^4	2.01
CO-Hb	9.6×10^4	2.00
Met-Hb	9.7×10^4	2.03
Deoxy-Hb	1.6×10^3	0.30
Deoxy-Hb + 2:1 IHP	1.1×10^3	0.06
CO-CP(A + B)-Hb	1.6×10^5	2.02
DeoxyCP(A + B)-Hb	1.5×10^5	1.99

[a] Binding data were obtained by equilibrium dialysis.

2. Preferential Binding to Liganded Hemoglobin

Viewed from the perspective of allosteric theory, Et_3Sn^+ could thus be an effector that shifts the R-T equilibrium toward R. If so, the affinity of cat hemoglobin for triethyltin would depend upon the conformational state of the protein, being higher for the liganded (oxy-, CO-, and met-) than for the unliganded (deoxy) hemoglobins. As seen from the results shown in Table 4, binding of Et_3Sn^+ indeed depends upon the state of heme ligation and, therefore, presumably upon the quaternary conformation of the protein. Two equivalents of Et_3Sn^+ are bound to the oxy-, CO-, and met-hemoglobins with affinity constants of about $9.5 \times 10^4 M^{-1}$ to $9.7 \times 10^4 M^{-1}$, whereas only about 0.30 equivalents are bound to cat deoxyhemoglobin with an affinity constant that is smaller by about $1^1/_2$ orders of magnitude. The influence of certain other parameters that affect the quaternary structure of the protein were likewise analyzed. They included the addition of the organic phosphate, inositol hexaphosphate (IHP), which is known to perturb the allosteric equilibrium of hemoglobin toward T[18,20] and digestion with carboxypeptidases A and B which removes the carboxyl terminal residues of hemoglobin and produces a protein whose allosteric equilibrium is biased toward R.[21-23] In the presence of saturating amounts of IHP (molar ratio of IHP/Hb = 2/1), little if any binding to deoxyhemoglobin was observed (0.06 equivalents per mole). On the other hand, two equivalents of Et_3Sn^+ were bound with a slight but significantly higher affinity to carboxypeptidase digested CO-hemoglobin than to the undigested CO-hemoglobin, and essentially the same results were obtained with the deoxygenated form of carboxypeptidase digested hemoglobin, apparently because the protein remains in the R form even when it is deoxygenated. These results indicate that there is significant structural alteration in the region of the Et_3Sn^+ binding sites when the protein undergoes tertiary and quaternary conformational changes associated with reversible heme ligation.

From the simulated three-dimensional structures of the deoxy- and carbonyl-derivatives of cat hemoglobin, Chu et al.[16,17] have been able to tentatively explain the decrease in affinity of triethyltin for the T-state hemoglobin molecule. They found that in the R state of the protein, the SG sulfur atom of Cys 13 and NE2 nitrogen atom of His 113 are separated by about 6 Å, an ideal separation for potential tin ligands. On changing to the deoxy state, the A and G helices rotate with respect to one another. The overall distance between the side chains of these donor amino acids remains approximately the same; however, the tin atom can now interact only through the ND1 nitrogen atom of His 113. Such an interaction is less sterically favorable and less stable from an energetic point of view than the interaction with the NE2 atom in the R state of the protein.[24] The low affinity of triethyltin for cat deoxyhemoglobin can be explained by this change in geometry.

B. Oxidation and Reduction of the Hemes

Since the putative triethyltin binding sites are at the external surfaces and far away from the hemes, the effects on oxygen binding evidently arise allosterically. There are Et_3Sn^+-induced changes in the rates of oxidation and reduction of the heme irons in cat hemoglobin which are also observed. The organotin promotes the oxidation of oxyhemoglobin by sodium nitrite and inhibits the reduction of methemoglobin by ascorbate,[25] effects that are opposite and antagonistic to those exerted by IHP.[26-28] Thus, these effects of the organotin are also in agreement with the conclusion that the compound binds preferentially to the R form of the protein. That such effects involve alterations in the quaternary structure of the protein is also indicated by studies on the oxidation and reduction of the valency hybrid hemoglobins, $\alpha_2\beta_2^+$ and $\alpha_2^+\beta_2$, in which only the α or β hemes can become oxidized or reduced. In the presence of Et_3Sn^+, the rates of oxidation of the two hybrid hemoglobins are stimulated to about the same extent,[26] indicating that changes are induced in the environment of the α as well as β hemes. Similarly, in the presence of Et_3Sn^+, the rate of reduction of the β hemes in the hybrid $\alpha_2\beta_2^+$ by ascorbate is reduced.[26] It can thus be concluded that triethyltin affects the functional properties of the α as well as the β subunits of cat hemoglobin, even though it is apparently bound exclusively to the α subunit and at sites that are far removed from the hemes and subunit contacts.

C. Changes in Heme Spectra

That binding of Et_3Sn^+ affects the heme environment is also shown by the development of difference absorption bands in the 500- to 650-nm region of the spectra of methemoglobin, with additions of increasing amounts of the organotin.[25] The three major negative difference peaks that occur at 500, 611, and 655 nm are in contrast to the three positive difference peaks that appear at 512, 600, and 649 nm in the spectrum of the IHP to methemoglobin complex.[29] The latter have been used as a diagnostic for the quaternary T conformation of the protein. The development of the negative difference peaks owing to Et_3Sn^+ is thus also in agreement with the interpretation that the compound induces a shift in the allosteric equilibrium of the protein toward R. This conclusion is further supported by the observation that the positive UV difference peaks at 294 and 302 nm, characteristic of the IHP/methemoglobin complex are absent in the spectrum of Et_3Sn^+/methemoglobin complex.[25]

IV. DISCUSSION

The suggestion that Cys 13α and His 113α provide side-chain donor ligands at the Et_3Sn^+ binding sites of cat and rat hemoglobins is in accord with the fact that these residues are found only in the two hemoglobins that bind triethyltin. Most other animal hemoglobins contain alanine at 13α and leucine at 113α,[13] residues whose side chains are clearly incapable of coordination with the organometal. The Cys 13 occurs uniquely in cat and rat hemoglobin and His 113α is found only in dog, mouse, and echidna hemoglobins besides the cat and rat. The absence of either residue evidently eliminates the ability of the protein to bind the trialkyltin. Residue 13α occupies a position within the A helix (A11), and residue 113α is at the beginning of the bend between the G and H helices (GH1) in the three-dimensional structure of hemoglobin.[15] These regions are juxtaposed so that the side chains of A11 and GH1 are close to each other. Insertion of cysteine at A11 and histidine at GH1 provides sulfur and nitrogen as potential ligands for pentacoordination of the trialkyltin, placing the triethyltin in a bridge between the A and G helices of the α subunit and at an external surface of hemoglobin.

Changes in the functional properties of cat hemoglobin induced by Et_3Sn^+ must arise from an allosteric mechanism since the binding sites are far removed from the hemes. The properties of the triethyltin/cat hemoglobin complex suggest that it occurs through alterations in the quaternary structure of the protein. Presumably, structural changes induced at the binding sites are transmitted through change in tertiary structure to the $\alpha_1\beta_2$ interface of the hemoglobin tetramer. Alteration at the $\alpha_1\beta_2$ interface affects the packing of the two $\alpha\beta$ dimers against each other, which, in turn, alters the geometry of the heme environment.[19] With triethyltin, changes in tertiary structure apparently favor the packing of $\alpha\beta$ dimers in the R conformation. That a change in structure in the region of the Et_3Sn^+ binding site can influence the functional parameters of hemoglobin is indicated by the observation that Hb Hopkins-2, a human variant with a His → Asp substitution at position 112 (G19), demonstrates increased oxygen affinity relative to normal human adult hemoglobin.[30] Whether variants with such radical amino-acid substitutions at positions 13α or 113α will also exhibit altered hemoglobin function is not known, since such mutant hemoglobins have not been found. It is of interest to note, however, that whereas most other hemoglobins contain nonpolar residues at these positions, the residues in cat and rat hemoglobins are polar. This may be functionally significant as both hemoglobins demonstrate intrinsically lower oxygen affinities[31,32] in comparison with other animal hemoglobins. The increased nonpolar character imparted by triethyltin binding to this region of the protein may thus be a factor in the induction of conformational and functional changes in these proteins.

The detailed description of the binding site for Et_3Sn^+ in cat hemoglobin should serve as a useful guide to evaluate similar sites in less well-characterized proteins in other tissues. It should be noted, however, that other types of trialkyltin binding sites may well occur in other proteins. For example, evidence for 4-coordinated tin binding in such sites in certain proteins have been found.[33]

ACKNOWLEDGMENTS

This work was supported by National Institutes of Health grant AM-15770 and Public Health Service grant BRSG-2-507-RR-5434-22 to F. Taketa and an MRC grant of Canada to A. G. Mauk.

REFERENCES

1. **Stoner, H. B., Barnes, J. M., and Duff, J. I.,** Studies on the toxicity of alkyl tin compounds, *Br. J. Pharmacol.*, 10, 16, 1955.
2. **Krigman, M. R. and Silverman, A. P.,** General toxicology of tin and its organic compounds, *Neurotoxicity*, 5, 129, 1984.
3. **Aldridge, W. N.,** The influence of organotin compounds on mitochondrial functions, in *Organotin Compounds: New Chemistry and Applications*, Zuckerman, J. J., Ed., Adv. Chem. Ser. No. 157, American Chemical Society, Washington, D.C., 1976, 186.
4. **Rose, M. S. and Aldridge, W. N.,** The interaction of triethyltin with components of animal tissues, *Biochem. J.*, 106, 821, 1968.
5. **Rose, M. S.,** Evidence of histidine in the triethyltin binding site of rat hemoglobin, *Biochem. J.*, 111, 129, 1969.
6. **Elliot, B. M. and Aldridge, W. N.,** Binding of triethyltin to cat hemoglobin and modification of the binding sites by diethylpyrocarbonate, *Biochem. J.*, 163, 583, 1977.
7. **Elliot, B. M., Aldridge, W. N., and Bridges, J. W.,** Triethyltin binding to cat hemoglobin: evidence for two chemically distinct sites and a role for both histidine and cysteine residues, *Biochem. J.*, 177, 461, 1979.
8. **Taketa, F., Siebenlist, K., Kasten-Jolly, J., and Palosaari, N.,** Interaction of triethyltin with cat hemoglobin: identification of binding sites and effects on hemoglobin function, *Arch. Biochem. Biophys.*, 203, 466, 1980.
9. **Taketa, F., Dibona, F., Smits, M. R., and Lessard, J. L.,** Studies on cat hemoglobin and hybrids with HbA, *Biochemistry*, 6, 3809, 1967.

10. **Lessard, J. L.**, Ph.D. dissertation, Marquette University, Milwaukee, 1970.
11. **Taketa, F., Mauk, A. G., Mauk, M. R., and Brimhall, B.**, The tryptic peptide composition of the beta chains of hemoglobins A and B of the domestic cat (*Felis catus*), *J. Mol. Evol.*, 9, 261, 1977.
12. **Brimhall, B., Stenzel, P., Dresler, S. L., Hermodson, M., Strangland, K., Joyce, J., and Jones, R. T.**, On the tryptic peptides from hemoglobin chains of six carnivores, *J. Mol. Evol.*, 9, 237, 1977.
13. **Dayhoff, M. D.**, *Atlas of Protein Sequence and Structure*, Vol. 5, Suppl. 2, National Biomedical Research Foundation, Washington, D.C., 1970.
14. **Taketa, F.**, unpublished data, 1982.
15. **Perutz, M. F. and Ten Eyck, L. F.**, Stereochemistry and cooperative effects in hemoglobin, *Cold Spring Harbor Symp. Quant. Biol.*, 36, 295, 1971.
16. **Chu, A. L., Taketa, F., Mauk, A. G., and Brayer, G. D.**, Trialkyltin binding to cat hemoglobin: a structural model, *Fed. Proc. Fed. Am. Soc. Exp. Biol.*, 44, 1779, 1985.
17. **Chu, A. L., Taketa, F., Mauk, A. G., and Brayer, G. D.**, Structural model for the trialkyltin binding site on cat hemoglobin, *J. Biomol. Struct.*, 3, 579, 1985.
18. **Perutz, M. F., Ladner, J. E., Simon, S. R., and Ho, C.**, Influence of globin structure on the state of the heme. I. Human deoxyhemoglobin, *Biochemistry*, 13, 2163, 1975.
19. **Baldwin, J. and Chothia, C.**, Haemoglobin: the structural changes related to ligand binding and its allosteric mechanism, *J. Mol. Biol.*, 129, 175, 1979.
20. **Perutz, M. F., Fersht, A. R., Simon, S. R., and Roberts, G. C. K.**, Influence of globin structure on the state of the heme. II. Allosteric transitions in methemoglobin, *Biochemistry*, 13, 2174, 1974.
21. **Antonini, E., Wyman, J., Zito, R., Rossi-Fanelli, A., and Caputo, A.**, Studies on carboxypeptidase digests of human hemoglobin, *J. Biol. Chem.*, 236, PC60, 1961.
22. **Kilmartin, J. V. and Wootton, J. F.**, Inhibition of Bohr effect after removal of C-terminal histidines from hemoglobin chains, *Nature*, 228, 766, 1970.
23. **Kilmartin, J. V., Fogg, J. H., and Perutz, M. F.**, Role of C-terminal histidine in the alkaline Bohr effect of human hemoglobin, *Biochemistry*, 19, 3189, 1980.
24. **Reynolds, W. F. and Tzeng, C. W.**, Determination of the preferred tautomeric form of histamine by ^{13}C NMR spectroscopy, *Can. J. Biochem.*, 55, 576, 1976.
25. **Siebenlist, K. R. and Taketa, F.**, Organotin protein interactions: binding of triethyltin bromide to cat hemoglobin, *Biochem. J.*, 233, 471, 1986.
26. **Tomoda, A., Matsukawa, S., Takeshita, M., and Yoneyama, Y.**, Effect of inositol hexaphosphate on hemoglobin oxidation by nitrite and ferricyamide, *Biochem. Biophys. Res. Commun.*, 74, 1469, 1977.
27. **Tomoda, A., Matsukawa, S., Takeshita, M., and Yoneyama, Y.**, Characterization of intermediate hemoglobin produced during methemoglobin, *J. Biol. Chem.*, 253, 7415, 1978.
28. **Tomoda, A., Matsukawa, S., Takeshita, M., and Yoneyama, Y.**, Effect of organic phosphates on methemoglobin reduction by ascorbic acid, *J. Biol. Chem.*, 251, 7494, 1976.
29. **Perutz, M. F., Heidner, E. J., Ladner, J. E., Beetlestone, J. G., Ho, C., and Slade, E. F.**, Influence of globin structure on the state of the heme. III. Changes in heme spectra accompanying allosteric transitions in methemoglobin and their implications for heme-heme interaction, *Biochemistry*, 13, 2187, 1974.
30. **Charache, S. and Ostertag, W.**, Hemoglobin Hopkins-2 (α_{112}Asp)$_2\beta_2$): "low-output" protects from potentially harmful effects, *Blood*, 36, 852, 1970.
31. **Taketa, F. and Morrell, S. A.**, Oxygen affinity of cat hemoglobin, *Biochem. Biophys. Res. Commun.*, 24, 705, 1966.
32. **Baumann, R., Bauer, C., and Bartels, H.**, Influence of chronic and acute hypoxia on O_2 affinity and red cell 2,3 diphosphoglycerate of rats and guinea pigs, *Respir. Physiol.*, 11, 135, 1971.
33. **Aldridge, W. N., Street, D. W., and Noltes, J. G.**, The action of 5-coordinate triorganotin compounds on rat liver mitochondria, *Chem. Biol. Interact.*, 34, 223, 1981.

Chapter 11

TRIETHYLTIN BROMIDE AND PROTEIN PHOSPHORYLATION IN SUBCELLULAR FRACTIONS FROM RAT AND RABBIT BRAIN

F. Taketa and P. E. Neumann

TABLE OF CONTENTS

I.	Introduction	118
II.	Methods	118
	A. Preparation of Subcellular Fractions	118
	B. Protein Phosphorylation, Sodium Dodecylsulfate-Polyacrylamide Gel Electrophoresis (SDS-PAGE), and Autoradiography	118
	C. Determination of Pyruvate Dehydrogenase (PDH) Activity	118
	D. Protein Concentration	119
III.	Results	119
IV.	Discussion	121
	Acknowledgments	123
	References	123

I. INTRODUCTION

The behavioral and neuropathological effects of triethyltin (Et_3Sn^+) intoxication have been well characterized,[1] but the biochemical basis for the development of these effects remains to be elucidated. Studies on the effects of organotins on tissue metabolism have shown that Et_3Sn^+ is a selective inhibitor of glucose oxidation and respiration in the brain and that they are associated with alterations in mitochondrial function.[2] Whether these effects are relevant to the selective neurotoxicity of Et_3Sn^+ is uncertain, however, since liver mitochondria are apparently as sensitive as brain mitochondria.

Much evidence has accumulated to support the hypothesis that neuroactive agents produce diverse types of responses in the nervous system by affecting the phosphorylation status of specific neuronal proteins.[3] Recent observations on the influence of the organotins on protein phosphorylation systems in brain membranes[4] suggest that such effects may underlie their mechanisms of neurotoxicity. Siebenlist and Taketa[5] have found that Et_3Sn^+ causes a rapid activation of partially purified red cell and bovine brain membrane-bound cAMP-dependent protein kinases followed by a slow irreversible loss of enzyme activity. The neurotoxicity of the organotin may thus be exerted through effects on specific protein kinases and on phosphorylation of target proteins in the brain. We report here the results of studies on the in vitro effects of Et_3SnBr on the phosphorylation of proteins in crude synaptosomes and other subcellular fractions from rat and rabbit brain.

II. METHODS

A. Preparation of Subcellular Fractions

Adult male Sprague-Dawley (Sprague-Dawley Co., Madison, Wis.) rats were sacrificed by decapitation and their brains removed and placed in ice-cold 0.32 M sucrose; 4 mM Tris (tris[tris-{hydroxymethyl}aminomethane])-HCl, pH 7.4; 0.1 mM PMSF (phenylmethanesulfonyl fluoride); 10 mg/ℓ leupeptin. Cerebral cortex tissue was homogenized in a Teflon® glass homogenizer and fractionated into subcellular components as described by Krueger et al.[6] Purified rat or rabbit (New Zealand White) mitochondria were prepared by the method of Clark and Nicklas.[7] Rabbits were sacrificed by intracardial injection of saturated KCl solution.

B. Protein Phosphorylation, Sodium Dodecylsulfate-Polyacrylamide Gel Electrophoresis (SDS-PAGE), and Autoradiography

Aliquots of each fraction were placed in 30 mM potassium-phosphate buffer, pH 7.2, containing 1 mM MgCl$_2$, 0.1 mM EGTA, and the indicated concentrations of other components. After preincubation for 1 min at 30°C, 5 $\mu\ell$ of 50 μM [γ^{32}P]ATP (5 μCi/nmol) was added (50 $\mu\ell$ final volume) and the reaction terminated 15 sec later by the addition of 25 $\mu\ell$ of an "SDS-stop solution" which contained 9% SDS, 6% mercaptoethanol, 15% glycerol, and a small amount of bromphenol blue in 0.186 M Tris-HCl, pH = 6.7. Aliquots (50 $\mu\ell$) were then subjected to SDS-PAGE (10% acrylamide)[8] and autoradiography. Relevant bands were excised from the dried gels and digested with H_2O_2.[9] Scintillation fluid (3.5 mℓ) was added to the digested gel pieces and ^{32}P counted in a Packard Tri-Carb scintillation counter.

C. Determination of Pyruvate Dehydrogenase (PDH) Activity

Isolated rabbit mitochondria were frozen and thawed, then diluted to a protein concentration of 4 mg/mℓ with 20 mM potassium phosphate buffer, pH 7.2, containing 2.5 mM β-mercaptoethanol, 0.1 mM PMSF, and 10 mg/ℓ leupeptin (buffer A). The mixture was incubated for 15 min at 30°C with 10 mM MgCl$_2$ and 1 mM CaCl$_2$ to convert PDH to its fully active dephosphorylated state.[10] Mg^{2+} and Ca^{2+} were then removed from the mixture by dialysis for 18 hr at 4°C against three changes of buffer A.

Phosphorylation of the proteins in this preparation was carried out by adding 35 µℓ of the dialyzed suspension to 45 µℓ of buffer A containing 2 mM $MgCl_2$, 0.2 mM EDTA. The Et_3SnBr was then added (10 µℓ) to give the indicated final concentrations. After preincubation for 1 min at 30°C, 10 µℓ of a solution containing 0.5 mM ATP, 0.2 M NaF, 0.2 mM $NaVO_4$, 1 mM $MgCl_2$, and 0.1 mM EDTA in buffer A was added, and the reaction quenched 30 sec later by the addition of 25 µℓ of 25 mM dichloroacetic acid in buffer A.

PDH activity was determined using the technique described by Browning et al.,[11] except that composition of the assay mixture was the same as that used by Leiter et al.[9] The [^{14}C]CO_2 liberated from [1-^{14}C]pyruvic acid (2.5 nCi/nmol) by the pyruvate decarboxylase reaction was trapped on a 1.5-cm^2 piece of Whatman 3MM paper saturated with TS-1 tissue solubilizer (Research Products International). The reaction was initiated by the addition of enzyme (25 µℓ) to the assay mixture. Buffer A was substituted for enzyme in blank determinations. All assays were performed in duplicate.

D. Protein Concentration

Protein concentrations were estimated by the method of Bradford[12] using bovine serum albumin as standard.

III. RESULTS

Preliminary studies on the phosphorylation of proteins in a crude synaptosome fraction[6] with [$\gamma^{32}P$]ATP indicated that phosphorylation of M_r = 42,000- (42-), 52,000- (52-) and 76,000- to 80,000 daltons (76 to 80 kdaltons) components was influenced by Et_3SnBr. In order to gain insight about the identity and subcellular distribution of these proteins, this preparation (P_2) was subfractionated[6] into fractions enriched in myelin, synaptosomes, or mitochondria and each fraction subjected to the phosphorylation assay. The autoradiograph of the gel from SDS-PAGE (Figure 1) indicates that the 42 kdaltons component, whose state of phosphorylation is increased by Et_3SnBr (50 µM), is concentrated in the mitochondrial fraction. The presence of Et_3SnBr also apparently reduces the phosphorylation of the 52-kdalton band and stimulates the phosphorylation of the 76- to 80-kdalton bands, most notably in the P_2 and synaptosomal fractions. Enhanced phosphorylation of material that comigrates with the dye front on SDS-PAGE is also observed in the P_2 and mitochondrial fractions. Among the affected phosphoproteins, the 42-kdalton component is the most sensitive to Et_3Sn^+. Stimulation of its phosphorylation is detected at 1 µM Et_3Sn^+ (not shown), whereas changes in the state of phosphorylation of the 52- and 76- to 80-kdalton components are found with 25 µM or higher concentrations of the organotin. Rat cerebral cortex mitochondria, prepared substantially free of synaptosomes and synaptic membrane fragments by an alternative procedure,[7] demonstrate further enrichment of the Et_3Sn^+-sensitive 42 k-dalton component (Figure 1), indicating that it is indeed of mitochondrial origin.

A rat brain mitochondrial protein (M_r = 40,000 to 42,000 daltons) whose phosphorylation is enhanced by electrical stimulation[13] or behavioral training[14] was identified earlier to be the α subunit of PDH.[15] The mobility of the Et_3Sn^+-sensitive 42-kdalton phosphoprotein on SDS-PAGE is similar to that of this protein. Since it is known that the activity of the PDH complex is regulated by phosphorylation (inactivation) and dephosphorylation (activation) of its α subunit,[9] the effects of various activators and inhibitors of PDH on the phosphorylation of the 42-kdalton component were examined. Figure 2 shows that phosphorylation of the 42-kdalton band is regulated in the predicted manner by these agents. In the presence of high concentrations of the PDH-kinase inhibitors, pyruvate and dichloroacetic acid,[16] phosphorylation of the band is reduced, whereas in the presence of Et_3SnBr and the

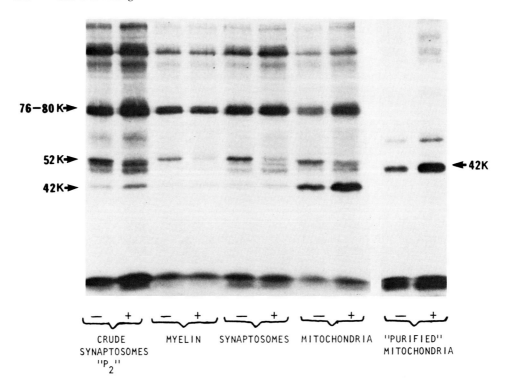

FIGURE 1. Effects of Et₃SnBr on protein phosphorylation in subcellular fractions from rat brain. In lanes 1 to 8 aliquots of each fraction (100 μg protein) were subjected to phosphorylating conditions in the presence (+) or absence (−) of 50 μM Et₃SnBr, followed by SDS-PAGE and autoradiography; lanes 1 and 2 crude synaptosomes (P₂); lanes 3 and 4 myelin; lanes 5 and 6 synaptosomes; lanes 7 and 8 mitochondria; in lanes 9 and 10, purified rat cerebral-cortex mitochondria (50 μg protein) were subjected to phosphorylating conditions in the presence (+) or absence (−) of 10 μM Et₃SnBr and treated similarly.

known activators of PDH kinase, NADH and acetyl CoA, phosphorylation is stimulated. The presence of NAD and CoA results in an intermediate level of phosphate incorporation probably due to their partial conversion to NADH and acetyl CoA, respectively, during the initial preincubation period. Morgan and Routtenberg[15] showed that with the exception of the α subunit of PDH, the phosphorylation of brain proteins is completely inhibited when EDTA is present in excess of Mg^{2+}. The Et_3Sn^+-sensitive 42-kdalton band demonstrates this property as well (Figure 1). That inhibition of brain mitochondrial PDH activity occurs in association with the Et_3Sn^+-induced phosphorylation of the 42-kdalton component is indicated by the results shown in Figure 3. With exposure of mitochondria to increasing concentrations of organotin, a progressive decrease in PDH activity is accompanied by a concomitant increase in the state of phosphorylation of the 42-kdalton protein. It can thus be concluded that the 42-kdalton, Et_3Sn^+-sensitive brain mitochondrial component is the α subunit of PDH and that Et_3Sn^+ produces inhibition of PDH by promoting its phosphorylation.

The 76 to 80 kdalton phosphoproteins are identified as "Synapsin Ia and Ib" on the basis of their molecular size (M_r) on SDS-PAGE, their occurrence as prominant components in synaptosomal fractions, and their selective phosphorylation in the presence of cAMP or Ca^{2+}/calmodulin (not shown), features that are characteristic of Synapsin.[3] The 52-kdalton component is tentatively identified as the regulatory subunit of cAMP-dependent protein kinase (type II) based on its molecular weight and on the fact that the latter is known to interact with triethyltin[5] and to become autophosphorylated when released from the holoen-

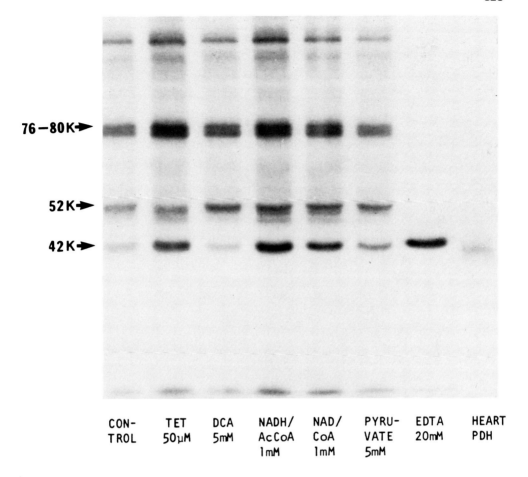

FIGURE 2. Effects of various PDH activators and inhibitors on phosphorylation of the 42kdalton band. Aliquots of the mitochondrial fraction from rat cerebral cortex (50 μg protein) and purified bovine-heart PDH (10 μg protein) were subjected to the phosphorylation assay with the indicated concentrations of activators or inhibitors, followed by SDS-PAGE and autoradiography. Lane 1, control (H$_2$O); lane 2, 50 μM Et$_3$SnBr; lane 3, 5 mM dichloroacetic acid; lane 4, 1 mM NADH and 1 mM acetylCoA; lane 5, 1 mM NAD and 1 mM CoA; lane 6, 5 mM pyruvate; lane 7, 20 mM EDTA; and lane 8, purified bovine heart PDH (2.67 μg protein).

zyme.[3] It should be noted that although the effects of Et$_3$SnBr on the phosphorylation of the 52- and 76- to 80-kdalton proteins have been observed in most preparations, there have been some preparations in which the effects were diminished or were absent (in contrast to the 42-kdalton protein where the effect is consistently observed). Whether this variability results from technical factors or from biologically significant differences in the various preparations is not known at this time.

IV. DISCUSSION

Although the in vivo effects of Et$_3$Sn$^+$ on brain PDH remain to be demonstrated, the in vitro effects described in this work suggest that the neurotoxicology of Et$_3$Sn$^+$ may be associated with its influence on the state of phosphorylation and activity of the enzyme complex. Brain, in contrast to other tissues, contains only a minimal excess of PDH above that needed for the normal flux of pyruvate through the TCA cycle.[17] Thus, profound effects on function can be expected with altered PDH activity, since the brain is almost entirely dependent upon the aerobic oxidation of glucose for its energy needs. Such effects are indeed

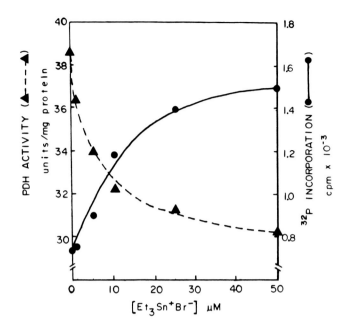

FIGURE 3. Effect of [Et$_3$SnBr] on ^{32}P incorporation into the α subunit of rabbit-brain PDH and resulting PDH activity. Purified rabbit-brain mitochondria were phosphorylated with [γ^{32}P] ATP in the presence of 0 to 50 μM Et$_3$SnBr and PDH activity determined.

observed in hereditary PDH deficiency and in thiamin deficiency.[17,18] Impairment of brain function resulting from a block in pyruvate oxidation may also be a consequence of reduced synthesis of the neurotransmitter, acetylcholine, owing to inadequate production of acetylCoA from pyruvate.[17] In addition, inhibition of pyruvate oxidation-dependent calcium sequestration in brain mitochondria may affect neurotransmitter release at nerve terminals.[11]

The influence of Et$_3$Sn$^+$ on the phosphorylation of the 52- and 76- to 80-kdalton (Synapsins) proteins may also be relevant to its mechanism of neurotoxicity. Greengard and associates have provided evidence that Synapsin plays a role in the release of neurotransmitters at the synaptic cleft.[3] Cyclic AMP promotes phosphorylation of Synapsin through the activation of cAMP-dependent protein kinase. The organotin may enhance phosphorylation of the 76- to 80-kdalton protein through such a mechanism since it is also known to activate this enzyme.[5] The identity of the 52-kdalton protein and the mechanism of its phosphorylation needs to be determined. If it is indeed the regulatory subunit of cAMP-dependent protein kinase, a plethora of effects associated with its phosphorylation may be expected since numerous substrate proteins of known and unknown function are normally regulated through the action of its partner catalytic subunit. The molecular basis for the reduced intensity of ^{32}P in the 52-kdalton band in the presence of Et$_3$Sn$^+$ is not known. Whether it is a reflection of a change in the structure or availability of the substrate protein or in the activity of the relevant kinase or phosphatase remains to be determined.

Preliminary studies on the comparative effects of Et$_3$Sn$^+$, Me$_3$Sn$^+$, and Et$_3$Pb$^+$ on protein phosphorylation in brain subcellular fractions have demonstrated structure-related specificities. For example, at 1- to 50-μM concentrations, only Et$_3$Sn$^+$ causes significant stimulation of phosphorylation of the α subunit of PDH. On the other hand, Et$_3$Pb$^+$ is somewhat more effective than Et$_3$Sn$^+$ as an inhibitor of the 52kdalton protein phosphorylation. Reduced phosphorylation of the protein is clearly observed at 5 μM Et$_3$Pb$^+$, whereas a similar effect is found only at 25 μM Et$_3$Sn$^+$. Under the same conditions, Me$_3$Sn$^+$ demonstrates no effect on the phosphorylation of either of these proteins. It would nevertheless be of interest to examine the effects of Me_3Sn^+ on brain protein phosphorylation in further detail, especially in the hippocampus, since its effects are said to be localized in this region of the brain.

ACKNOWLEDGMENTS

This work was supported by National Institutes of Health grants ES-04005 and AM-15770 and by Public Health Service grant BRSG 2-507-RR-5434-22. We thank Carl G. Kolvenbach for expert technical assistance.

REFERENCES

1. **Krigman, M. R. and Silverman, A. P.**, General toxicology of tin and its organic compounds, *Neurotoxicology*, 5, 129, 1981.
2. **Aldridge, W. N., Street, B. W., and Noltes, J. G.**, The action of 5-coordinate triorganotin compounds on rat liver mitochondria, *Chem. Biol. Interact.*, 34, 223, 1981.
3. **Nestler, E. J. and Greengard, P.**, *Protein Phosphorylation in the Nervous System*, John Wiley & Sons, New York, 1984.
4. **Taketa, F. and Siebenlist, K. R.**, Activation of protein kinases by triethyltin, *Neurotoxicology*, 3, 132, 1982.
5. **Siebenlist, K. R. and Taketa, F.**, The effects of triethyltin bromide on red cell and brain cyclic AMP-dependent protein kinases, *J. Biol. Chem.*, 258, 11384, 1983.
6. **Krueger, B. K., Forn, J., and Greengard, P.**, Depolarization-induced phosphorylation of specific proteins, mediated by calcium ion influx, in rat brain synaptosomes, *J. Biol. Chem.*, 252, 2764, 1977.
7. **Clark, J. B. and Nicklas, W. J.**, The metabolism of rat brain mitochondria, *J. Biol. Chem.*, 245, 4724, 1970.
8. **Laemmli, U. K.**, Cleavage of structural proteins during the assembly of the head of bacteriophage T4, *Nature*, 227, 680, 1970.
9. **Leiter, A. B., Weinberg, M., Isohashi, F., Utter, M. F., and Linn, T.**, Relationship between phosphorylation and activity of pyruvate dehydrogenase in rat liver mitochondria and the absense of such a relationship for pyruvate carboxylase, *J. Biol. Chem.*, 253, 2716, 1978.
10. **Booth, R. F. and Clark, J. B.**, The control of pyruvate dehydrogenase in isolated brain mitochondria, *J. Neurochem.*, 30, 1003, 1978.
11. **Browning, M., Baudry, M., Bennet, W. F., and Lynch, G.**, Phosphorylation-mediated changes in pyruvate dehydrogenase activity influence pyruvate-supported calcium accumulation by brain mitochondria, *J. Neurochem.*, 36, 1932, 1981.
12. **Bradford, M. M.**, A rapid and sensitive method for the quantitation of microgram quantities of protein utilizing the principle of protein-dye binding, *Anal. Biochem.*, 72, 248, 1976.
13. **Browning, M., Dunwiddie, T., Bennet, W., Gispen, W., and Lynch, G.**, Synaptic phosphoproteins: specific changes after repetitive stimulation of the hippocampal slice, *Science*, 203, 60, 1979.
14. **Routtenberg, A.**, Participation of brain stimulation reward substrates in memory: anatomical and biochemical evidence, *Fed. Proc. Fed. Am. Soc. Exp. Biol.*, 38, 2446, 1979.
15. **Morgan, D. G. and Routtenberg, A.**, Evidence that a 41,000 dalton brain phosphoprotein is pyruvate dehydrogenase, *Biochem. Biophys. Res. Commun.*, 95, 569, 1980.
16. **Whitehouse, S., Cooper, R. H., Randle, R. J.**, Mechanism of activation of pyruvate dehydrogenase by dichloroacetate and other halogenated carboxylic acids, *Biochem. J.*, 141, 761, 1974.
17. **Blass, J. P. and Gibson, G. E.**, Studies of the pathophysiology of pyruvate dehydrogenase deficiency, *Adv. Neurol.*, 21, 181, 1978.
18. **Victor, M., Adams, R. D., and Collins, G. H.**, *The Wernicke-Korsakoff Syndrome*, F. A. Davis, Philadelphia, 1971, 148.

Chapter 12

TOXICOLOGICAL PROPERTIES OF ORGANIC DERIVATIVES OF TIN: PRODUCTION OF MARKED ALTERATIONS OF HEPATIC AND EXTRA-HEPATIC HEME METABOLISM

Daniel W. Rosenberg and Attallah Kappas

TABLE OF CONTENTS

I.	Introduction	126
II.	Experimental	126
III.	Results and Discussion	127
IV.	Conclusions	133
	Acknowledgments	133
	References	135

I. INTRODUCTION

Recent biochemical and toxicological interest in organotin compounds reflects the increasing importance of these agents in numerous agricultural and industrial[1] applications. Such wide use of organotins has prompted an extensive evaluation of the general toxicology of these compounds. A depression of thymus-dependent immunity and thymus-atrophy[2,3] production of edematous lesions in the white matter of the central nervous system[4] and inhibition of oxidative phosphorylation[5,6] are among the various biological effects of these organometallic compounds which have been described.

The rate-limiting steps in heme synthesis and heme degradation represent highly sensitive enzymatic determinants with which to evaluate the potential toxicity of various environmental and industrial chemicals. Since many inorganic metals have been shown to affect these enzymes[7] and evidence exists for the metabolism and dealkylation of organotin compounds in vivo[8] as well as their direct effects on cytochrome P-450 in vitro,[9] we have examined the toxicity of a number of organotin compounds (Figure 1) with respect to heme metabolism in hepatic and extrahepatic organs. These effects have been compared to those produced by the inorganic metal constituent, tin. To evaluate the potential for alterations to occur in the gastrointestinal tract and to compare different routes of administration, the effects of TBTO, a commercially important biocidal agent, have been examined in further detail in the rat small intestine following oral administration of this compound.

II. EXPERIMENTAL

Male Sprague-Dawley rats (200 to 250 g) were purchased from Taconic Farms (Germantown, N.Y.). Tricyclohexyltin hydroxide (TCHH), triphenyltin acetate (TPTA), and diethyltin dichloride (DEDC) were a generous gift of the M & T Chemical Company (Rahway, N.J.). Di-*n*-butyltin dichloride (DBDC), mono-*n*-butyltin trichloride (MBTC), bis(tri-*n*-butyltin)oxide(TBTO), and DEDC were purchased from Ventron Corp., (Danvers, Mass.). The organotins were at least 95% pure as determined by the manufacturer. All other reagents were of the highest grade commercially obtainable and were purchased from Sigma Chemical Co. (St. Louis, Mo.).

Rats were maintained on Standard Purina Rodent Laboratory Chow (Ralston Purina Co., St. Louis, Mo.), and allowed to acclimatize to a light-cycled room (12-hr light/dark cycle) for at least 1 week prior to study. Rats were injected subcutaneously with the organometallic compounds (in 95% ethanol) in a single dose of 15 mg/kg body weight unless otherwise indicated. Control rats received an equal volume of the vehicle ethanol (1.0 mℓ/kg) and were identical to saline-treated animals in all parameters studied. Inorganic tin ($SnCl_2$) was given as a saline suspension in a single s.c. injection (8.78 mg/kg). In studies of intestinal heme metabolism, TBTO was dissolved in corn oil (60 mg/kg) and administered by gavage using a Perfektum (Popper and Sons, Inc., New Hyde Park, N.Y.) stainless steel 18-guage animal-feeding needle. Control rats received an equivalent amount of corn oil (1.0 mℓ/kg).

Heme oxygenase (EC 1.14.99.3) was measured in the microsomal fraction (pellet from $105,000 \times g$ centrifugation) as previously described,[10] with the $105,000 \times g$ supernatant fraction derived from normal rat liver serums or the source of biliverdin reductase. Bilirubin formation was calculated using an extinction coefficient of 40 mM^{-1} cm^{-1} between 464 and 530 nm. Cytochrome P-450 content was measured in liver microsomes by the method of Omura and Sato.[11] Renal and intestinal cytochrome P-450 was measured in microsomal suspensions from the dithionite-reduced difference spectrum of CO-bubbled samples, using a molar absorptivity coefficient of 104 mM^{-1} cm^{-1} for the absorption difference between 450 and 490 nm.[12] δ-Aminolevulinate (ALA) synthase (EC 2.31.37) activity was measured in the washed $9000 \times g$ pellet by the method of Sassa et al.[13] Benzo(a)pyrene hydroxylase

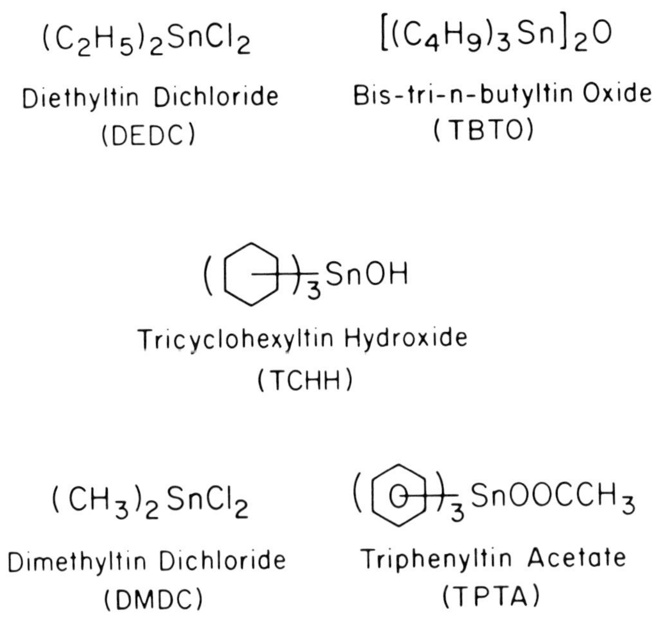

$(C_2H_5)_2SnCl_2$
Diethyltin Dichloride
(DEDC)

$[(C_4H_9)_3Sn]_2O$
Bis-tri-n-butyltin Oxide
(TBTO)

$(\text{C}_6\text{H}_{11})_3SnOH$
Tricyclohexyltin Hydroxide
(TCHH)

$(CH_3)_2SnCl_2$
Dimethyltin Dichloride
(DMDC)

$(\text{C}_6\text{H}_5)_3SnOOCCH_3$
Triphenyltin Acetate
(TPTA)

FIGURE 1. Five representative organotin compounds.

activity was measured in microsomes by the procedure of Nebert and Gelboin,[14] modified for small samples as described by Proia et al.[15] The content of liver mitochondrial cytochromes aa_3,b,c and c_1 was determined spectrally by the procedure of Williams.[16] Protein content was determined by the method of Lowry et al.,[17] using crystalline bovine serum albumin as standard. Sections of rat small intestine were prepared for light microscopy by staining with hematoxylin and eosin. The data were analyzed by student's t-test, and a p value <0.05 was regarded as statistically significant.

III. RESULTS AND DISCUSSION

The effects of a single dose (15 mg/kg body weight) of various di- and trialkyltin compounds of differing structure on heme oxygenase activity and cytochrome P-450 content in liver at 72 hr are shown in Figures 2 and 3. For comparison, included in Figures 2 and 3 are the effects of the inorganic metal constituent, tin, at a dose equimolar to the tin content of TCHH. The three water-insoluble trialkyltin compounds, TPTA, TCHH, and TBTO, all produced a substantial (four- to fivefold) induction of heme-oxygenase activity in liver (Figure 2), although these compounds are without effect on this enzyme in kidney at this and earlier time points.[25] Also effective in inducing the activity of this enzyme was DBDC, while the water-soluble dialkyltin compound, DEDC, was less effective at this time point, as was MBTC. $SnCl_2$ was essentially without effect on heme oxygenase activity at 72 hr in liver although this metal has been shown in earlier studies[18] to be an extremely potent inducer of heme oxygenase activity in kidney at 16 hr.

The induction of heme oxygenase, the rate-limiting enzyme in heme catabolism to bile pigment, is generally accompanied by significant and sustained decreases in cytochrome P-450 content. Therefore, cytochrome P-450 content in liver was also measured (Figure 3). The content of this hemeprotein at 72 hr was most dramatically lowered by a single dose of the two trialkyltin compounds, TCHH and TBTO. Each produced an ~70% decrease in the levels of cytochrome P-450, while TPTA treatment resulted in a 35% decline, although these trialkyltin compounds were all without effect on renal cytochrome P-450.[25] A 45%

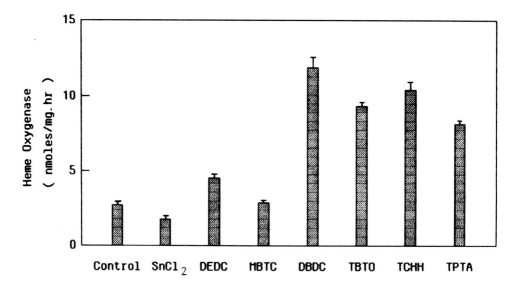

FIGURE 2. The effects of inorganic tin and organotins on hepatic heme oxygenase activity at 72 hr. Rats were injected subcutaneously with 15 mg of the organotin compounds per kilogram of body weight or 8.78 mg $SnCl_2$/kg at 72 hr prior to sacrifice. Hepatic microsomal fractions were prepared and heme oxygenase activity measured as described in the Experimental Section. Values reported are means ± SE for at least two separate experiments involving a minimum of four to six animals.

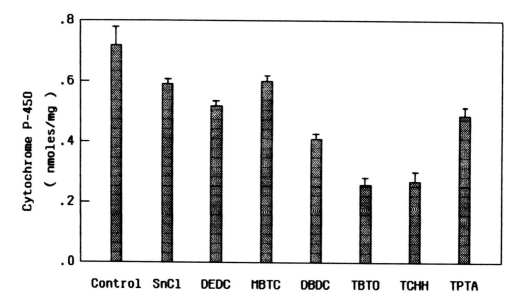

FIGURE 3. The effects of inorganic tin and organotins on hepatic cytochrome P-450 content at 72 hr. Rats were injected subcutaneously with 15 mg of the organotin compounds per kilogram of body weight or 8.78 mg $SnCl_2$/kg at 72 hr prior to sacrifice. Hepatic microsomal fractions were prepared and cytochrome P-450 content measured as described in the Experimental Section. Values reported are means ± SE for at least two separate experiments involving a minimum of four to six animals.

Table 1
THE EFFECTS OF DIALKYLTIN COMPOUNDS ON HEME-OXYGENASE ACTIVITY AND CYTOCHROME P-450 CONTENT IN LIVER AND KIDNEY AT 16 Hr[a]

Treatment	Heme oxygenase (nmol bilirubin/mg protein · hr)	Cytochrome P-450 (nmol/mg protein)
Controls	3.75 ± 021	0.74 ± 0.03
Liver		
DMDC	9.78 ± 2.58[b]	0.52 ± 0.04[b]
DEDC	11.27 ± 0.47[b]	0.47 ± 0.01[b]
Controls	1.65 ± 0.11	0.072 ± 0.004
Kidney		
DMDC	8.03 ± 0.65[b]	0.052 ± 0.001[b]
DEDC	12.93 ± 0.60[b]	0.048 ± 0.003[b]

[a] Organotins were administered subcutaneously in a single injection (15 mg/kg body weight). Animals were sacrificed 16 hr later. Hepatic and renal microsomal fractions were prepared and assays performed as described in the Experimental Section. Values reported are means ± standard error (SE) for two separate experiments involving a minimum of six animals.

[b] These values were significantly different from the controls treated with ethanol alone ($p < 0.01$, Student's t test).

reduction in cytochrome P-450 content in liver was produced by DBDC, while DEDC was somewhat less effective than DBDC (~30% below controls) at this time point, as were MBTC and inorganic tin.

Since the maximum perturbations of heme metabolism produced by various inorganic metal compounds are generally observed at 16 hr after treatment,[8,9] the effects of two water-soluble divalent tin compounds, DMDC and DEDC, on heme oxygenase activity and cytochrome P-450 content were examined at this time point in liver and in kidney (Table 1). Both compounds produced an elevation in heme oxygenase activity in liver and kidney, DEDC being somewhat more potent than DMDC in both organs examined. Similarly, cytochrome P-450 content was lowered significantly ($p < 0.01$) in liver by treatment with both organotins. In kidney, where cytochrome P-450 levels are approximately 10% of that found in liver microsomes, similar decreases were produced.

Therefore, the water-soluble diorganotins DMDC and DEDC differ from the water-insoluble trialkyltins in that they not only induce heme oxygenase in liver, but also significantly induce the enzyme in kidney. In this respect, DMDC and DEDC mimic the inducing action of inorganic tin in kidney,[18] although they do not induce the enzyme to the same extent in this organ as does the inorganic metal; however, at a dose calculated in relation to their actual content of tin, DMDC and DEDC appear to be more potent than inorganic tin as inducers of renal heme oxygenase. Thus, in the case of TPTA, TBTO, and TCHH, organic derivativization of tin shifts the site of action of the metal from kidney to liver; and in the case of DMDC and DEDC, not only does enzyme induction occur in liver, but the potency of enzyme induction in kidney is enhanced as well.

The prolonged elevation of microsomal heme oxygenase that occurs following organotin treatment might sufficiently deplete the cellular heme pool by diverting newly synthesized heme towards a catabolic pathway to such an extent that the ability of the cell to synthesize hemeproteins might become severely impaired. The dramatic and sustained depletion of hepatic microsomal cytochrome P-450 following organotin treatment suggested that these effects might extend to other hemeprotein pools in the liver as well. The content of the mitochondrial cytochromes aa_3,b,c, and c_1, integrally involved in cellular respiration, were, therefore, examined at 5 and 10 days after a single dose (30 mg/kg) of either TCHH or TBTO. These results are shown in Tables 2 and 3. A minimum 5-day interval was chosen to exceed the reported 3- to 5-day half-life of these mitochondrial cytochromes.[19]

At 5 days, heme oxygenase activity was still elevated (2.5 × controls) in response to treatment with either organotin compound, while cytochrome P-450 content was approximately 50 to 60% below controls. The content of cytochromes c and aa_3, however, were unaffected by either organotin, whereas the level of cytochrome b was significantly below controls following treatment with TCHH ($p < 0.05$) or TBTO ($p < 0.02$). Cytochrome c_1 content was ~15% below controls in TBTO treated rats at this time point (Table 1), suggesting a differential vulnerability of the heme moiety of respiratory cytochromes to organotin-induced alterations of hepatic heme metabolism.

At 10 days after treatment, there were no significant alterations in the content of any of the mitochondrial cytochromes (Table 3). Thus, the levels of these mitochondrial cytochromes had returned to normal despite the presence of a continued elevation in heme-oxygenase activity (~150% of controls) and a sustained depletion of cytochrome P-450, at least in the case of TCHH (~80% of controls).

These sustained perturbations of heme metabolism produced by trialkyltin compounds, such as TBTO, prompted further examination of the effects of this commercially important biocidal agent on a likely target organ, the gastrointestinal tract. Since the epithelial cells of the proximal small intestine have been shown to exhibit a highly active cytochrome P-450-dependent monooxygenase system,[20-22] the effects of oral administration of TBTO on various aspects of heme metabolism were examined in this segment of the gut. These results are shown in Table 4.

At 48 hr after a single dose of TBTO, heme-oxygenase activity in the intestinal mucosa was elevated. Together with this induced-enzyme activity, cytochrome P-450 content was markedly reduced (50% of controls). The activity of benzo(a)pyrene hydroxylase, an extremely sensitive index of cytochrome P-450-dependent functional activity, was dramatically reduced at this time point (<30% of controls). The ALA-synthase activity, the rate-limiting enzyme in heme biosynthesis, which has been found in previous studies to exhibit a biphasic response to metal[7] and organometal treatment,[23] was slightly (~175% of controls) elevated in these eipithelial cells at 48 hr (Table 4). The cells of the proximal epithelium therefore act in a manner analogous to the liver in terms of their response to TBTO treatment.[23]

Upon exposure to a number of organic chemicals as well as certain inorganic metals,[24] a depletion of cytochrome P-450 has often been associated with gross histopathological abnormalities. To determine whether TBTO might also produce evidence of histopathology, a single dose of the organotin (60 mg/kg) was given by gavage to rats. Sections of stomach, duodenum, and jejunum were taken from animals prior to and 72 hr after TBTO treatment. Sections of duodenum, stained with hematoxylin and eosin (magnification × 347), are shown in Figures 4A and B. At the light microscopic level, there were no differences between controls (A) and TBTO-treated (B) animals, and there was no evidence of any cellular lesions in either group. Following TBTO treatment, the intestinal villi did not significantly differ in appearance from normal animals. Villus epithelial cells (v) and crypt epithelial cells (c) were intact and normal in appearance. There was, in fact, no evidence of cellular injury in the stomach or jejunum as well,[25] confirming the high degree of specificity with which this organotin compound interacts with and perturbs the heme-metabolic system in the gut.

The results of these studies describe a novel toxicological action of organotins, i.e., the ability of these compounds to produce prolonged alterations in critical steps in the heme-

Table 2
THE EFFECTS OF TCHH AND TBTO ON THE CONTENT OF MITOCHONDRIAL CYTOCHROMES, CYTOCHROME P-450, AND HEME-OXYGENASE ACTIVITY IN LIVER AT 5 DAYS AFTER TREATMENT[a]

Treatment	Mitochondrial cytochromes (nmol/mg protein)				Cytochrome P-450 (nmol/mg protein)	Heme oxygenase activity (nmol bilirubin/mg protein · hr)
	c	c_1	b	aa_3		
Controls	0.098 ± 0.005	0.135 ± 0.007	0.112 ± 0.003	0.198 ± 0.008	0.76 ± 0.06	2.10 ± 0.05
TCHH	0.098 ± 0.004	0.126 ± 0.004	0.103 ± 0.003[b]	0.179 ± 0.014	0.30 ± 0.02[c]	5.39 ± 0.06[c]
TBTO	0.095 ± 0.005	0.115 ± 0.005	0.093 ± 0.003[c]	0.189 ± 0.011	0.36 ± 0.03[c]	4.14 ± 0.22[c]

[a] TCHH and TBTO were administered subcutaneously in a single injection (30 mg/kg body weight). Animals were sacrificed 5 days later. Hepatic microsomal and mitochondrial fractions were prepared and assays performed as described in the Experimental Section. Values reported are means ± SE for two separate experiments involving a minimum of eight animals.
[b] These values were significantly different from the control treated with ethanol alone ($p < 0.05$, Student's t test)

Table 3
THE EFFECTS OF TCHH AND TBTO ON THE CONTENT OF MITOCHONDRIAL CYTOCHROMES, CYTOCHROME P-450, AND HEME-OXYGENASE ACTIVITY IN LIVER AT 10 DAYS AFTER TREATMENT[a]

Treatment	Mitochondrial cytochromes (nmol/mg protein)			Cytochrome P-450 (nmol/mg protein)	Heme oxygenase activity (nmol bilirubin/mg protein·hr)
	c	c_1	b	aa_3		
Controls	0.114 ± 0.004	0.143 ± 0.010	0.121 ± 0.008	0.215 ± 0.010	0.69 ± 0.01	3.49 ± 0.26
TCHH	0.098 ± 0.007	0.132 ± 0.011	0.110 ± 0.007	0.230 ± 0.012	0.55 ± 0.03[b]	5.44 ± 0.29
TBTO	0.111 ± 0.004	0.147 ± 0.004	0.117 ± 0.006	0.246 ± 0.010	0.62 ± 0.05	3.39 ± 0.16

[a] TCHH and TBTO were administered subcutaneously in a single injection (30 mg/kg body weight). Animals were sacrificed 10 days later. Hepatic microsomal and mitochondrial fractions were prepared and assays performed as described in the Experimental Section. Values reported are means ± SE for two separate experiments involving a minimum of eight animals.

[b] These values were significantly different from the control treated with ethanol alone ($p < 0.05$, Student's t test)

Table 4
THE EFFECTS OF ORAL ADMINISTRATION OF TBTO ON HEME METABOLISM IN SMALL INTESTINAL MUCOSA AT 48 Hr[a]

Treatment	Heme oxygenase (nmol bilirubin/mg protein · hr)	Cytochrome P-450 (nmol/mg protein)	Benzo(a)pyrene hydroxylase (nmol 8-hydroxy-benzo(a)pyrene/mg protein · hr)	ALA-synthase (nmol ALA/mg protein · hr)
Control	5.03 ± 0.16	0.032 ± 0.002	7.34 ± 0.83	0.153 ± 0.008
TBTO	8.33 ± 0.24[b]	0.016 ± 0.002[b]	2.20 ± 0.58[b]	0.253 ± 0.047[b]

[a] TBTO was dissolved in corn oil and administered by gavage in a single dose (60 mg/kg body weight). The animals were sacrificed 48 hr later and assays performed as described in the Experimental Section. Values reported are means ± SE for at least two separate experiments including a total of at least six animals.

[b] These values were significantly different from the controls treated with corn oil alone ($p < 0.01$, Student's t test).

metabolic pathway that ultimately leads to a sustained depression of cytochrome P-450 content and related functional activities. Depending on the organic constituents covalently attached to the tin atom as well as the resultant water solubilities, these compounds can affect several important parameters of heme metabolism, namely cytochrome P-450 and heme oxygenase, in liver and/or kidney, and depending on the route of administration, in the gastrointestinal tract as well. The widespread agricultural applications of trialkyltin biocidal agents have greatly increased the exposure risks to workers associated with commercial applications of these compounds. Given this potential for exposure and the subsequent toxicological aberrations produced by these compounds, a clearer understanding of how these potent actions of organotins on heme metabolism can ultimately affect human health is necessary.

IV. CONCLUSIONS

1. A number of organotin compounds of differing structure produced elevated heme-oxygenase activity and reduced cytochrome P-450 content in liver at 72 hr after a single dose.
2. The water-soluble dialkyltins, DMDC and DEDC, produced a substantial induction of heme-oxygenase activity at 16 hr in both liver and kidney.
3. TBTO and TCHH, although producing a prolonged induction of heme oxygenase in liver (longer than 1 week after a single dose), did not markedly affect mitochondrial cytochrome content in this organ when measured at 5 and 10 days after a single dose of either compound.
4. When given by gavage, TBTO produced dramatic alterations in heme metabolism in small intestinal mucosa at 48 hr without any evidence of cellular lesions at the light microscopic level.

ACKNOWLEDGMENTS

The authors wish to thank Dr. Thomas Donnelly for the preparation and interpretation of tissue sections. The authors also thank Mr. David Markowitz for his skillful and dedicated technical assistance. The assistance of Mrs. Heidi Robinson and Ms. Jill Brighton for preparation of this manuscript is gratefully acknowledged. These studies were supported in part by U.S. Public Health Service Grant ES-5-01055 and a gift from The Ogden Corporation, New York.

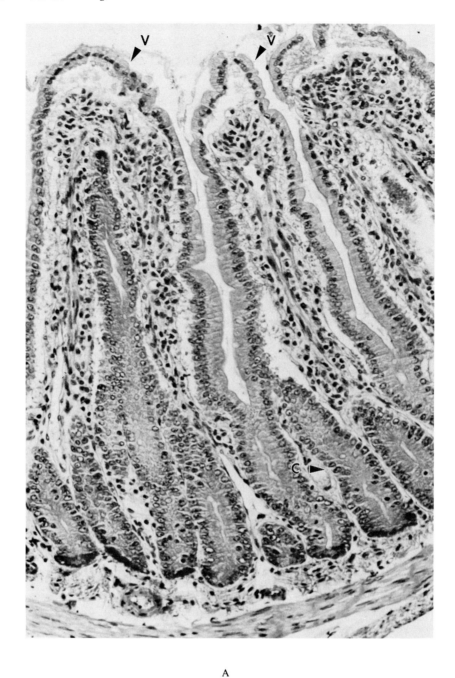

A

FIGURE 4. Sections of rat duodenum stained with hematoxylin and eosin taken from controls and animals receiving oral administration of TBTO. TBTO was dissolved in corn oil and administered by gavage in a single dose (60 mg/kg body weight). The animals were sacrificed prior to (A) and 72 hr after TBTO treatment (B) and sections of proximal small intestine prepared for light microscopy (magnification × 347) as described in the Experimental Section. Villus epithelial cells (V) and crypt epithelial cells (C) are indicated by the arrows.

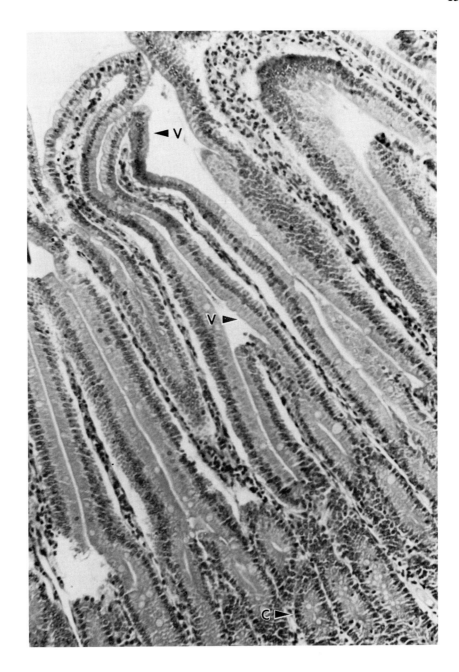

FIGURE 4B

REFERENCES

1. **Zuckerman, J. J., Ed.**, *Organotin Compounds: New Chemistry and Applications*, Adv. Chem. Ser. No. 157, American Chemical Society, Washington, D.C., 1976.
2. **Seinen, W., Vos, J. G., Brands, R., and Hooykaas, H.**, Lymphocytotoxicity and immunosuppression by organotin compounds. Suppression of graft-versis-host reactivity, blast transformation, and E-rosette formation by di-*n*-butyltin dichloride and di-*n*-octyltin dichloride, *Immunopharmacology*, 1, 343, 1979.

3. **Miller, R. R., Hartung, R., and Cornish, H. H.**, Effects of diethyltin dichloride on aminoacid and nucleoside transport in suspended rat thymocytes, *Toxicol. Appl. Pharmacol.*, 55, 564, 1980.
4. **Magee, P. N., Stoner, H. R., and Barnes, J. M.**, The experimental production of oedema in the central nervous system of the rat by triethyltin compounds, *J. Pathol. Bacteriol.*, 73, 107, 1957.
5. **Aldridge, W. N., Street, B. W., and Skilleter, D. N.**, Oxidative phosphorylation. Halide-dependent and halide-independent effects of triorganotin and triorganolead compounds on mitochondrial functions, *Biochem. J.*, 168, 353, 1977.
6. **Aldridge, W. N., Casida, J. E., Fish, R. M., Kimmel, E. C., and Street, B. W.**, Action on mitochondria and toxicity of metabolites of tri-*n*-butyltin derivatives, *Biochem. Pharmacol.*, 26, 1997, 1977.
7. **Maines, M. D. and Kappas, A.**, Metals as regulators of heme metabolism, *Science*, 198, 1215, 1977.
8. **Fish, R. H., Kimmel, E. C., and Casida, J. E.**, Bioorganotin chemistry: reactions of tributyltin derivatives with a cytochrome P-450 dependent monooxygenase enzyme system, *J. Organomet. Chem.*, 118, 41, 1976.
9. **Rosenberg, D. W. and Drummond, G. S.**, Direct *in vitro* effects of bis(tri-n-butyltin)oxide on hepatic cytochrome P-450, *Biochem. Pharmacol.*, 32, 3823, 1983.
10. **Maines, M. D. and Kappas, A.**, Cobalt stimulation of heme degradation in the liver, *J. Biol. Chem.*, 250, 4171, 1975.
11. **Omura, T. and Sato, R.**, The carbon monoxide-binding pigment of liver microsomes. I. Evidence for its hemoprotein nature, *J. Biol. Chem.*, 239, 2370, 1964.
12. **Matsubara, T., Koike, M., Touchi, A., Tochino, Y., and Sugeno, K.**, Quantitative determination of cytochrome P-450 in rat liver homogenate, *Anal. Biochem.*, 75, 596, 1976.
13. **Sassa, S., Kappas, A., Bernstein, S. E., and Alvares, A. P.**, Heme biosynthesis and drug metabolism in mice with hereditary hemolytic anemia, *J. Biol. Chem.*, 254, 729, 1979.
14. **Nebert, D. W. and Gelboin, H. V.**, Substrate-inducible microsomal aryl hydroxylase in mammalian cell culture. I. Assay and properties of induced enzyme, *J. Biol. Chem.*, 243, 6242, 1968.
15. **Proia, A. D., McNamara, D. J., Edwards, K. D. G., and Anderson, K. E.**, Effects of dietary protein and cellulose on hepatic and intestinal mixed-function oxidations and hepatic HMG-CoA reductase in the rat, *Biochem. Pharmacol.*, 30, 2553, 1981.
16. **Williams, J. N.**, A method for the simultaneous quantitative estimation of cytochromes a,b,c_1, and c in mitochondria, *Arch. Biochem. Biophys.*, 107, 537, 1964.
17. **Lowry, O. H., Rosebrough, N. J., Farr, A. L., and Randall, R. J.**, Protein measurement with the Folin phenol reagent, *J. Biol. Chem.*, 193, 265, 1951.
18. **Kappas, A. and Maines, M. D.**, Tin: a potent inducer of heme oxygenase in kidney, *Science*, 192, 60, 1976.
19. **Druyan, R., De Bernard, B., and Rabinowitz, M.**, Turnover of cytochromes labeled with δ-aminolevulinic acid-^{3}H in rat liver, *J. Biol. Chem.*, 244, 5874, 1969.
20. **Wattenberg, L. W.**, Dietary modification of intestinal and culmonary aryl hydrocarbon hydroxylase activity, *Toxicol. Appl. Pharmacol.*, 23, 741, 1972.
21. **Hoensch, H., Woo, C. H., Raffin, S. B., and Schmid, R.**, Oxidative metabolism of foreign compounds in rat small intestine: cellular localization and dependence on dietary iron, *Gastroenterology*, 70, 1063, 1976.
22. **Stohs, S. J., Grafstrom, R. C., Burke, M. D., Moldeus, P. W., and Orrenius, S. G.**, The isolation of rat intestinal microsomes with stable cytochrome P-450 and their metabolism of benzo(α)pyrene, *Arch. Biochem. Biophys.*, 177, 105, 1976.
23. **Rosenberg, D. W., Drummond, G. S., and Kappas, A.**, The influence of organometals on heme metabolism: *in vivo* and *in vitro* studies with organotins, *Mol. Pharmacol.*, 21, 150, 1981.
24. **DeMatteis, F.**, Loss of microsomal components in drug-induced liver damage, in cholestasis and after administration of chemicals which stimulate heme catabolism, *Pharmacol. Ther. (A)*, 2, 693, 1978.
25. **Rosenberg, D. W.**, unpublished observations.

Chapter 13

THE IMMUNE FUNCTIONS OF THE THYMUS AND THEIR ALTERATION BY TOXIC CHEMICALS AND RADIATION

Christine E. McDermott

TABLE OF CONTENTS

I.	Introduction	138
II.	Phylogeny	138
III.	Thymus Anatomy	139
	A. Macroscopic Anatomy	139
	B. Microscopic Anatomy	139
	1. The Capsule	139
	2. Central Cell Types	139
	a. Epithelial Cells	139
	b. Lymphoid Cells	139
	c. Others	139
	3. Cortex	139
	a. Subcapsular Cortex	140
	b. Inner Cortex	140
	4. Medulla	140
	5. Vascular and Lymphatic Connections	141
IV.	T-Cell Differentiation	141
	A. Thymocyte Origins	141
	B. Thymocyte Surface Antigens	142
	1. Terminal Deoxynucleotide Transferase (TdT)	142
	2. Thy-1	142
	3. Thymic Leukemia (TL)	142
	4. Histocompatibility Antigens	142
	5. Peanut Agglutinin (PNA)	142
	6. Miscellaneous	142
	7. Lyt Antigens	142
	C. Immunocompetence of Thymocyte Subclasses	142
	D. Developmental Pathways	143
V.	Thymic Hormones and Microenvironment	143
	A. Thymic Microenvironment	143
	B. Thymic Hormones	144
	1. Chemical and Biological Characterization	145
	a. Thymosin	145
	b. Thymopoietin	145
	c. Thymic Humoral Factor (THF)	145
	d. Thymulin	146
	2. Target Cells	146
	3. Induction of Differentiation Antigens	146

		4.	Subcellular Mechanism	146
	C.	Thymic Growth Factors		147

VI. Functions of T-Derived Lymphocytes..147
  A. Effector T Cells 147
    1. Lyt 1$^+$ Cells 147
    2. Lyt 23$^+$ Cells..148
    3. Significance of Effector T Cells 148
  B. Regulatory T Cells 148

VII. Thymic Involution 149

VIII. Radiation and Chemical Effects...150
  A. Radiation 150
  B. Toxic Chemicals Other Than Tin...150
    1. Cytotoxic Drugs 150
    2. Halogenated Hydrocarbons..150
    3. Metals and Metal Compounds 151
  C. Tin 151

IX. Tin, the Thymus, and Tumors 152

References..152

I. INTRODUCTION

For many years the thymus was considered an organ of uncertain function, probably associated with the endocrine system. Until the early 1960s it was generally assumed that the thymus was not essential to life, because removing the organ from mature animals seemed to have little effect on them. However, early in the 1960s, Miller showed that if the thymus was removed from a newborn animal, the animal subsequently did not develop immunologic competence and soon died.[1]

This essential character of the thymus derives largely from its role in providing an appropriate microenvironment for the differentiation and maturation of the lymphoid cells participating in humoral and cell-mediated immunity.[2] In addition, there is considerable evidence that the thymus produces internal secretions (hormones) necessary for lymphocytes in other lymphoid organs to function properly.[3]

II. PHYLOGENY

The thymus, found in all jawed vertebrates, is phylogenetically the first distinct lymphoid organ. It probably had its origin in lymphocytic accumulations present in the pharynx of more primitive chordates which were filter feeders and thus susceptible to infection by bacteria entering the pharynx. Certainly, T-cell-like functions extend much farther back than the chordates: specific alloimmune memory responses have been described even in sponges and coelenterates.[4]

III. THYMUS ANATOMY

A. Macroscopic Anatomy

The thymus is located in the thorax just beneath the upper part of the sternum, above the heart and below the thyroid in most species. Depending upon the species, it can consist of two, three, four, or multiple lobes, separate or interconnected.[5,6]

The size of the thymus varies greatly with age. In humans, it is largest in relation to body weight during fetal life and the first 2 years of neonatal life. From the second year until the time of puberty it continues to increase in size, but less rapidly than the remainder of the body. After puberty it begins to involute and, as a consequence, becomes smaller as the individual ages. For many years the size of the thymus was probably underestimated, since it was studied primarily at autopsy, and many diseases cause premature or increased involution. Modern estimates say that the gland in humans probably weighs 10 to 15 g at birth and 30 to 40 g at puberty. From then on it declines in weight, but is still identifiable in old people.[5,6]

B. Microscopic Anatomy

Anatomically the thymus can be divided into four regions: (1) the fibrous capsule and interlobular septa, (2) the subcapsular cortex, (3) the inner or deep cortex, and (4) the medulla.

1. The Capsule

The lobes of the thymus are joined and covered by a thin connective tissue capsule which extends into each lobe to form cross walls called septa or trabeculae. The septa partially separate the inner thymus into lobules 1 to 2 mm in width.[5,6] Although the capsule is composed of fibrous connective tissue it is freely permeable, at least at certain times, to lymphocytes coming from outside.[7]

2. Central Cell Types

In the three regions beneath the connective tissue capsule there are two major and several minor cellular components.

a. Epithelial Cells

The thymus epithelial reticular cells form a three-dimensional sponge-like network, in which neighboring cells are linked by desmosomes. Both "light" and "dark" epithelial cells are seen in electron micrographs, with dark ones containing keratin and other fibrous proteins and light ones probably being responsible for thymic hormone secretion.[2,8]

b. Lymphoid Cells

Lymphoid cells, or "thymocytes", fill the interstices between the reticular epithelial cells. There are large "blast" type cells and smaller cells typically considered to be mature nondividing cells.[7]

c. Others

Other cells found within the connective tissue capsule are macrophages, fat cells, mast cells, and, rarely, plasma cells, eosinophils, and myoid cells. Several of these cell types are actually found in the perivascular space surrounding the blood vessels, which is barriered from the interior of the thymus proper by an epithelial sheath.[2,7]

3. Cortex

The lymphocytes are not spread evenly through the substance of each lobule; instead, they tend to be concentrated toward the borders near the capsule or interlobular septa. The peripheral part of each lobule, heavily infiltrated with lymphocytes, is called the cortex, while the more central part of the lobule containing fewer lymphocytes is called the medulla.

Several investigators have described the ultrastructural differences between cortical and medullary epithelial cells. Two types of epithelial cells have been found in the cortex: flattened and stellate. Flattened cells form a continuous layer along the inner surface of the thymus capsule, interlobular septa, and perivascular connective tissue spaces. Stellate cells form a meshwork within which the lymphocytes are embedded.[8]

a. Subcapsular Cortex

The subcapsular cortex is the chief site of thymic lymphopoiesis and is thus the zone of greatest mitotic activity. Lymphocytes here are numerous; they are large lymphocytes which are rapidly dividing (6 to 9 hr/cycle).[8] The origin of the precursors of thymic lymphocytes is still somewhat unclear: some electron microscopists used to claim that early lymphocytes originated from direct transformation of epithelial cells of the primordial thymus,[9] but most feel that the lymphocytes arise from hematopoietic stem cells or some immediate progenitor cell with which the thymus is seeded. It is not at all clear where such stem cells would enter the thymus (except that it is not through lymphatic circulation since no afferent lymphatics enter the thymus), but one suggested route has been through the capillaries of the subcapsular region by the process of diapedesis (squeezing between the cells forming the capillary wall).[7] In addition, it has been suggested that subcapsular cortical epithelial cells stimulate the mitotic process; interestingly, these epithelial cells are antigenically different from those in other thymic regions and produce different thymic hormones.[8]

b. Inner Cortex

Within the inner cortex there are numerous small, nonproliferating lymphocytes that are interspersed with large dividing lymphocytes. These inner cortical thymocytes are generally immunologically incompetent and short-lived, and 95% of them die within the thymus.[8,10] Also, there are characteristic epithelial cells called interdigitating reticular cells, which may be of monocyte or macrophage lineage. These wrap their long processes around thymocytes and in some studies have been shown to be phagocytic (capable of engulfing solid particles, i.e., foreign cells).[7]

Today most workers agree that most inner cortical thymocytes arise within the thymus from subcapsular cortical precursors. In murine systems, the cortical thymocytes have been shown to move slowly from the subcapsular cortex toward the thymic medulla, with the movement process taking apparently about 3 days. The movement is thought to be due to mitotic pressure. Traditionally, the inner cortex has been regarded as the site of thymic lymphocyte differentiation, but little is actually known about the T-cell differentiation process.[7]

4. Medulla

The medulla has far fewer lymphocytes than either of the two cortical regions. Only about 10 to 15% of thymic lymphocytes are medullary.[8] Other cells found in the medulla include macrophages, fat cells, and occasionally plasma cells. Another peculiarity of the medulla is the presence of Hassal's corpuscles, which are aggregates of epithelial reticular cells. They are more numerous in animals which have undergone antigenic stimulation and in older animals. The function of Hassal's corpuscles is unknown; suggested functions include (1) accumulation and disposal of unwanted antigens and (2) disposal of dead thymocytes.[7]

As mentioned, there are relatively few lymphocytes in the medulla. In contrast to cortical lymphocytes, medullary lymphocytes are smaller, more dense, and in general, immunocompetent. In these characteristics they resemble lymphocytes in peripheral lymphoid organs, such as spleen and lymph nodes, more than they do cortical (central lymphoid) thymocytes.[8] Until recently it was thought that thymic lymphocytes moved under mitotic pressure from the cortex to the medulla and that on the way and under the influence of thymic hormones, they differentiated into mature immunocompetent cells, ready to move out to the peripheral lymphoid organs. However, recent studies suggest that only a minor population of the medullary thymocytes actually arises from subcapsular cortical thymocytes. The major medullary thymocyte pool may be a resident population of mature T cells, not derived from cortical cells and not the main source of short-lived thymocytes destined for export to the peripheral lymphoid organs.[8,11]

Thus, to some extent, the cortex and medulla behave as separate entities. As T-lymphocyte progenitors proliferate and differentiate in the cortex, their progeny migrate from outer to inner cortex and possibly from there to the rest of the body, without entering the medulla. It is not known whether they leave the cortex via the blood circulation or the lymphatics. T lymphocytes in the medulla, on the other hand, represent part of the recirculating pool of T lymphocytes, as they exchange freely with T lymphocytes in other organs, probably by migrating through the walls of postcapillary venules.[6,11]

5. Vascular and Lymphatic Connections

The thymus is fairly well vascularized. Arteries supplying the thymus follow the connective tissue septa and branch off into the lobular cortex, where at the corticomedullary junction they break up into capillaries that supply both cortex and medulla. The arteries and capillaries loop back into thin veins, passing back into the connective tissue septa. The cortical capillaries are unusual in that they are surrounded by a perivascular space and further covered by a thick endothelial layer, the "blood-thymus barrier", which may prevent blood-borne antigens from reaching the cortex. The medullary arteries and capillaries are, in contrast, highly permeable to blood-borne proteins. The cortical or medullary venules may be one route for the exit of developed T cells from the thymus.[5,7]

The thymus, in contrast to the lymph nodes, contains no lymph sinuses or afferent lymphatic vessels. Lymphocytes thus could not enter the thymus via lymphatics. The thymus does contain efferent lymphatics, which arise within the lobules and join to form longer lymphatic vessels, which accompany the arteries and veins into the tissue septa.[5,7]

IV. T-CELL DIFFERENTIATION

A. Thymocyte Origins

Originally it was envisaged that thymic lymphocytes arose by direct transformation of thymic epithelial cells. However, thymic lymphoid populations are regularly replaced by progeny of immigrant hematopoietic cells, and most workers now consider that thymic lymphoid cells are in fact derived from stem cells of bone marrow origin. This importation presumably continues throughout life, though evidence for this is not especially convincing yet.[10] It is still questionable as to whether these colonizing stem cells are homogeneous or already "committed" in some way to the T-cell lineage. Certainly they are not yet detectably different from other lymphoid precursors in, for instance, surface antigens.[12]

Once in the thymus, prethymic progenitor cells are converted into T-precursor cells and from there on to more mature T cells. The main difference between the progenitor and precursor cells is the detection on precursors of the first tissue-specific markers. In the T-cell lineage this occurs (as far as we know) in the thymus, which permits various intrathymic cell-cell interactions. The prethymic progenitors proliferate intensively to generate many thymocyte precursors. Most of the cell division takes place in the subcapsular cortex. This is where ^{3}T-labeled cells first appear and subsequently accumulate at the corticomedullary junction. Later a small proportion migrate to the medulla.[12] The visible differentiative steps can be defined by the sequential expression of a set of different differentiation antigens or by following development of immune functions.[10,12,13]

B. Thymocyte Surface Antigens

Surface antigen changes (especially in the mouse) have been used to define differentiation pathways, and different biologic functions have been correlated with the various antigens.[10,12,13]

1. Terminal Deoxynucleotide Transferase (TdT)

The earliest phenotypic marker is the enzyme TdT, which is present in a few lymphoid progenitors in bone marrow and in the majority of cortical thymocytes. It is absent in later stages.[12]

2. Thy-1

The earliest intrathymic precursor stage is defined by the appearance of the Thy-1 antigen, which is first detected on mouse thymocytes at 13 days gestation and which by day 17 is found on more than 95% of thymocytes. Medullary thymocytes as well as peripheral T cells express it, but less intensely than the less "mature" cortical thymocytes.[10,12]

3. Thymic Leukemia (TL)

Another thymus-specific marker, the TL antigen, also appears during early gestation, so that by 19 days 90% of mouse thymocytes are TL^+. The expression of TL, unlike that of Thy-1, is completely lost in medullary cells and peripheral lymphocytes.[12] It is a glycoprotein which bears considerable structural homology to the MHC class I (H-2 K and D) antigens.[10]

4. Histocompatibility Antigens

Products of the mouse MHC (H-2) locus are also expressed on intrathymic precursors. All thymocytes express H-2 D antigens, medullary cells more intensely than cortical cells. Only medullary cells express detectable H-2 K.[10] The H-2 I (Ia) antigens appear only on a few classes of T lymphocytes, specifically suppressor T cells, and are probably acquired from other nonlymphoid cells such as thymic macrophages or thymic epithelial cells, which show high Ia levels.[12,14]

5. Peanut Agglutinin (PNA)

Another marker that has been used to separate "mature" (i.e., medullary and peripheral) thymocytes from "immature" (i.e., subcapsular and cortical) lymphocytes is the ability to bind PNA.[10,13]

6. Miscellaneous

A number of other antigens such as ALA-1 and Qa 1, 2, and 3, have been described on T-derived cells. So far, most of these have been used as phenotypic markers of postthymic differentiation events.[12]

7. Lyt Antigens

The most useful series of differentiation antigens to date are the Lyt antigens. The Lyt 1, 2, and 3 antigens have been especially valuable because they correllate with certain functional properties of the lymphocytes and because their acquisition can be correllated with maturational events in the thymus. $Ly1^+23^-$ cells are T-helper cells, and $Ly1^-23^+$ are cytotoxic and suppressor T cells.[12,14]

In spite of the value of differentiation antigens as markers, their functions are largely unknown. It has been suggested that TdT may function as a somatic mutagen, Thy-1 may be involved in cell traffic phenomena, and Lyt 2 may be related to antigen receptors on $T_{C/S}$ cells.[12]

C. Immunocompetence of Thymocyte Subclasses

In studying differentiation pathways, immunocompetence must, of course, also be considered. Three major functional T-lymphocyte subclasses have been identified: T_H or helper cells, T_C or cytotoxic cells, and T_S or suppressor cells. Mature thymocytes of these classes are found in newborn thymus, localized in the medulla (which first appears as an anatomically distinct region around the time of birth). Some of these may migrate to peripheral lymphoid organs, but most peripheral T lymphocytes are functionally incompetent Ly123$^+$ T cells, which presumably migrated from the inner cortex without entering the medulla on the way. Some immature cells, for instance, Ly123$^+$ cortical thymocytes, can be induced to differentiate into Ly23$^+$ cytotoxic cells by contact with antigen, concanavalin A treatment, or thymic hormones. Thus, cortical thymocytes may give rise to some (though not all) mature medullary subsets as well as to most peripheral T cells.[12]

D. Developmental Pathways

Using Lyt antisera, peripheral T cells, and a variety of experimental approaches, an early model of T-cell differentiation was proposed in which precursor cells expressing all three antigens gave rise to either Ly1$^+$ or Ly23$^+$ effector cells. This model was then applied to the thymus. Most cortical thymocytes appeared to be Ly123$^+$ and thus immature.[10] This model has since had to be modified. Using more sensitive antibodies it has been shown that all T lymphocytes are Ly1$^+$, as are some malignant cells and normal B cells.[14] Also, the earliest cells appearing are in fact those expressing only Lyt 1, which are seen before the Ly123$^+$ T cells.[12]

Correlating function with Lyt antigens enables proposal of a modified two-lineage model with T_H and $T_{C/S}$ pursuing different maturation pathways beginning in the subcapsular cortex. This model proposes that Ly1$^+$ progenitors in the subcapsular cortex differentiate to give two lines, an Ly1$^+$-only (T_H) line and an Ly123$^+$ ($T_{C/S}$) line. These large cells in the subcapsular areas divide and give rise to small cortical cells of the two types. Some of these migrate from the thymus to contribute to the peripheral T_e (immature "early" T cells), $T_{C/S}$, and T_H pools. Others may migrate to the medulla, where they represent probably a minority of medullary cells. The majority of medullary cells either have an intramedullary or perhaps a peripheral origin.[10,12]

The multitude of cell types and functions so far discovered makes elucidation of their developmental interrelationships extremely difficult; much work still remains to be done. Scollay, in a recent essay,[11] says that "if cellular events in the thymus can be likened to a jigsaw puzzle, then a few critical pieces are obviously missing!"

V. THYMIC HORMONES AND MICROENVIRONMENT

The main function of the thymus is production of T cells. The maturation of T cells within the thymus is a complex process. It was initially assumed that the main maturational effect of the thymus was mediated by humoral thymic factors and later thought that direct contact with the epithelial environment played the major role. It is now believed that both these signals operate, with thymic microenvironment important in the earlier stages and hormones in the later stages. Exposure of T-cell precursors to MHC products on epithelial cells and to the action of lymphokines produced by medullary T cells also plays a part.[15]

A. Thymic Microenvironment

T-lymphocyte differentiation, as we have mentioned, begins with the hematopoietic stem cells and ends with the production of terminally differentiated effector cells, some of which are derived from long-lived memory cells.[11] From experimental data in rodent models, as well as data from studies of human immunodeficiency diseases, it appears that passage through the thymus is an obligatory step for the generation of immunocompetent cells. Thymic events are complex. First, since hematopoietic cells migrate to the thymus, embryonic thymus must signal them in some way to come to the thymus. Once in the fetal or neonatal thymic environment, these precursor cells undergo cell division and functional and phenotypic changes. Later, a portion of intrathymic cells emigrate from the thymus and appear in lymph nodes and the thoracic duct. Emigration is mostly unidirectional, though recent evidence indicates that in some instances long-lived memory T cells can migrate back to the thymic medulla.[8] The adult probably continues to receive periodic influxes of new precursors from the bone marrow through life.[12]

A number of investigators have shown that the maturation of T cells in the thymus requires direct contact between lymphocytes and the thymic epithelium. Most of these experiments involved isolating thymic epithelium from the T-cell precursors to be influenced by putting one or the other into cell-impermeable diffusion chambers.[15] A developing thymocyte is exposed to a number of different cell types that could influence it. During embryogenesis the thymus arises in the pharyngeal region, and there is evidence that both the endoderm and the ectoderm in that region contribute to the thymic epithelium. In addition to these two epithelial types, the developing thymus contains macrophages, the mesenchymal tissues forming the capsule and septa, and a poorly defined Langerhans-type cell (a nonphagocytic dendritic antigen-binding cell found in the skin and gastrointestinal tract), as well as other miscellaneous cells.[16]

Using monoclonal antibodies, Haynes has been able to identify four major regions of the human thymic microenvironment, which, logically enough, correspond to the four major anatomic regions: (1) the capsule and septa, which stain with an antibody called TE 7; (2) the subcapsular cortex, which is TE 4^+, TE 3^+, Thy-1^+, and A2B5$^+$; (3) the inner cortex, which is TE3^+, and (4) the medulla, which is TE 4^+ and A2B5$^+$. Certain of these tissue areas have been further identified with particular steps of thymus maturation. The TE 7^+ layer is probably the mesoderm-derived (capsular connective tissue) component that induces thymic-epithelial differentiation. The TE 4^+ epithelia are also carriers of HLA antigens and are thus believed to be involved in conferring MHC restriction on developing T lymphocytes.[8]

Using these monoclonal antibodies, three phases of thymic microenvironment development can be defined: (1) early in fetal development (4 to 8 weeks in humans) the mesodermal-derived fibrous tissues induce endodermal- and ectodermal-derived thymic epithelia to proliferate and mature. The TE 7^+ mesenchymal stroma causes invagination of the TE 4^+ thymic epithelium and thus produces lobulation;[8] (2) at 9 to 15 weeks development, the thymic primordia are colonized by blood-borne lymphocyte precursors, large basophilic cells from yolk sac, fetal liver, and bone marrow.[12] Presumably these are attracted to the thymus by epithelial-produced chemoattractants, whose identity is still a complete mystery. By the end of this period the subcapsular cortex, inner cortex, and medulla with Hassal's corpuscles (see Section III.B.4) are recognizable;[8] (3) the thymic environment continues to contribute to intrathymic T-cell functional maturation. This is perhaps the most studied but least well-understood phase.[8]

In addition to the intrathymic differentiation phases, there is evidence of prethymic differentiation of T cells in the bone marrow (ability of nude mice to respond to certain thymic hormones) as well as evidence for postthymic immunologically incompetent T-cell precursors, so that postthymic differentiation, perhaps by circulating hormones, would also be necessary.[8]

B. Thymic Hormones

The production of thymic hormones is now well established. Reconstitution of immune functions was attempted experimentally as early as 1896, when Abelous and Bellard described restoration of muscle tone in thymectomized frogs given crude thymus extracts. These sorts of studies demonstrated diverse effects of thymus extracts, including induction of lymphocytosis, prevention of wasting in newborn thymectomized mice, induction of thymocyte division, etc. However, until the early 1970s these studies were done with crude extracts, and thus the results were not clean. Since 1970 a number of thymic-humoral factors have been isolated and characterized chemically. Their biologic activities have been assayed in three main systems: (1) ability to reconstitute cellular immunity in thymus-deprived animals, (2) effects on in vitro maturation of immature precursor cells to functional thymus-derived lymphocytes, and (3) ability to enhance T-cell function and/or alter the course of disease in man. Some of the thymic factors so far examined include thymosin, thymopoietin, thymic humoral factor, and thymulin.[17]

All the thymic hormones found so far are acidic peptide hormones. Little amino acid sequence homology has yet been observed among the peptides whose sequences have been established. Also, although not all have been purified to homogeneity, the variety of physical and chemical properties suggests the existence of a family of thymus hormones, not just one. Not all of these hormones have so far been proven to be of exclusively thymic origin, although all have been isolated from the thymus.[15]

1. Chemical and Biological Characterization
a. Thymosin

Goldstein extracted from calf thymus a crude fraction called thymosin fraction V. Upon further purification 12 peptides have been isolated: 8 acidic alpha thymosins and 4 neutral beta thymosins. Of these the best studied is alpha-1 thymosin, whose primary sequence is now established.[3,18] There is strong evidence for its thymic origin, since antibodies raised against it bind to thymic epithelium in two regions, the subcapsular cortex and the medulla, to cells of a particular antigenic type.[8,15,18] Also, alpha-1 thymosin can be produced by in vitro translation of poly-A-mRNA extracted from the thymus.[19] Thymosin beta-1 is identical in sequence to ubiquitin, a common nonhistone protein. The sequence of thymosin beta-4 has also been elucidated.[18,19] In contrast to alpha-1, beta-3 and beta-4 are found only in the subcapsular cortical region and not in the medulla. In addition, beta-4 is produced by thymic macrophages.[8]

Fraction V thymosins are active in a number of assays. They can act in lieu of the thymus gland to reconstitute certain immune functions in thymus-deprived individuals; for instance, they have been used to induce T-cell surface marker differentiation in congenitally athymic mice. In vitro they can induce formation of macrophage migration inhibition factor (MIF) and increased production of antibody-forming cells. They are active in several assays measuring differentiation of murine lymphocytes in vitro, including mixed lymphocyte culture (MLC), E-rosette, and mouse mitogen assays. Also, they have been shown to induce TdT activity, found almost exclusively in cortical thymocytes.[18]

b. Thymopoietin

Goldstein also first isolated the thymic hormone called thymopoietin, which exists in three variant forms with almost identical sequences. The active site has been localized to a particular pentapeptide. Thymopoietin has been localized to the thymus by bioassay and by immunofluorescence,[3] in particular to the same epithelial cells in the subcapsular cortex and medulla as thymosin alpha-1.[8] The major activity of thymopoietin, so far, is in the induction of differentiation of prothymocytes into functional thymocytes, displaying such functions as T-cell cytotoxicity and suppressor T-cell function.[17,19,20]

c. Thymic Humoral Factor (THF)

This was isolated by Trainin; its amino-acid composition is known, but its sequence is not yet known. This factor is able to restore to lymphoid cells from thymectomized mice the ability to participate in mixed-lymphocyte reactions, to kill tumor cells, and to react to T-cell lectins. In vivo it increases T-helper activity, restores graft-vs.-host (GvH) reactivity against tumors and cellular immunocompetence, and gives clinical improvement in patients suffering from immunodeficiencies.[3,15,20]

d. Thymulin

Thymulin, or thymic serum factor (FTS), was isolated by Bach from human serum. This factor, though found in serum, is thymic-related because it is absent in thymectomized animals and reappears after thymic grafting. It is a neutral nonapeptide of known sequence containing zinc.[20] Thymulin has been traced to the thymus by observing localization of antibodies directed against the synthetic hormone on thymic epithelium (as well as epithelial cells in other tissues). Thymulin induces T-cell markers to appear on T-cell precursors. It can enhance T-cell cytotoxicity in thymectomized mice, acts on T cells involved in delayed hypersensitivity (DTH), and has significant enhancing effects on T-suppressor cells.[15]

2. Target Cells

Thymic factors do not act identically on the various lymphocyte subsets, as is obvious from the variety of biological actions already mentioned: lymphocytosis, prevention of wasting, enhancement of skin graft rejection, tumor rejection, GvH reactivity, lymphocyte-mediated cytotoxicity, helper- and suppressor-cell activity, concanavalin A reactivity, MLC reactivity, decreased autoimmunity, and development of a whole spectrum of T-cell differentiation antigens. Except for the induction of differentiation antigens, thymic factors typically work poorly on the congenitally athymic nude mouse, which has led to the postulate that thymic factors act primarily on "postthymic" cells, cells, perhaps in the spleen, that have already encountered thymic influence by direct contact with thymic epithelium. Thymic hormones in vitro do not work well on mature normal T cells and are thus always assayed on splenocytes derived from thymus-deprived animals (either nude or neonatally thymectomized). Thus it seems that the target cells cannot be completely mature either.[3,15,17]

3. Induction of Differentiation Antigens

Induction of differentiation markers is perhaps the most common assay for thymic hormone activity. Some of the markers induced include the Lyt 1, 2, and 3 antigens, TL antigens, Thy-1 antigens, and xenogeneic T-cell antigens, as well as E-rosette forming ability and TdT activity. These are commonly used to indicate maturity of the T cell. However, unless they are correlated with functional studies, we do not know whether thymic hormones are truly inducing functional maturation. In splenocytes from nude mice, thymic hormones frequently induce differentiation antigens, but no T-cell functions.[3,15]

4. Subcellular Mechanism

The subcellular bases for thymic hormone action are not yet known with certainty, especially with regard to the actual induction of mature T-cell functions. With regard to differentiation marker induction (which may not correlate to true functional maturation), the hormones probably act by a second messenger phenomenon,[18] such as that proposed by Sutherland[21] for many other peptide hormones. A second messenger system, of course, involves binding of the hormone to a receptor on a cell membrane, affecting membrane molecules such as adenyl or guanyl cyclase or ion pumps, and thus changing levels of cAMP, cGMP, or intracellular ions that, in turn, act as intracellular signals.

Bach has demonstrated that receptors for thymulin exist on at least certain T-leukemia cells. Evidence for receptors for other thymic hormones is as yet lacking.[3] The relationship of cAMP and cGMP to thymic hormones is still controversial. Adding cAMP to cells tends to mimic the effect of certain thymic hormones in the induction of differentiation markers. THF has been reported to increase cAMP levels and thymopoietin to increase cGMP levels.[3,17,18] Since different systems have produced very different results, careful investigation is still needed to produce a coherent molecular mechanism of thymic hormone action.

C. Thymic Growth Factors

Direct contact between potential T cells and other thymic cells is needed for T-cell development. Thymic hormones are also needed. One more necessity appears to be thymic growth factors, specifically a molecule called interleukin (IL) 2, produced by Ly1$^+$ thymic medullary cells. Allogeneically activated medullary cells can, by production of IL 2, induce certain immune responses (Con A- and allo-reactivity) in spleen cells from congenitally athymic-nude or T-deprived mice. Of course, this IL 2 is produced by an already mature medullary lymphocyte, itself previously stimulated by direct or indirect contact with the thymic microenvironment.[14,15] Thus, its production is not independent of either thymic microenvironment or thymic hormones.

VI. FUNCTIONS OF T-DERIVED LYMPHOCYTES

The function of the vertebrate immune system is to react to foreign antigens and remove or destroy them through the action of either specific antibodies or specifically activated lymphocytes. Upon entry into the body, an antigen is trapped by accessory cells, commonly considered to be macrophages,[14] and concentrated in the peripheral lymphoid organs. After the macrophage accessory cells bind antigen on their surfaces, it is internalized by phagocytosis and then digested within phagolysosomes. Digestion degrades most of the antigen to nonantigenic components. However, some is returned undigested to the macrophage surface. These antigenic "determinants" can be efficiently presented, in conjunction with accessory cell major histocompatibility (Ia, H-2 K, H-2 D) antigens, to antigen-reactive T and B lymphocytes.[14,22,23]

A number of T-derived effector cells can be stimulated or activated by contact with antigen presented by accessory cells. These belong to both the Ly 1$^+$ and to the Ly 2,3$^+$ categories.

A. Effector T Cells
1. Lyt 1$^+$ Cells

One major group of Lyt 1$^+$ effector lymphocytes are the T_H or helper T cells. The T_H precursors recognize antigen bound to the surface of the macrophage and respond to it by blast transformation, cell division, and differentiation to mature T_H cells. Effector T_H cells interact with mature B cells, enabling them to produce antibody.[14,22,24]

Stimulation of T_H cells by antigen-charged accessory cells normally occurs only if the T cell and the accessory cell share MHC (usually Ia) antigens. In order to become fully activated, the T cells must recognize at the same time on the accessory-cell surface both the foreign antigen and their self-Ia molecule. This phenomenon of "MHC restriction" extends to other subclasses of T cells as well.[14,22,25]

Antigen binding to B-cell surface receptors in the presence of activated effector T cells and accessory cells activates the B cells, but the molecular mechanism is not well understood. It is likely that cross-linking and rearrangement of B-cell surface molecules is one of the events that signal the B-cell nucleus to begin cell proliferation and differentiation to antibody-producing plasma cells. There is also evidence that T_H cells may secrete antigen-specific helper factors, consisting of antigenic determinants plus antigen-receptor molecules plus, perhaps, MHC (Ia) antigens. The T_H cells (or possibly other types of T cells in the vicinity) may also secrete B-cell growth and differentiation factors that are not antigen specific.[14,22,26]

A second type of Lyt 1$^+$ cells that are stimulated by antigen-charged accessory cells are the T_A, or activator T cells. Activator T cells (considered as a T_H subclass by many workers) are thought to secrete growth factors, in particular, those grouped together as IL 2, that aid in the development of cellular immunity.[14] Activation of T_A cells requires presentation of antigen in conjunction with self-Ia antigens on the surface of accessory cells, and continued activation requires continued antigen contact.[22]

Another relatively less well-known class of Ly 1^+ effector T cells are the T_D cells. Immature T_D cells recognize antigen and self-Ia molecules on antigen-charged accessory cells and undergo blast transformation, like T_A cells. After differentiation to mature T_D cells they are carried by the circulatory system to sites of peripheral antigen deposition, such as lymph nodes or skin. There the T_D effector cell recognizes macrophage-like cells bearing antigen and Ia molecules and, by releasing a variety of lymphokines, initiates the local inflammatory response we call delayed hypersensitivity.[22,25]

2. Lyt 23$^+$ cells

Another major group of effector T cells are the Lyt 23$^+$ T_C cells. These cells are also activated by contact with antigen-charged accessory cells. They differ from T_H, T_A, and T_D in that they, in order to become stimulated, must recognize the antigen in conjunction with MHC D or K antigens, rather than I antigens. They are also different from T_A cells in their ability to remain stimulated without further antigen contact. The T_C cells form a complete positive regulatory loop. The T_C blast cells develop a new surface receptor for the T-cell growth factor IL 2, which is produced and secreted by effector T_A cells. IL 2 is not antigen-specific; thus, after T_C cells have been activated by specific antigen once, any generalized activation of T_A keeps the T_C activated. After blast transformation T_C precursors become mature T_C cytotoxic effector cells. The cytotoxic function is also MHC restricted. T_C cells recognize target cells bearing the stimulatory antigen and their own MHC K or D surface molecules and kill them by an as yet poorly understood mechanism.[14,22,25]

3. Significance of Effector T Cells

What do all these cells mean to the organism? Mature T_A and T_H, by cooperating with B cells, allow production of specific antibodies. Antibodies have a multiplicity of functions, including killing invading microorganisms, preventing infection by blocking attachment of viruses or bacteria to tissues, inactivating viruses and toxins, rendering foreign cells susceptible to complement lysis (cell breakage mediated by antibodies and the group of serum proteins collectively called complement; lymphocytes are not directly involved), etc. T_A, T_D, and T_C cooperate to provide cell-mediated immunity. The lymphokines released by T_D and other effector T cells attract macrophages to the site of an infection and activate them, prevent intracellular-virus replication, kill cells other than lymphocytes, etc. T_C cells kill foreign target cells, such as virus-infected cells, tumor cells, and grafted cells, by contact lysis (cell breakage mediated directly by a T lymphocyte or other cell by an unknown mechanism; neither complement nor antibodies are involved).[22,27] Thus, it is fairly obvious that an adequate supply of T cells of these various effector types is necessary for good health.

B. Regulatory T Cells

The T cells mentioned so far are basically effector T cells, that is, T cells that directly do something. However, T cells also fulfill regulatory roles. The major regulatory T cells are the T_S, or suppressor T cells. The details of T_S induction are not clear, but a much-simplified tentative pathway can be established. The T_S cells (possibly a cascade of several different T_S cells) are activated by interaction with T_H or T_A cells (whether with the same T_H as interact with B cells is not certain) which were, in turn, induced by antigen-specific interactions with antigen-charged accessory cells. The antigen-charged accessory cells also seem to be directly necessary at later stages in T_S induction. The T_S cells seem to be MHC restricted at the I-J gene locus.[14] Effector T_S cells act directly or via secreted suppressor proteins to suppress immune responses by inhibiting antigen-specific T_H cells to thus inhibit antibody formation and, possibly, by inhibiting other classes of T cells and even B cells directly.[14,26,28]

During the course of an immune response the T_S-cell population changes, due to antibody linkages forming an "immune network". Antibodies produced in the first wave of an immune response serve as antigens to elicit a second wave of antibodies, and so forth. Presumably also, second and third wave antibodies serve as antigens to elicit new species of T_S cells. Complex immunoregulatory circuits based upon these linkages have been postulated, but considerable work remains to be done in this area.[29,30] An added complexity is the discovery of "contrasuppressor" T cells, which interfere with the T_S-induced suppression of various target cells. Very little is known about these as yet.[14,25,28]

At this point I will recall the jigsaw puzzle with the missing pieces mentioned earlier. Scollay also said in that paper, "if you have read this far and are confused, then you were following me all right!"[11]

VII. THYMIC INVOLUTION

At puberty or in response to catastrophic or prolonged illness, the thymus will shrink considerably in size. It will lose many of its cortical lymphocytes and subsequently become infiltrated with adipose cells among the reticular cells.[31] The mechanism of the fat-cell deposition is not understood, but the loss of lymphocytes and consequent mild to severe shrinkage in size we do understand.

The reduction in size is due primarily to loss of inner-cortical lymphocytes by steroid-induced death. Cortical lymphocytes (not medullary lymphocytes) lack the enzyme 20-alpha-hydroxyl-steroid dehydrogenase, which is involved in steroid hormone catabolism.[32] As a result, cortical cells are particularly sensitive to circulating levels of testosterone and adrenal steroid hormones. At puberty, sex hormone and adrenocorticosteroid levels increase, resulting in a slow decrease in thymus size. Levels also increase mildly during pregnancy and during any stressfull situation, such as severe illness; thymus size has been shown to respond to most of these situations.[5,6,32,33] Correspondingly, a decrease in circulating steroids, for instance, brought about by removing the glands secreting them, is associated with apparent hypertrophy of the thymus or failure to involute.[6]

Age involution is a normal process, but a highly variable one among individuals. Some elderly persons have as many cortical lymphocytes as a postpubertal youth.[33] The involution process is gradual, not particularly even, but overall, irreversible. In animals, in addition to age involution similar to that in humans, reversible involution is apparent. Seasonal changes, probably day length, will cyclically affect thymic size and lymphocyte density. Both males and females may undergo temporary involution during breeding season and rapid recovery thereafter. Hibernation may also affect the thymus, though it has not yet been investigated independently of breeding status.[31] Reversible involution is seen in certain situations in man, Acute or stress involution in children is caused by increased endogenous corticosteroid-hormone production due to severe illness. Stress involution is reversible, if the child survives the stressfull situation. The reversal takes several weeks or even months, and the thymus size may rebound beyond normal.[34]

The involuted thymus is commonly considered to be nonfunctional due to reduced lymphocyte numbers and fat accumulation, but this is not very logical. Bone marrow also has reduced lymphocyte numbers and increased fat with age, yet no one doubts that its continued activity is necessary to the organism.[33] All of the recent reports show that the thymus remains functional and continues to produce virgin T cells, albeit in reduced numbers, throughout life.[32] Adult thymectomy has been considered to have little effect on an organism, and this is true in the short run. However, if immune responses are followed for extended periods after thymectomy, an effect is obvious. For instance, 9 months after thymectomy of 2-month-old mice, the anti-SRBC antibody response is considerably lowered.[35] The reasons why the effect is more subtle are fairly obvious. In neonatal thymectomy, the establishment of an adequate initial pool of immunocompetent cells is abrogated and at a time when the animal is growing rapidly and, presumably, seriously needs to be increasing its lymphoid-cell pool size. Later thymectomy interferes only with the maintenance of the adequate pool. Since many lymphocytes, especially memory cells, are fairly long-lived, it takes a longer period of time for the immune deficiency to become obvious. It is also possible that later thymectomy interferes with continued production of thymic hormones necessary for differentiation outside the thymus of immature T cells populating the spleen, Peyer's patches (small accumulations of lymphocytes in the intestinal lining), etc.[33,35]

VIII. RADIATION AND CHEMICAL EFFECTS

As discussed above, the thymus is an organ essential for the proper functioning of the immune system. A number of environmental influences can inhibit proper thymic or T-cell function, and some can cause a reduction in thymic size and cellularity that is superficially similar to natural involution.[33]

A. Radiation

Lymphoid cells are among the most radiosensitive of all mammalian tissues because radiation damages nucleic acids, thus causing death during mitosis, and lymphoid cells are among the most rapidly dividing cells. Within a few days after exposure to significant doses of ionizing radiation the lymphoid tissues, including the thymus, will be almost devoid of viable lymphocytes and much reduced in size.[36-38]

There are differences among lymphocyte classes in radiosensitivity. In general, B lymphocytes are considerably more radiosensitive than T lymphocytes (which are still very sensitive compared to nonlymphoid cells).[36-38] Virgin or naive T and B cells are more sensitive than antigen- or mitogen-activated cells, which have presumably completed their required cell divisions.[36,37] Among T cells, T_S cells appear to be extremely radiosensitive, while T_H cells have both a sensitive and a resistant subpopulation.[37]

Direct radiation-induced cytotoxicity probably accounts for most radiation-induced immunosuppression, alterations in the balance between differentially radiosensitive subpopulations for the rest, and also for some reports of radiation-induced immune augmentation.[39] Logically enough, considering the relative radiosensitivities of T and B cells, the antibody response is usually more suppressed than DTH or other mainly T-cell immune responses.[37]

B. Toxic Chemicals Other Than Tin

1. Cytotoxic Drugs

A great many compounds exist that could be classified as immunosuppressive drugs, agents deliberately given to a human being generally as either a cancer treatment or as a deliberate immunosuppressant in cases of autoimmune disease or organ transplantation. Some examples of these drugs are cyclophosphamide, azathioprine, and amethopterin. Most immunosuppressive drugs are chemicals that damage nucleic acids or interfere with their replication. Thus, like radiation, they cause the death of cells attempting to divide, with rapidly dividing lymphocytes as prime target. The immunosuppressive effects of these drugs are so similar to those of radiation that they have been called radiomimetic drugs. Like radiation, they are not particularly thymus-specific.[40-42]

2. Halogenated Hydrocarbons

A number of halogenated hydrocarbons have been examined for their effects upon the immune system. Low levels of polychlorinated and polybrominated biphenyls cause cortical thymus atrophy, lymphocyte depletion of T-dependent areas of spleen and lymph nodes, reduced levels of circulating lymphocytes, and suppression of both antibody production and cell-mediated immune responses such as DTH and mitogen responsiveness. Compounds such as 2,3,7,8-tetrachlorodibenzo-*p*-dioxin and similar compounds are interesting in that they cause severe suppression of most cell-mediated immune reactions, including T-cell mitogen responsiveness, DTH, graft-vs-host (G$_v$H) reactivity, and allograft rejection, as well as profound thymic atrophy, but have little or no effect on T$_H$ activity.[43]

3. Metals and Metal Compounds

Most of the heavy metals, including lead, cadmium, mercury, nickel, gold, silver, and platinum, will, in moderate doses, suppress both humoral and cell-mediated immunity. Lead, for instance, reduces thymic weight, antibody production, mitogen responsiveness of both T and B cells, and DTH, but not mixed-lymphocyte reactivity. Cadmium's immunosuppressive effects are less well defined, but include decreased antibody synthesis, mitogen responsiveness, and delayed hypersensitivity. However, cadmium seems to enhance cell-mediated cytotoxicity against tumors, and thus impairs tumor growth. Inorganic mercury and methylmercury have been shown to reduce antibody responses and lymphocyte mitogen responsiveness, but the data are as yet scanty. Cobalt, chromium, silica, arsenic, and nickel have all been reported to suppress one aspect or another of the immune response.[43,44]

Other metals have been examined primarily with regard to deficiencies rather than toxicities. Zinc is a major example here; zinc deficiency results in significant thymic atrophy and reduced T$_C$ and T$_H$ activity.[44,45] This is possibly due to the fact that thymulin, or FTS, actually contains zinc.[20] Copper and selenium deficiencies also reduce thymic activity.[46]

C. Tin

Humans can come into contact with tin or tin compounds in a number of situations, due to the incorporation of tin and tin chemicals into cans, plastics, fungicides, etc.[47] The toxicity of elemental and inorganic tin has generally been considered to be low.[48-56] Large doses of elemental tin (i.p. injection of tin powder suspended in normal saline through a large needle) will cause lymph-node plasma-cell proliferation which is inhibited by soluble inorganic tin salts.[57-59] A slight reduction in IgM antibody-forming cells after administration of inorganic tin salts has also been reported.[58] Thus, soluble inorganic tin may have some immunosuppressive effects.

However, the compounds of particular interest with respect to the thymus are the organotin compounds, used as stabilizers for plastics, agricultural and industrial biocides, and industrial catalysts.[48-56] Monoorganotins have no major toxic effects.[60,61] Diorganotins are moderately toxic, especially when injected, producing liver and bile duct abnormalities.[62] Triorganotin compounds are potent neurotoxins.[61]

Recent studies have indicated that di- and triorganotin compounds have considerable immunosuppressive effects, especially upon the thymus, at doses lower than those producing systemic toxicity. Oral or i.v. administration of di- and trialkyltin compounds reduces thymus and spleen weight significantly and causes lymphocyte depletion in the thymus and thymus-dependent lymphoid tissues.[60,63-65] It has been suggested that the organotins act as mitotic inhibitors, since no obvious histological evidence of in vivo cytotoxicity is seen.[60] However, direct cytotoxicity is not ruled out by lack of obvious histopathology. In vitro, both direct cytotoxicity[62,66,67] and mitotic inhibition[60] have been demonstrated. In addition, several groups have shown organotin-mediated suppression of such aspects of T-dependent immunity as DTH, skin graft rejection, GvH reactivity, reactivity to T-cell mitogens, macrophage migration, and the anti-SRBC (anti-sheep red-blood cell) plaque-forming cell response.[60,64-68] It seems likely that all these immunosuppressive effects are secondary to the loss of T cells due either to mitotic inhibition or direct cytotoxicity.

IX. TIN, THE THYMUS, AND TUMORS

Since the major function of the immune system is elimination of foreign materials and since many tumors bear foreign antigens, the immune system has long been postulated to be involved in prevention or control of neoplasms.[69] At least some degree of immune involvement is seen in many model tumor systems. Most tumors are not susceptible to attack by antibody alone or to antibody plus complement. They are susceptible to attack by T_C cells, and leukemias are quite susceptible to attack by K cells (antibody-dependent cell-mediated cytotoxicity) and NK (natural killer) cells, which are probably not T cells.[70]

Animals deprived of their thymus early in life are extremely sensitive to oncogenic viruses. Congenitally, athymic nude mice, however, after improved husbandry, have reduced their expsoure to viruses and do not have increased cancers; perhaps this is because they have increased NK-cell levels.[70]

Tumor cells could escape the postulated immune surveillance by a variety of mechanisms:[70] through induction of immune tolerance (either early low-dose or late high-dose), through selection for nonantigenic or different antigenic variants or temporary antigenic modulation,[71] through immunosuppression due to chemical treatments, immunosuppressive viruses like the AIDS virus, or tumor-produced immunosuppressive agents such as that which occurs in Hodgkin's disease (cancer of lymph-node cells in the microphage lineage),[70,72] through immunostimulation, where the cellular immune response for unknown reasons promotes tumor growth,[73] and through immunological enhancement, where serum factors (antitumor antibodies or solubilized tumor cell antigens) inhibit T_C cytotoxic action.[74,75]

Clearly, anything that alters the immune system has at least the potential for altering the balance between an incipient tumor and its host animal. The immunosuppressive effects of tin compounds form the basis for postulating that tin may have an effect upon tumors. In fact, a number of recently studied tin compounds have been shown to concentrate in the thymus and to reduce the rates of tumor growth in mice.[76,77] Thus, the interaction of tin with the thymus may be of considerable clinical significance. The details of this interaction are as yet unknown, and considerable work by chemists, immunologists, and tumor biologists will be necessary for its elucidation. In this jigsaw puzzle, we have barely put the edges together!

REFERENCES

1. **Miller, J. F. A. P., Marshall, A. H. E., and White, R. G.,** The immunological function of the thymus, *Adv. Immunol.*, 2, 111, 1962.
2. **Singh, J.,** The ultrastructure of epithelial reticular cells, in *The Thymus Gland*, Kendall, M. D., Ed., Academic Press, London, 1981, 133.
3. **Bach, J.-F.,** Thymic hormones, *J. Immunopharmacol.*, 1, 277, 1979.
4. **Manning, M. J.,** A comparative view of the thymus in vertebrates, in *The Thymus Gland*, Kendall, M. D., Ed., Academic Press, London, 1981, 7.
5. **Cooper, E. L.,** *General Immunology*, 1st ed., Pergamon Press, Oxford, 1982, chap. 7.
6. **Ham, A. W. and Cormack, D. H.,** *Histology*, 8th ed., Lippincott, Philadelphia, 1979, chap. 13.
7. **Kendall, M. D., Ed.,** The cells of the thymus, in *The Thymus Gland*, Academic Press, London, 1981, 63.
8. **Haynes, B. F.,** The human thymic microenvironment, *Adv. Immunol.*, 36, 87, 1984.
9. **Volpe, E. P., Tomkins, R., and Reinschmidt, D.,** Experimental studies on the embryonic derivation of thymic lymphocytes, in *Developmental Immunobiology*, Solomon, J. B. and Horton, J. D., Eds., Elsevier/North-Holland, Amsterdam, 1977, 109.
10. **Ceredig, R., Lopez-Botet, M., and Moretta, L.,** Phenotypic and functional properties of mouse and human thymocytes, *Semin. Hematol.*, 21, 244, 1984.

11. **Scollay, R.,** Intrathymic events in the differentiation of T lymphocytes: a continuing enigma, *Immunol. Today,* 4, 282, 1983.
12. **Jordan, R. K. and Robinson, J. H.,** T lymphocyte differentiation, in *The Thymus Gland,* Kendall, M. D., Ed., Academic Press, London, 1981, 151.
13. **Scollay, R. and Shortman, K.,** Thymocyte subpopulations: an experimental review including flow cytometric cross correlations between the major murine thymocyte markers, *Thymus,* 5, 245, 1983.
14. **Dutton, R. W. and Swain, S. L.,** Regulation of the immune response: T-cell interactions, *CRC Crit. Rev. Immunol.,* 3, 209, 1982.
15. **Bach, J.-F.,** The thymus in immunodeficiency diseases, *Birth Defects,* 19, 245, 1983.
16. **Jenkinson, E. J.,** Thymus, T-cell differentiation, and the T-cell system, *Adv. Exp. Med. Biol.,* 149, 237, 1982.
17. **Wara, D. W.,** Thymic hormones and the immune system, *Adv. Pediatr.,* 28, 229, 1981.
18. **Goldstein, A. L., Low, T. L. K., Thurman, G. B., Zatz, M. M., Hall, N., Chen, J., Hu, S.-H., Naylor, P. B., and McClure, J. E.,** Current status of thymosin and other hormones of the immune system, *Recent Prog. Horm. Res.,* 37, 369, 1981.
19. **Trainin, N., Pecht, M., and Handzel, Z. T.,** Thymic hormones: inducers and regulators of the T-cell system, *Immunol. Today,* 4, 16, 1983.
20. **Dardenne, M. and Bach, J.-F.,** Thymic hormones, in *The Thymus Gland,* Kendall, M. D., Ed., Academic Press, London, 1981, 113.
21. **Sutherland, E. W.,** Studies on the mechanism of hormone action, *Science,* 177, 401, 1972.
22. **Hood, L. E., Weissman, I. L., Wood, W. B., and Wilson, J. H.,** *Immunology,* Benjamin/Cummings Publishing, Menlo Park, Calif., 1984, chap. 8.
23. **Unanue, E. R.,** The regulation of lymphocyte functions by the macrophage, *Immunol. Rev.,* 40, 227, 1978.
24. **Cantor, H. and Boyse, E. A.,** Regulation of cellular and humoral responses by T-cell subclasses, *Cold Spring Harbor Symp. Quant. Biol.,* 41, 23, 1976.
25. **Miller, J. F. A. P.,** The biology of the T cell in the mouse, *Pathology,* 14, 395, 1982.
26. **Tada, T. and Okumura, K.,** The role of antigen-specific T cell factors in the immune response, *Adv. Immunol.,* 28, 1, 1979.
27. **Cooper, E. L.,** *General Immunology,* 1st ed., Pergamon Press, Oxford, 1982, chap. 2.
28. **Hood, L. E., Weissman, I. L., Wood, W. B., and Wilson, J. H.,** *Immunology,* Benjamin/Cummings Publishing, Menlo Park, Calif., 1984, chap. 10.
29. **Green, D. R., Flood, P. M., and Gershon, R. K.,** Immunoregulatory T-cell pathways, *Annu. Rev. Immunol.,* 1, 439, 1983.
30. **Herzenberg, L. A., Tokuhisa, T., and Hayakawa, K.,** Epitope-specific regulation, *Annu. Rev. Immunol.,* 1, 609, 1983.
31. **Kendall, M. D., Ed.,** Age and seasonal changes in the thymus, in *The Thymus Gland,* Academic Press, London, 1981, 21.
32. **Hood, L. E., Weissman, I. L., Wood, W. B., and Wilson, J. H.,** *Immunology,* Benjamin/Cummings Publishing, Menlo Park, Calif., 1984, chap. 7.
33. **Kendall, M. D.,** Have we underestimated the importance of the thymus in man?, *Experientia,* 40, 1181, 1984.
34. **Day, D. L. and Gedgaudas, E.,** The thymus, *Radiol. Clin. North Am.,* 22, 519, 1984.
35. **Miller, J. F. A. P.,** The thymus in relation to the development of immunological capacity, in *The Thymus,* Wolstenholme, G. E. W. and Porter, R., Eds., Little, Brown, Boston, 1966, 153.
36. **Anderson, R. E. and Warner, N. L.,** Ionizing radiation and the immune response, *Adv. Immunol.,* 24, 215, 1976.
37. **Doria, G., Agarossi, G., and Adorini, L.,** Selective effects of ionizing radiations on immunoregulatory cells, *Immunol. Rev.,* 65, 23, 1982.
38. **McDermott, C. E. and Gengozian, N.,** The effect of low exposure-rate gamma irradiation on T and B lymphocyte function in the mouse, *Int. J. Radiat. Biol.,* 37, 415, 1980.
39. **Anderson, R. E., Lefkovits, I., and Troup, G. M.,** Radiation-induced augmentation of the immune response, *Contemp. Top. Immunobiol.,* 11, 245, 1980.
40. **Bach, J.-F.,** The pharmacological and immunological basis for the use of immunosuppressive drugs, *Drugs,* 11, 1, 1976.
41. **Kaplan, S. R.,** Immunosuppressive agents, *N. Engl. J. Med.,* 289, 952, 1976.
42. **Lance, E. M.,** Immunosuppression, *Clin. Immunobiol.,* 1, 193, 1972.
43. **Faith, R. E., Luster, M. I., and Vos, J. G.,** Effects on immunocompetence by chemicals of environmental concern, *Rev. Biochem. Toxicol.,* 2, 173, 1980.
44. **Koller, L. D.,** Immunotoxicology of heavy metals, *Int. J. Immunopharmacol.,* 2, 269, 1980.
45. **Beisel, W. R.,** Single nutrients and immunity, *Am. J. Clin. Nutr.,* 35(Suppl. 2), 417, 1982.

46. **Chandra, R. K.,** Trace elements and immune responses, *Immunol. Today*, 4, 322, 1983.
47. **Hedges, E. S.,** *Tin in Social and Economic History*, Edward Arnold, London, 1964.
48. **Zuckerman, J. J., Ed.,** *Organotin Compounds: New Chemistry and Applications*, Adv. Chem. Ser. No. 157, American Chemical Society, Washington, D.C., 1976.
49. **Zuckerman, J. J., Reisdorf, R. P., Ellis, H. V., III, and Wilkinson, R. R.,** *Chemical Problems in the Environment: Occurrence and Fate of the Organoelements*, Bellama, J. M. and Brinckman, F. E., Eds., ACS Symp. Ser. No. 82, American Chemical Society, Washington, D.C., 1978, 388.
50. **Neumann, W. P.,** *The Organic Chemistry of Tin*, Wiley-Interscience, New York, 1970.
51. **Poller, R. C.,** *The Chemistry of Organotin Compounds*, Academic Press, New York, 1970.
52. **Sawyer, A. W., Ed.,** *Organotin Compounds*, Vol. 1 to 3, Marcel Dekker, New York, 1971/1972.
53. **Davies, A. G. and Smith, P. J.,** *Comprehensive Organometallic Chemistry*, Vol. 2, Wilkinson, G., Stone, F. G. A., and Abel, E. W., Eds., Pergamon Press, Oxford, 1982, 519.
54. **Thayer, J. S.,** *Organometallic Compounds and Living Organisms*, Academic Press, New York, 1984.
55. **Craig, P. C.,** *Comprehensive Organometallic Chemistry*, Vol. 2, Wilkinson, G., Stone, F. G. A., and Abel, E. W., Eds., Pergamon Press, Oxford, 1982, 979.
56. **Zuckerman, J. J.,** Organotin chemistry: a brief primer with comments on organometallic chemotherapy, in *Tin as a Vital Nutrient: Implications in Cancer Prophylaxis and Other Physiological Processes*, Cardarelli, N. F., Ed., CRC Press, Boca Raton, Fla., 1986, 289.
57. **Levine, S. and Sowinski, R.,** Plasmacellular lymphadenopathy produced in rats by tin, *Exp. Mol. Pathol.*, 36, 86, 1982.
58. **Hayashi, O., Chiba, M., and Masakazu, K.,** The effects of stannous chloride on the humoral immune response of mice, *Toxicol. Lett.*, 21, 279, 1984.
59. **Levine, S. and Sowinski, R.,** Tin salts prevent the plasma cell response to metallic tin in Lewis rats, *Toxicol. Appl. Pharmacol.*, 68, 110, 1983.
60. **Penninks, A. H. and Seinen, W.,** Mechanisms of dialkyltin induced immunopathology, *Vet. Q.*, 6, 209, 1984.
61. **Seinen, W.,** Immunotoxicity of alkyltin compounds, *Immunol. Consid. Toxicol.*, 1, 103, 1981.
62. **Penninks, A. H. and Seinen, W.,** The lymphocyte as target of toxicity: a biochemical approach to dialkyltin induced immunosuppression, *Adv. Immunopharmacol.*, 2, 41, 1983.
63. **Krajnc, E. I., Wester, P. W., Loeber, J. G., van Leeuwen, F. X. R., Vos, J. G., Vaessen, H. A. M. G., and van der Heijden, C. A.,** Toxicity of bis(tri-n-butyltin)oxide in the rat. I. Short-term effects on general parameters and on the endocrine and lymphoid systems, *Toxicol. Appl. Pharmacol.*, 75, 363, 1984.
64. **Hioe, K. M. and Jones, J. M.,** Effects of trimethyltin on the immune system of rats, *Toxicol. Lett.*, 20, 317, 1984.
65. **Henninghausen, G. and Lange, P.,** Immunotoxic effects of dialkyltins used for stabilization of plastics, *Pol. J. Pharmacol. Pharm.*, 32, 119, 1980.
66. **Li, A. P., Dahl, A. R., and Hill, J. O.,** In vitro cytotoxicity and genotoxicity of dibutyltin dichloride and dibutyl-germanium dichloride, *Toxicol. Appl. Pharmacol.*, 64, 482, 1982.
67. **Vos, J. G., Van Logten, M. J., Kreeftenberg, J. G., and Kruizinga, W.,** Effect of triphenyltin hydroxide on the immune system of the rat, *Toxicology*, 29, 325, 1984.
68. **Vos, J. G., de Klerk, A., Krajnc, E. I., Kruisinga, W., van Ommen, B., and Rozing, J.,** Toxicity of bis(tri-n-butyltin)oxide in the rat. II. Suppression of thymus dependent immune responses and of parameters of nonspecific resistance after short term exposure, *Toxicol. Appl. Pharmacol.*, 75, 387, 1984.
69. **Burnet, F. M.,** Immunological surveillance in neoplasia, *Transplant Rev.*, 7, 3, 1971.
70. **Hood, L. E., Weissman, I. L., Wood, W. B., and Wilson, J. H.,** *Immunology*, Benjamin/Cummings Publishing, Menlo Park, Calif., 1984, chap. 12.
71. **Gold, P.,** Antigenic reversion in human cancer, *Annu. Rev. Med.*, 22, 85, 1971.
72. **Penn, I.,** Depressed immunity and the development of cancer, *Clin. Exp. Immunol.*, 46, 459, 1981.
73. **Prehn, R. T.,** Do tumors grow because of the immune response of the host?, *Transplant Rev.*, 28, 34, 1976.
74. **Feldman, J. D.,** Immunological enhancement: a study of blocking antibodies, *Adv. Immunol.*, 15, 167, 1972.
75. **Hellström, K. E. and Hellström, I.,** Lymphocyte-mediated cytotoxicity and blocking serum activity to tumor antigens, *Adv. Immunol.*, 18, 209, 1974.
76. **Cardarelli, N. F., Quitter, B. M., Allen, A., Dobbins, E., Libby, E. P., Hager, P., and Sherman, L. R.,** Organotin implications in anticarcinogenesis. Background and thymus involvement, II, *Aust. J. Exp. Biol. Med. Sci.*, 62, 199, 1984.
77. **Cardarelli, N. F., Cardarelli, B. M., Libby, E. P., and Dobbins, E.,** Organotin implications in anticarcinogenesis. Effects of several organotins on tumor growth rate in mice. II, *Aust. J. Exp. Biol. Med. Sci.*, 62, 209, 1984.

Chapter 14

HOMEOSTATIC THYMIC HORMONE: CHEMICAL PROPERTIES AND BIOLOGICAL ACTION

M. Zeppezauer, R. Reichhart, and H. Jörnvall

TABLE OF CONTENTS

I. Introduction 156

II. Biological Interactions of HTH 156
    A. Substitutive Therapy 156
    B. Hormonal Properties 156
    C. Endocrine Functions of HTH 157
    D. Thymus-Thyroid Interactions 157
    E. Thymus-Adrenal Interactions 157
    F. Thymus-Pituitary Interactions 157
    G. Thymus-Gonad Interactions 157
    H. Thymus and Radiation 158

III. Chemical Properties of HTH 159
    A. Purification and Sequence Determination 159
    B. Possible Hormone Character and Novel Functions of Histones 160
    C. Sequence Comparison with Other Thymic Hormones and Related Proteins 162
    D. Prohormone Analogies 165
    E. Chemical Modifications 165
    F. Functional Implications 165
    G. Correlations with a Binding Region 167

IV. Conclusions 167

References 167

I. INTRODUCTION

One of the most thoroughly studied thymus hormone preparations is the homeostatic thymus hormone (HTH) of Comsa. Originally, it was enriched in a procedure worked out by Bezssonoff and Comsa[1] which consisted of acid extraction and subsequent precipitation steps with ammonium sulfate and ethanol. This preparation was used for numerous studies by Comsa and co-workers which proved the substitutive effect of the HTH on thymectomized animals[2] and revealed a network of interactions between HTH and various endocrine glands.[3]

Further purification was achieved by Bernardi and Comsa by subjecting the Bezssonoff-Comsa preparation to successive chromatographic steps such as gel filtration and ion-exchange chromatography on hydroxyapatite.[4] Bioassays developed on the basis of the endocrine interactions of HTH showed that the different biological activities were enriched in one fraction. The designation HTH was given to this preparation by Bernardi and Comsa which was subsequently used to further establish the endocrine interactions of the thymus and to investigate potential therapeutic applications of the thymic hormones.[5]

II. BIOLOGICAL INTERACTIONS OF HTH

A. Substitutive Therapy

Both the extract of Bezssonoff and Comsa and HTH were tested extensively on thymectomized animals. When given in daily s.c. injections, these preparations completely suppress the consequences of the thymectomy in guinea pigs. Histological examination of the thyroid, testes, lymph nodes, and anterior pituitary revealed that administration of the thymus extract or HTH to thymectomized guinea pigs completely prevented the previously described histological changes of thyroid stimulation, the testes stimulation followed by degenerative changes, the lymph node atrophy, and the pituitary cellular changes which have been uniformly noted in thymoprivic animals. Thymic extracts or HTH maintained the ascorbic acid level in the adrenal of thymectomized guinea pigs and the percentage of lymphocytes in blood, spleen, and bone marrow. These determinations were repeated at 5, 11, 18, 27, 35, and 45 days after the thymectomy. Finally, it could be demonstrated that antibody production was restored by the extract of Bezssonoff and Comsa and by HTH. No toxic effects of the preparations were noted.[2,3]

B. Hormonal Properties

A hormone, in a classical sense, is a substance delivered from a specific tissue or gland into the circulating blood. This implies that secretion has to be demonstrated in order to prove the hormone character of a given biological substance. In the case of HTH, the hormone-like activity could be detected in the thymus, the lymph nodes, and the spleen, whereas it was absent in other organs, e.g., the liver, the lung, the kidney, the testes, and the muscles.

In both rats and guinea pigs, this hormone-like activity was demonstrated to be carried by the HTH isolated from the lymphatic organs by the method of Bernardi and Comsa. The HTH had disappeared 3 days after thymectomy from the spleen and lymph nodes. Furthermore, extract from human thymus prepared by the Bezssonoff-Comsa method was active as shown by bioassay; it was found to decrease in activity in dystrophic infants. When the thymus weights decreased to about 0.02% of the total body weight, the hormone content of the thymus tended toward zero. From desiccated human urine, a fraction could be prepared by the method of Bezssonoff and Comsa which prevented the consequences of thymectomy in guinea pigs. On the other hand, this fraction was missing in the urine of a 9-year-old girl who had undergone total thymectomy 1 year before.[2]

C. Endocrine Functions of HTH

This part of the work of Comsa represents the most thorough characterization of the multiple endocrine functions of a substance produced by the thymus gland. It was based mainly on the extirpation of the thymus and of other endocrine glands simultaneously and substitutive therapy with thymus hormone and the relevant hormones.[2,3,5]

D. Thymus-Thyroid Interactions

The thymus and the thyroid function as antagonists. Starting from earlier observations of other workers with crude thymus extracts, Comsa described the influence of HTH on creatine excretion and glucose uptake mediated by thyroxine. These parameters were used to develop a semiquantitative assay for HTH. Male infantile guinea pigs are thymectomized, thyroidectomized, and castrated. Thyroxine and thymic extract or hormone are injected simultaneously.

From the 24th to the 48th hour following the injection, the animals are placed in individual metabolism cages. They are fed lettuce and oats. Creatine is determined in the urine separately from creatinine. The thyroxine influence on creatine excretion is considered to be suppressed if (1) the average excretion rate of the animals (usually groups of four) is equal to or smaller than the excretion rate in untreated thymus-thyroidectomized castrates (0.8 ± 0.07 mg/100 g of body weight per 24 hr) and (2) none of these treated animals excreted 1.0 mg/100 g or more. At thyroxine doses below 25 μg/100 g of body weight, the thymus dose sufficient to suppress the influence of a thyroxine dose of 5 to 24 μg/100 g body weight has been found to obey the relationship

$$ax = y$$

where x is the thyroxine dose and y is the corresponding dose of the thymic preparation. The constant 'a' was used as a measure of the purity of the thymus extract. In various samples of the Bezssonoff-Comsa extract, values from 2.6 to 18 were found; with various samples of the HTH preparation of Bernardi and Comsa, the values of 'a' were found to lie between 0.97 and 1.09. The constant 'a' was defined as a guinea-pig unit of thymus hormone, corresponding to the amount of hormone sufficient to suppress the influence of 1 μg of thyroxine (see References 3 and 5 and references therein).

E. Thymus-Adrenal Interactions

In numerous experiments with adrenectomized and thymectomized animals, Comsa and co-workers found that the thymus probably exerts a moderating influence on the adrenal gland, whereas the adrenal seems to stimulate the thymus.[3,5]

F. Thymus-Pituitary Interactions

The thymus involutes after hypophysectomy and brings about a decrease in the content of HTH in thymus, spleen, and lymph nodes. Substitution with growth hormone restores the HTH production and restores the immune response. HTH and growth hormone act synergistically.[3,5,6] The endocrine interactions between thymus and pituitary are still intricate and also seem to involve the action of ACTH.[3,5]

G. Thymus-Gonad Interactions

Comsa found experimental evidence for the suppressive influence of estradiol and testosterone on the thymus which also involved the interaction with thyroxine, whereas the thymus became hyperplastic in castrates. Also in these systems the interactions are complicated and this mechanism is not well understood.[3,5] Figure 1 gives a summary of the hormonal coordination of the immune response according to Comsa et al.[5]

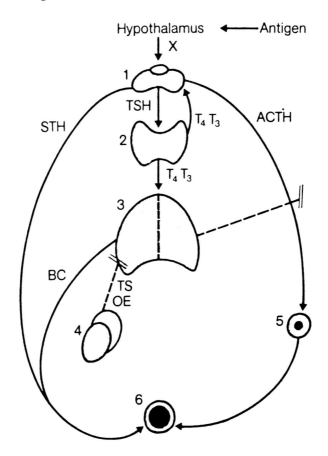

FIGURE 1. Summary of the hormonal coordination of the immune response. Stimulating influences (- - - -), inhibiting influences (||). (1) Adenohypophysis; (2) thyroid; (3) thymus; (4) gonads; (5) adrenal; (6) lymphocytes. Abbreviations: BC, thymic hormone (Bernardi-Comsa); TS, testosterone; OE, estradiol; X, unknown; STH, growth hormone; TSH, thyreotropin; ACTH, corticotropin; T_4T_3, thyroid hormone. (From Comsa, J., Leonhardt, H., and Wekerle, H., *Rev. Physiol. Biochem. Pharmacol.*, 92, 115, 1982. With permission.)

H. Thymus and Radiation

The nearly complete involution of the thymus in irradiated animals is well known, and the various lesions are well described. Treatment of irradiated animals with thymus extract did not prevent the initial lesions, but it accelerated significantly their restoration.[3] The HTH was administered to X-irradiated C57 bl mice in daily doses varying from 0 to 100 μg per animal and day. Untreated animals consistently had developed leukemia between 80 and 240 days, and all of the animals died. In contrast, a daily dose of 100 μg per animal completely prevented the outbreak of the disease (Figures 2 and 3). Thymoprive animals treated with the extract of Bezssonoff and Comsa still showed a significant mortality. From these experiments two conclusions were drawn.[7] First, the HTH has a distinct protective effect. Second, the impure extract contains a substance or substances which seem to promote leukemia to some extent and which are eliminated in the purification of HTH. The nature of these components still remains to be elucidated. Also, it has to be shown whether HTH protects the animals from the effect of X-irradiation or whether it has a specific influence on the development of the neoplastic disease. Nevertheless, these experiments indicate a therapeutic potential of HTH and related compounds in the treatment of neoplastic diseases and/or immune deficiencies.[8]

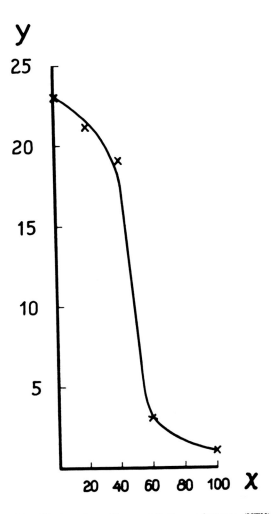

FIGURE 2. Abscissa: dose of homeostatic thymus hormone (HTH) (μg/day). Ordinate: number of leukemia deaths in each group (25 animals per group). (Data from Comsa, J., Baumann, B., Zeppezauer, M., Leonhardt, H., and Weber, N., *C. R. Acad. Sci. Ser. D*, 288, 185, 1979.)

III. CHEMICAL PROPERTIES OF HTH

A. Purification and Sequence Determination

The HTH was prepared from calf thymus according to Bernardi and Comsa,[4] but it was purified in the presence of phenyl methylsulfonyl fluoride to decrease proteolysis. Upon sodium dodecyl sulfate (SDS) polyacrylamide gel electrophoresis in a 7.5% gel under reducing and nonreducing conditions, this preparation revealed two peptide bands consistently present, corresponding to M_r 15,000 and 16,500 daltons (Figure 4A). Molecular weight determination of native HTH by Sephadex® exclusion chromatography gave an M_r value of about 30,000 daltons, suggesting the original presence of dimers. In contrast to previous reports from purifications without use of protease inhibitors, we found no evidence for the presence of small peptides nonprecipitable with trichloroacetic acid or of carbohydrate[2] in the preparation.

In order to separate the two major polypeptide chains from minor and variable impurities, the HTH preparations were submitted to reversed-phase high-performance liquid chroma-

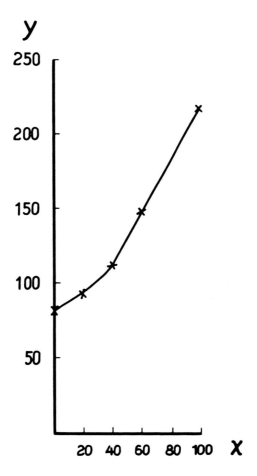

FIGURE 3. Abscissa: dose of HTH (μg/day). Ordinate: day of first leukemia death in each group, counted from the last irradiation. (Data from Comsa, J., Baumann, B., Zeppezauer, M., Leonhardt, H., and Weber, N., *C. R. Acad. Sci. Ser. D,* 288, 185, 1979.)

tography (HPLC) using an isopropanol gradient. The two components were eluted in a major peak, marked C in Figure 4. This was preceded by two minor peaks (A and B). The latter correspond to several components in variable yield and with electrophoretic positions (Figure 4A) identical to those of components that have been found to be inactive during preceding purification steps. The SDS polyacrylamide gel electrophoresis under reducing and nonreducing conditions of samples from fraction C confirmed the presence of two constituent peptide components (Figure 4A). However, end-group determination with the dansyl method showed only proline as N-terminal residue (the second polypeptide chain has a blocked N-terminus, cf. below). Reversed-phase HPLC using a shallow acetonitrile gradient gave separation (Figure 4B) of fraction C into the two components, HTH_α and HTH_β, in pure form, as judged by SDS polyacrylamide gel electrophoresis (Figure 4A). The amino acid sequences of the two proteins were determined by sequence degradations coupled with fragmentations with CNBr and proteolytic enzymes as detailed elsewhere,[9] and establish that HTH_α is identical to histone H2A, and HTH_β to histone H2B.[9,10] No evidence was detected for modification of residues in HTH.[9]

B. Possible Hormone Character and Novel Functions of Histones

The finding that HTH preparations yield the histone polypeptide chains H2A and H2B in

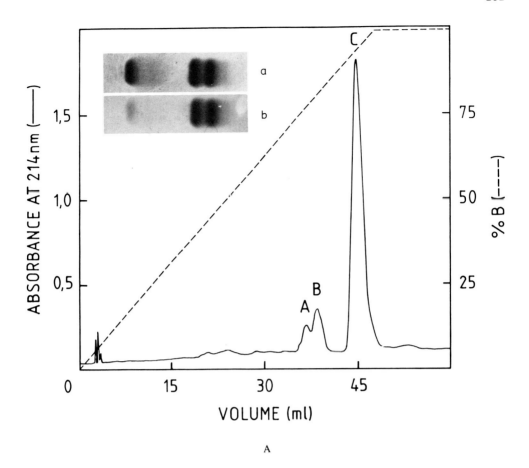

A

FIGURE 4. (A) Purification of the HTH preparation of Bernardi and Comsa[4] by reversed-phase high-performance liquid chromatography (HPLC) on μBondapak C18 in 0.1% trifluoroacetic acid with a steep gradient (% B) of isopropanol. Inset: SDS polyacrylamide gel electrophoresis of (a) the starting material and (b) HTH$_\alpha$ and HTH$_\beta$ in fraction C. (B) Separation of the HTH fraction C (A) into two components, HTH$_\alpha$ and HTH$_\beta$, by reversed-phase HPLC on μBondapak C18 in 0.1% trifluoroacetic acid with a shallow gradient (% B) of acetonitrile. (From Reichhart, R., Zeppezauer, M., and Jörnvall, H., *Proc. Natl. Acad. Sci. U.S.A.*, 82, 4871, 1985.)

apparent dimeric configurations as the major constituents suggests previously unknown possibilities of novel functions for histones. If HTH is not a trace component attached to the complex H2A:H2B, then all biological properties described for HTH should apply to one of these two components or to both, acting either additively or in synergism.

The biological effects in all tests[2-7] of HTH$_\alpha$ and HTH$_\beta$ now purified will require detailed studies in subsequent investigations. Structural analysis of HTH$_\alpha$ and HTH$_\beta$ reveal them to contain 129 and 125 residues, respectively, in good agreement with the values of about 15,000 daltons estimated by SDS polyacrylamide gel electrophoresis. The analyses also show that the HTH$_\alpha$ and HTH$_\beta$ structures are identical to those of calf and human histones H2A and H2B, respectively.[9] This explains the molecular weight of about M_r 30,000 daltons for HTH as determined by exclusion chromatography, because the inner histones interact leading to the dimer H2A:H2B. No evidence for amino acid exchanges or other modifications of the histone structures were obtained in HTH.[9]

The histone structures were analyzed for elements of structural similarities with other thymus hormones, histones, and functionally related molecules; for possible signals of protein cleavage, since peptide hormones are frequently liberated from larger proforms; and for correlations with histone modifications and other properties. Although individual observa-

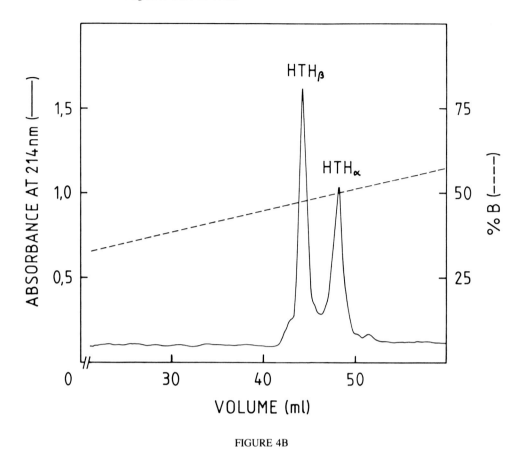

FIGURE 4B

tions are not significant by themselves, they are discussed below in order to summarize the new functional possibilities now apparent and open for future studies.

C. Sequence Comparison with Other Thymic Hormones and Related Proteins

The amino acid sequences determined of HTH_α/H2A and HTH_β/H2B were compared with those of histone H3,[11,12] thymosins,[13-16] thymopoietins,[17] FTS,[18] ubiquitin,[19] and prealbumin[20] in order to cover proteins that may be functionally related to either thymic hormones or to histones. A computer program was utilized employing variable span sizes to detect similarities independent of gaps and using randomly generated structures with the same compositions to estimate levels of chance occurrence.[21] It was found that no outstanding similarities exist and that none of the pairs reveal similarities that alone are significant. However, 7 of a total of 15 best fits (those with 6 and 7 identities per 15 residues) between H2A and H2B, H2A and H3, and H2B and H3 independently align the C-terminal regions of these histones in the same phase as shown in Figure 5.

Attempts at direct alignments in the N-terminal regions of the histone/HTH structures reveal fewer identities in the pair-wise comparisons (5 or fewer per 15 residues). However, by introduction of gaps, several of the maximal fits between different pairs can be accounted for in one alignment. Because of the gaps, the statistics are difficult to evaluate, and slightly different alignments can be constructed. The N-terminal alignment maximizing identities and still minimizing total gaps shows three other independent coincidences. These are shown in Figure 6A. One of the further coincidences is that this match, with only minor shifts, aligns with the areas of maximal C-terminal similarities among histones alone (cf. Figure 5). Another is that the region in Figure 6A detected by the multiple matches also involves

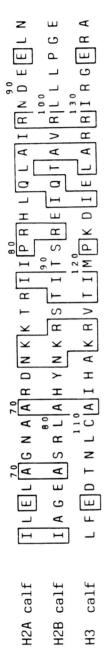

FIGURE 5. Alignments of C-terminal segments of histones H2A, H2B, and H3 according to the maximal matches in the pairwise comparisons. Only the region corresponding to the C-terminal end of H3 is shown (numbers indicate positions in H2A, top, and H3, bottom). Segments of H2A and H2B used are identical between man and calf, whereas for H3 the calf structure is shown. Identical residues are boxed. (From Reichhart, R., Zeppezauer, M., and Jörnvall, H., *Proc. Natl. Acad. Sci. U.S.A.*, 82, 4871, 1985.)

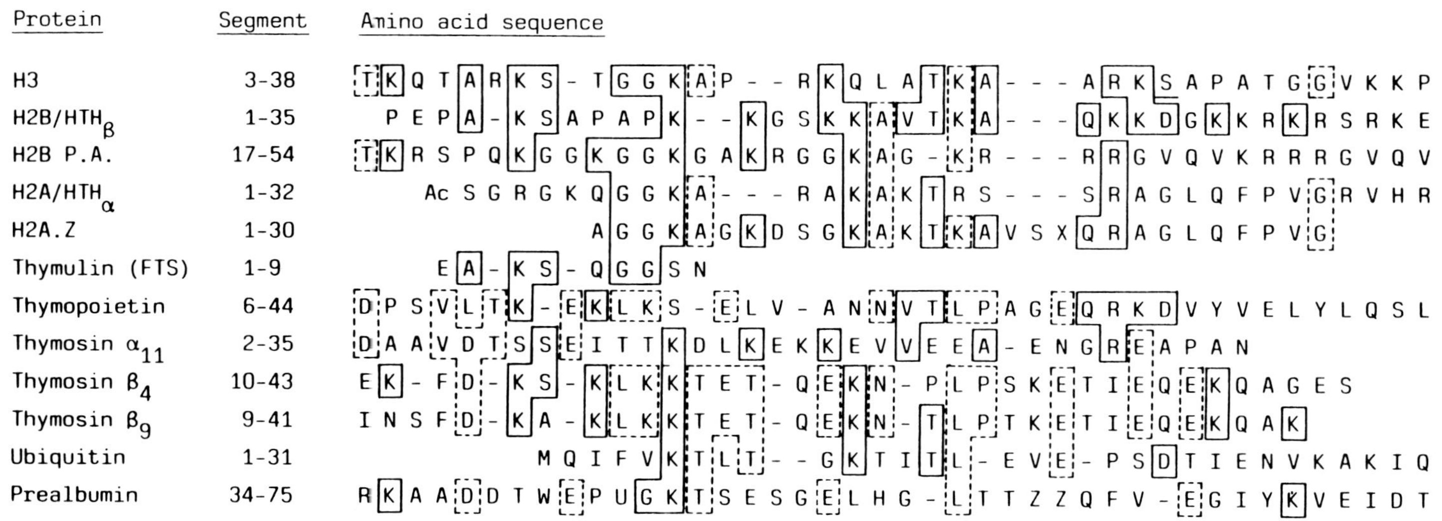

Protein	Segment	Amino acid sequence
H3	3-38	T K Q T A R K S - T G G K A P - - R K Q L A T K A - - - A R K S A P A T G G V K K P
H2B/HTH$_\beta$	1-35	P E P A - K S A P A P K - - K G S K K A V T K A - - Q K K D G K K R K R S R K E
H2B P.A.	17-54	T K R S P Q K G G K G G K G A K R G G A G - K R - - R R G V Q V K R R R G V Q V
H2A/HTH$_\alpha$	1-32	Ac S G R G K Q G G K - - - R A K A K T R S - - S R A G L Q F P V G R V H R
H2A.Z	1-30	A G G K A G K D S G K A K T K A V S X Q R A G L Q F P V G
Thymulin (FTS)	1-9	E A - K S - Q G G S N
Thymopoietin	6-44	D P S V L T K - E K L K S - E L V - A N N V T L P A G E Q R K D V Y V E L Y L Q S L
Thymosin α_{11}	2-35	D A A V D T S S E I T T K D L K E K K E V V E E A - E N G R E A P A N
Thymosin β_4	10-43	E K - F D - K S - K L K K T E T - Q E K N - P L P S K E T I E Q E K Q A G E S
Thymosin β_9	9-41	I N S F D - K A - K L K K T E T - Q E K N - T L P T K E T I E Q E K Q A K
Ubiquitin	1-31	M Q I F V K T L T - G K T I T L - E V E - P S D T I E N V K A K I Q
Prealbumin	34-75	R K A A D D T W E P U G K T S E S G E L H G - L T T Z Z Q F V - E G I Y K V E I D T

A

FIGURE 6. (A) Comparison of the amino acid sequences of two protein groups, representing histones and thymus hormones. Histones are H3 from calf, H2B from calf and man, H2B P.A. from sea urchin sperm, *Parechinus angulosus*, H2A from calf and man, and H2A.Z variant from calf. FTS indicates serum thymic factor from pig. The thymopoietin shown is bovine, thymosins α_{11}, β_4 and β_9 are from calf, ubiquitin is bovine, and prealbumin is from man. Residues identical between the two groups are indicated by solid boxes, residues identical only within the histone or the other group by dotted boxes. Gaps are inserted in order to maximize homology, X indicating a two-residue insertion R-S, and U a three-residue insertion F-A-S. The multiresidue gaps in histones are supported already by the histone subtype H2A.Z., which is internally elongated as shown. Numerical positions of the first and last residue in each segment are given. (B) Comparison of segments of the two protein groups in A with postulated binding regions in proteins of the immune system, using an alignment scheme suggested previously.[22] Outside the regions shown, no similar large homology is discerned. Structures containing postulated binding regions are from Thy-1 cell-surface antigen (Thy-1), immunoglobulin ε- and γ-chains (IgE and IgG), histocompatibility antigen heavy chain (HLA-B7), and β$_2$-microglobulin (β$_2$-m). Identical residues are boxed. (From Reichhart, R., Zeppezauer, M., and Jörnvall, H., *Proc. Natl. Acad. Sci. U.S.A.*, 82, 4871, 1985.)

those regions that previously have been postulated to participate in binding interactions[22] (cf. Figure 6B). Consequently, *maximal structural fits, now apparent, couple with independently suggested functional similarities*. Finally, adjacent to the end of the region shown in Figure 6A, HTH_α and HTH_β have Lys-Arg and other dibasic structures typical of signals for proteases liberating active hormone structures from proforms.

Nevertheless, undue emphasis should not be placed on the similarities, and they should not, for example, be presumed to indicate ancestral connections. Related binding interactions[22] and other functional properties might suffice to explain the similarities. Notably, in relation to the apparent identity between HTH and histones and to previous comparisons,[22] the structural coincidences of Figure 6 would even be compatible with the two histones themselves being prohormones. The structures in Figure 6A are further compatible with the existence of proforms of thymosins and thymopoietin, in agreement with the demonstration of a precursor of thymosin α_1.[23]

D. Prohormone Analogies

The two regions in H2B resemble structures typical of prohormone cleavage sites, i.e., a dibasic amino acid sequence, most often Lys-Arg.[24] One such region is Lys-Arg-Lys-Arg starting at position 28, the other Lys-Arg starting at position 85, both without a following proline antisignal[25] and both predicted in β-turns of secondary structure outside α-helices[26] and, therefore, without apparent stabilization against proteolytic cleavage.[27,28]

Dibasic structures at similar positions are also present in H2A. The first region is at about the end of the structural coincidences between histones and thymus hormones (Figure 6A). The second region is in the C-terminal part that, with the alignment of Figure 6A, would correspond to the region of prealbumin that has previously been suggested to match cleavage sites in gastrointestinal hormones.[29]

Apart from these theoretical analogies, tryptic digestion of histones H2A and H2B in vitro is known to produce limited cleavages. Thus H2B is cleaved essentially after Lys-20 and Lys-23[30] and H2A essentially after Arg-11 and Lys-118.[31] Consequently, native conformations protect the histone molecules against complete proteolysis in a way analogous to the selective cleavages in prohormones. Endogenous proteases have been found to cleave in the same N- and C-terminal regions,[32,33] and corresponding fragments liberated from H2B would have a molecular weight of about 2000 daltons, which corresponds to the size originally reported for HTH.[2] Consequently, the possibility of a thymic-hormone active part of HTH_β/H2B in the N-terminal region, compatible with the structures in Figure 6A, cannot be excluded. The existence of thymus hormone precursors is also supported by the Lys-Arg structure at the C-terminus of thymopoietin.[17]

E. Chemical Modifications

Histones are known to occur in chemically modified forms.[34] The serine-6 of histone H2B is accessible to phosphorylation in vivo, and Ser-32 and Ser-36 may be phosphorylated by cyclic AMP-dependent protein kinase in vitro.[35] Both these phosphorylation sites are in the N-terminal region discussed above. Hypothetically, it therefore appears possible that serine phosphorylation/dephosphorylation may not only be involved in regulation of the conformational properties of histones in chromatin, but perhaps also in signal regulations at sites potentially sensitive to cleavages.

F. Functional Implications

About 5 to 15% of H2A and a few percent of H2B are linked to ubiquitin.[36,37] A relationship between the binding of ubiquitin to proteins and the regulation of protein breakdown has been observed.[38] Therefore, apart from the presumed functions of ubiquitin in chromatin condensation or in nucleosomal gene expression, ubiquitin could participate as a signal for

Protein	Species	Segment	Amino acid sequence
H3	(calf)	16-32	P - - R K Q L A T K A - - - A R K S A P A T
H2B/HTH$_\beta$	(calf)	12-29	- K G S K K A V T K A - - - Q K K D G K K R
H2A/HTH$_\alpha$	(calf)	11-26	- - - R A K A K T R S - - S R A G L Q F P
H2A.Z.	(calf)	6-28	G K D S G K A K T K A V S X Q R A G L Q F P
Thymopoietin	(bovine)	18-38	E L V - A N N V T L P A G E Q R K D V Y V E
Thymosin α_{11}	(calf)	16-35	L K E K K E V V E E A - E N G R E A P A N
Thymosin β_9	(calf)	21-40	E E T - Q E K N - T L P T K E T I E Q E K Q A
Ubiquitin	(bovine)	8-25	L T - G K T I T L - E V E - P S D T I E N
Thy-1	(rat)	63-83	S D R F I K V L T L A - N F T T K D E G D Y
IgE	(human)	494-514	F V F S R L E V T R A - E W Q E K D E F I C
IgG	(rabbit)	405-425	F L Y S K L S V P T S - E W Q R G D V F T C
HLA	(human)	242-262	E K W A A V V P S G - E E Q R Y T C H V Q
β_2-m	(human)	61-81	S F Y L L Y S Y T E F - T P T E K D E Y A C

FIGURE 6B

unfolding and selective HTH cleavage. As ubiquitin is found in the nuclei of nearly all cell types, thymus tissue-specific proteases and chemical modifications may be necessary for HTH cleavages and activities. An influence on protein catabolism and ubiquitin functions would offer a direct correlation with several effects of HTH on regulating systems. Additional functions of H2A and H2B, apart from their role as structural proteins of chromatin, are also implicated by their turnover (significantly higher than for H3, H4, and DNA[39]) and by the possible reconstitution of core histones after removal of H2A and H2B.[40]

G. Correlations with a Binding Region

A homology of a region within thymopoietin and the binding regions of molecules with an immunoglobulin-fold domain structure has been suggested.[22] This previous alignment is extended by the present structures (Figure 6A). For H2B, this region is one of an internal repeat (regions 16 to 20 and 116 to 120 being identical) in the same way as immunoglobulin structures are repetitive with a spacing of similar size. Such a structural similarity is also compatible with the known cross reaction of antihistone antibodies with the Fc portion of immunoglobulin heavy chains[41] or with a cell-surface protein present on human leukocytes.[42]

IV. CONCLUSIONS

In view of possible identities between HTH activities and histones H2A and H2B, the concept of previously unrecognized histone functions can now be tested. The crucial point appears to be whether histones H2A and H2B can explain the bioactivities known for HTH preparations. If so, the present observations of different similarities can offer correlations with ubiquitin that may indicate molecular mechanisms for the HTH functions in regulating protein breakdown.

Finally, the present observations may be considered in relation to evolution. An ancestral connection between the molecules involved could be one explanation of the observed similarities, extending previous suggestions of a superfamily.[43] However, the facts that binding regions may be affected (Figure 6B) and that biological HTH-histone activities may be carried out via ubiquitin or other common proteins also make it possible that similarities are explained by convergent evolution. Whatever the origin of the relationships, they provide new possibilities of understanding HTH-histone-ubiquitin interactions and of testing new hypothetical relationships.

REFERENCES

1. **Bezssonoff, N. A. and Comsa, J.,** Preparation d'un extrait purifie de thymus, application a l'urine humaine, *Ann. Endocrinol.,* 19, 222, 1958.
2. **Comsa, J.,** Thymus substitiution and HTH, in *Thymic Hormones,* Luckey, T. D., Ed., University Park Press, Baltimore, 1973, 39.
3. **Comsa, J.,** Hormonal interactions of the thymus, in *Thymic Hormones,* Luckey, T. D., Ed., University Park Press, Baltimore, 1973, 59.
4. **Bernardi, G. and Comsa, J.,** Purification chromatographique d'une preparation de thymus donée d'activite hormonale, *Experientia,* 21, 416, 1965.
5. **Comsa, J., Leonhardt, H., and Wekerle, H.,** Hormonal coordination of the immune response, *Rev. Physiol. Biochem. Pharmacol.,* 92, 115, 1982.
6. **Luckey, T. D. and Comsa, J.,** A synergistic effect of thymic preparations upon growth hormone, *Thymus,* 2, 49, 1980.
7. **Comsa, J., Baumann, B., Zeppezauer, M., Leonhardt, H., and Weber, N.,** Influence de l'hormone thymique sur la radioleucose de la souris, *C. R. Acad. Sci. Ser. D,* 288, 185, 1979.

8. **Comsa, J. and Zeppezauer, M.**, Therapeutical use of thymic hormones, *Microecol. Ther.*, 11, 131, 1981.
9. **Reichhart, R., Jörnvall, H., Carlquist, M., and Zeppezauer, M.**, The primary structure of two polypeptide chains from preparations of homeostatic thymus hormone (HTH$_\alpha$ and HTH$_\beta$), *FEBS Lett.*, 188, 63, 1985.
10. **Reichhart, R., Zeppezauer, M., and Jörnvall, H.**, Preparations of homeostatic thymus hormone consist predominantly of histones H2A and H2B and suggest additional histone functions, *Proc. Natl. Acad. Sci. U.S.A.*, 82, 4871, 1985.
11. **DeLange, R. J., Hooper, J. A., and Smith, E. L.**, Complete amino-acid sequence of calf-thymus histone III, *Proc. Natl. Acad. Sci. U.S.A.*, 69, 882, 1972.
12. **Olson, M. O. J., Jordan, J., and Busch, H.**, The amino terminal sequence of calf thymus histone III, *Biochem. Biophys. Res. Commun.*, 46, 50, 1972.
13. **Low, T. L. K. and Goldstein, A. L.**, The chemistry and biology of thymosin, *J. Biol. Chem.*, 254, 987, 1979.
14. **Caldarella, J., Goodall, G. J., Felix, A. M., Heimer, E. P., Salvin, S. B., and Horecker, B. L.**, Thymosin α_{11}: a peptide related to thymosin α_1 isolated from calf thymosin fraction 5, *Proc. Natl. Acad. Sci. U.S.A.*, 80, 7424, 1983.
15. **Low, T. L. K., Hu, S.-K., and Goldstein, A. L.**, Complete amino acid sequence of bovine thymosin β_4: a thymic hormone that induces terminal deoxynucleotidyl transferase activity in thymocyte populations, *Proc. Natl. Acad. Sci. U.S.A.*, 78, 1162, 1981.
16. **Hannappel, E., Davoust, S., and Horecker, B. L.**, Thymosins β_8 and β_9: two new peptides isolated from calf thymus homologous to thymosin β_4, *Proc. Natl. Acad. Sci. U.S.A.*, 79, 1708, 1982.
17. **Audhya, T., Schlesinger, D. H., and Goldstein, G.**, Complete amino acid sequence of bovine thymopoietins I, II, and III: closely homologous polypeptides, *Biochemistry*, 20, 6195, 1981.
18. **Pleau, J.-M., Dardenne, M., Blouquit, Y., and Bach, J.-F.**, Structural study of circulating thymic factor: a peptide isolated from pig serum. II. Amino acid sequence, *J. Biol. Chem.*, 252, 8045, 1977.
19. **Schlesinger, D. H., Goldstein, G., and Niall, H. D.**, The complete amino acid sequence of ubiquitin, an adenylate cyclase stimulating polypeptide probably universal in living cells, *Biochemistry*, 14, 2214, 1975.
20. **Kanda, Y., Goodmann, D. S., Canfield, R. E., and Morgan, F. J.**, The amino acid sequence of human plasma prealbumin, *J. Biol. Chem.*, 249, 6796, 1974.
21. **Jörnvall, H., Mutt, V., and Persson, M.**, Structural similarities among gastrointestinal hormones and related active peptides, *Hoppe Seyler's Z. Physiol. Chem.*, 363, 475, 1982.
22. **Hahn, G. S. and Hamburger, R. N.**, Evolutionary relationship of thymopoietin to immunoglobins and cellular recognition molecules, *J. Immunol.*, 126, 459, 1981.
23. **Haritos, A. A., Goodall, G. J., and Horecker, B. L.**, Prothymosin α: isolation and properties of the major immunoreactive form of thymosin α_1 in rat thymus, *Proc. Natl. Acad. Sci. U.S.A.*, 81, 1008, 1984.
24. **Pradayrol, L., Jörnvall, H., Mutt, V., and Ribet, A.**, N-terminally extended somatostatin: the primary structure of somatostatin-28, *FEBS Lett.*, 109, 55, 1980.
25. **Jornvall, H. and Persson, B.**, Amino acid sequence restriction in relation to proteolysis, *Biosci. Rep.*, 3, 225, 1983.
26. **Moss, T., Cary, D. P., Abercrombie, B. D., Crane-Robinson, C., and Bradbury, E. M.**, A pH-dependent interaction between histones H2A and H2B involving secondary and tertiary folding, *Eur. J. Biochem.*, 71, 337, 1976.
27. **Geisow, M. J. and Smyth, D. G.**, in *The Enzymology of Post Translational Modification of Proteins*, Vol. 1, Freedman, R. B. and Hawkins, H. C., Eds., Academic Press, London, 1980, 259.
28. **Jörnvall, H., Ekman, R., Carlquist, M., and Persson, B.**, in *Biogenetics of Neurohormonal Peptides*, Hakanson, R. and Thorell, J., Eds., Academic Press, London, in press.
29. **Jörnvall, H., Carlström, A., Pettersson, T., Jacobsson, B., Persson, M., and Mutt, V.**, Structural homologies between prealbumin, gastrointestinal prohormones and other proteins, *Nature*, 291, 261, 1981.
30. **Bohm, L., Briand, G., Sautiere, P., and Crane-Robinson, C.**, Proteolytic digestion studies of chromatin core-histone structure. Identification of limit peptides from histone H2B, *Eur. J. Biochem.*, 123, 299, 1982.
31. **Bohm, L., Crane-Robinson, C., and Sautiere, P.**, Proteolytic digestion studies of chromatin core-histone structure. Identification of limit peptides of histone H2A, *Eur. J. Biochem.*, 106, 525, 1980.
32. **Rill, R. L. and Osterhof, D. K.**, The accessibilities of histones in nucleosome cores to an arginine-specific protease, *J. Biol. Chem.*, 257, 14875, 1982.
33. **Eickbush, T. H., Watson, D. K., and Moudrianakis, E. N.**, A chromatin-bound proteolytic activity with unique specificity for histone H2A, *Cell*, 9, 785, 1976.
34. **Isenberg, I.**, Histones, *Annu. Rev. Biochem.*, 48, 159, 1979.
35. **Yeaman, S. J., Cohen, P., Watson, D. C., and Dixon, G. H.**, The substrate specificity of adenosine 3':5'-cyclic monophosphate-dependent protein kinase of rabbit skeletal muscle, *Biochem. J.*, 162, 411, 1977.

36. **Busch, H., Ballal, N. R., Busch, R. K., Choi, Y. C., Davis, F., Goldknopf, I. L., Matsui, S. I., Rao, M. S., and Rothblum, L. I.,** The nucleosones, a model for analysis of chromatin controls, *Cold Spring Harbor Symp. Quant. Biol.,* 42, 665, 1978.
37. **West, M. H. P. and Bonner, W. M.,** Histone H2B can be modified by the attachment of ubiquitin, *Nucl. Acids Res.,* 8, 4671, 1980.
38. **Hershko, A.,** Ubiquitin: roles in protein modification and breakdown, *Cell,* 34, 11, 1983.
39. **Grove, G. W. and Zweidler, A.,** Regulation of nucleosomal core histone variant levels in differentiating murine erythroleukemia cells, *Biochemistry,* 23, 4436, 1984.
40. **Louters, L. and Chalkley, R.,** In vitro exchange of nucleosomal hostones H2a and H2b, *Biochemistry,* 23, 547, 1984.
41. **Hannestad, K. and Stollar, B. D.,** Certain rheumatoid factors react with nucleosomes, *Nature,* 275, 671, 1976.
42. **Rekvig, O. P. and Hannestad, K.,** Human autoantibodies that react with both cell nuclei and plasma membranes display specificity for the octamer of histones H2A, H2B, H3, and H4 in high salt, *J. Exp. Med.,* 152, 1720, 1980.
43. **Williams, A. F.,** The immunoglobulin superfamily takes shape, *Nature,* 308, 12, 1984.

Chapter 15

REFINEMENT AND EVALUATION OF THE CROWN-GALL TUMOR DISC BIOASSAY AS A PRIMARY SCREEN FOR DIORGANOTIN COMPOUNDS WITH ANTITUMOR ACTIVITY

A. A. Mascio, A. D. Montelius, and B. A. King

TABLE OF CONTENTS

I.	Introduction	172
II.	Crown-Gall Tumor Disc Bioassay	172
III.	Metallic Compounds as Antitumor Agents	174
IV.	Methods and Materials	174
V.	Results and Discussion	175
	References	176

INTRODUCTION

In 1907, two American plant pathologists, Smith and Townsend,[1] reported that *Agrobacterium tumefaciens*, a Gram-negative bacterium, was responsible for a neoplastic condition in plants known as crown-gall disease. It was later established unequivocally that crown-gall tumor cells were truly autonomous and that the bacterium was only needed to transform host cells into tumor cells. Continued abnormal growth was completely independent of the bacterium.[2-4] *A. tumefaciens* is known to infect a wide variety of dicotyledenous (broad-leaved) plants including apple, pear, and grapefruit trees as well as herbacious plants such as carrots, tomatoes, and potatoes.[5] Its tumorigenic activity is associated with the presence of a large TI (tumor-inducing) DNA plasmid and its ability to incorporate itself into the plant-cell DNA.[6-10] The intracellular incorporation of extraneous nucleic acids into the genome of a normal cell is indeed one of the mechanisms of tumorigenesis.[11] This is true in both plants and animals, and thus it is very likely that some antitumor drugs might inhibit tumor initiation and growth in both plant and animal systems.

The crown-gall tumor as a possible screening system for antitumor agents has been developed by Galsky et al.[12,13] They found that the tumor could be initiated by *A. tumefaciens* on potato discs and that, once initiated, the growth of the resulting tumors could be inhibited by treatment with certain antitumor agents. Their results showed that there was a definite correlation between the ability of these agents to inhibit crown-gall formation and the activity of these same compounds against the P-388 leukemia system in mice. Galsky's technique has come to be known as the crown-gall potato disc bioassay. In 1982, Ferrigni and colleagues[14,15] modified Galsky's bioassay and found it to be a simple, accurate, safe, rapid, low-cost, in-house prescreen for antitumor activity. This bioassay has the potential to reduce the need for, and the expense of, animal subjects in the initial stages of antitumor screening.

We have successfully modified and extended Galsky's bioassay method in our laboratories and have generated crown-gall tumor cells on both potato and carrot slices. Our preliminary results on the kinetics of tumor inception, development, and growth as well as on the effects of a few diorganotin(IV) compounds with known antitumor activity on these processes have demonstrated the viability of this approach.

II. CROWN-GALL TUMOR DISC BIOASSAY

Crown-gall was one of the first tumors induced experimentally, but it was not until 1942 that researchers documented that crown-gall tumor cells were truly autonomous and thus comparable to animal tumors.[2,3,11] This discovery came about when, following initial infection through a wound, secondary galls were formed which did not contain the bacterial pathogen. Tumor research could now be conducted in plants, and information obtained from these studies could be related, albeit theoretically, to tumors in animals.

A great deal of research has been conducted in an attempt to determine the mechanisms of tumorigenesis of *A. tumefaciens*. Upon discovering that the bacterium is rarely found intracellularly and then only in terminally wounded cells, Braun[11,16] hypothesized the TI principle. According to this hypothesis, a specific bacterium initiates the disease by transmitting a tumorigenic substance to the susceptible plant cell. Subsequent research in this area has concentrated on the search for and characterization of this TI principle.

In the 1960s, Morel and colleagues[17] reported that crown-gall cells synthesized unique chemical compounds which are not present in normal plant cells. They named these compounds opines and found that they are derivatives of common metabolic intermediates. Their studies were conducted on octopine and nopaline, both of which are opines containing amino acids. The synthesis of octopine or nopaline by the crown-gall cell depends upon the strain of bacterium which transforms the cells. Morel proposed that the gene governing octopine or nopaline synthesis must be inserted by the bacterium into the host cell. The TI principle must, therefore, be DNA.

Based upon the assumption that the TI principle was DNA, Kerr[18,19] conducted research on the transfer of virulence from a virulent strain of *Agrobacterium* to an avirulent strain. Finding that the transfer of virulence occurred even between distantly related species, Kerr proposed that the virulence genes were carried by a bacterial virus or a plasmid.

Studies of DNA to DNA hybridization brought about the discovery of common sequences between bacterial plasmid DNA and crown-gall tumor cell DNA.[20,21] These findings gave further support to the belief that plasmid is the mobile carrier of tumor genes into the plant cell. The putative plasmid, now referred to as the TI plasmid, enables the bacterium to divert the plant cell's metabolism into the synthesis of substances required for the bacterium to grow. In this process, the plasmid transforms the normal plant cell into a crown-gall tumor cell.[9,22] Further studies have succeeded in the characterization of the TI plasmid and partial elucidation of the actual transformation process.[7,9,23,24]

There are two distinct phases in the crown-gall disease. These phases were first described by Braun and Stonier[25] in 1958 and expanded upon by Laetsch and Cleland.[26] The first phase is called the inception phase and involves the transformation of normal cells into tumor cells. For the inception phase to reach completion, two requirements must be met. The first requirement is conditioning. Normal cells can be altered, i.e., conditioned, to tumor cells by the irritation accompanying a wound. This renders the cell susceptible to subsequent induction. The need for a wound is essential because the pathogen lacks initial invasiveness. The wound also makes available sites at which the bacterium can attach and provides a medium that can support the metabolic activities of the bacterium.[27]

The second requirement, induction, involves the actual conversion of a conditioned host cell into a crown-gall tumor cell by a TI principle which is transferred into the host cell by means of the TI plasmid.

Once conditioning and induction have taken place, the disease progresses into its second phase of tumor formation. The second phase is characterized by the unregulated and autonomous growth of the tumor cell which occurs continuously once cellular alteration has taken place. These phases have been studied and documented in depth by Beardsley.[28]

The idea of utilizing the crown-gall tumor system as a means of elucidating the mechanisms of tumor induction and host cell transformation in animal tissues was first proposed by Braun.[11] Support for these comparative studies is found in the characteristics of both plant and animal tumors. Tumor tissue from both kingdoms displays the three main characteristics of all cancers: abnormal cellular multiplication, autonomy, and invasiveness. The transformation of both animal and plant cells involves a major reorganization of biosynthetic metabolism. A normal cell has a differentiated, orderly metabolism which synthesizes only those substances required by the resting cell. The tumor cell displays a highly undifferentiated metabolism with excessive synthesis of hormones, nucleic acids, and enzymatic proteins. The excessive production of these and other substances related to cell growth and division lead to the tumor cell's rapid multiplication, autonomy, and invasiveness. The energy of the tumor cell is channeled primarily into its proliferating system.

The underlying basis for autonomous growth in both plant and animal cells is similar at the physiologic and biochemical levels, regardless of the specific mode of tumor induction. Braun provides a comprehensive review of the relevence of plant tumor systems to the general cancer problem.[3,11] The similarities between plant and animal tumorigenesis led Galsky and colleagues to investigate the crown-gall disease as a means of testing antitumor activity of different compounds.[12,13] Obviously, the development of a simple, convenient, and inexpensive plant tumor system as a primary screen offers numerous advantages over the extensive animal testing protocols.

III. METALLIC COMPOUNDS AS ANTITUMOR AGENTS

The process of drug development is an elaborate and expensive endeavor. This is particularly true with antineoplastic chemotherapeutic agents since most of the differences on which selective toxicity is based are quantitative rather than qualitative. Also, in order to effect cure, all tumor cells must be killed. The most fundamental problem in developing clinically useful antitumor agents continues to be the lack of selectivity between tumor cells and normal cells. Despite this fact, great strides have been achieved in cancer chemotherapy and many new types of compounds are continuously being explored and tested for their biological activity. Only within the last 20 years, however, have metallic compounds been investigated as anticancer agents. Rosenberg and colleagues conducted the original experiments which indicated that certain platinum compounds were potent antitumor agents.[29] Extensive studies have been done on the antitumor activity of platinum and other transition metal complexes and a number of nontransition metal compounds. A review of the chemistry of platinum compounds and their relation to antitumor activity is presented by Cleare.[30]

A number of metallic derivatives have been found to exhibit antitumor activity when tested in vivo utilizing the P-388 lymphocytic-leukemia system in mice. In particular, diethyltin dihalide and dipseudohalide complexes have shown reproducible therapeutic activity.[31] The T/C values (median survival time of the treated group divided by that of the untreated control group) for diethyltin complexes in the P-388 tumor system are somewhat lower than those for platinum compounds. However, organotin compounds have not been shown to have a high toxicity in the nephron of the kidney, as is seen with platinum compounds.[32]

Recently, it has been shown that the diorganotin(IV) derivatives also exhibit antitumor activity. The antitumor activity of certain diorganotin complexes including adenine (R_2SnAd_2)[33] and glycylglycine ($R_2SnGlyGly$)[33] has been documented, and several hypotheses have been proposed concerning the anti-tumor action of these compounds.[31-34]

IV. METHODS AND MATERIALS

All starting materials were purchased from Aldrich Chemical. Diphenyltin(IV) dichloride, and triphenyltin(IV) chloride were recrystallized from hexanes. Benzotriazole (Bz) was purified by recrystallization from chloroform, carbon tetrachloride (5:95%) mixed solvent. Tetrahydrofuran (THF) was purified by first distilling from triphenylphosphine and potassium hydroxide, then twice distilling from sodium hydride (NaH). Adenine and sodium hydride (99%) were used as received.

All syntheses were carried out under dry nitrogen. Benzotriazolatotriphenyltin(IV) was prepared by a variation of the method of Gassend et al.[35] A tetrahydrofuran solution of benzotriazole was added slowly to a suspension of NaH in THF at room temperature and stirred until evolution of H_2 gas had ceased. A solution of triphenyltin(IV) chloride in THF was then added and the mixture refluxed for 3 hr. The THF was removed *in vacuo,* and the resulting solid was leached with boiling ethanol, then filtered hot. On cooling, white crystals precipitated from the filtrate and were collected by suction filtration. Bis(adeninato)diphenyltin(IV) was prepared by the method of Pellerito et al.[36] However, unlike Pellerito's product, our solid was insoluble in hot ethanol and in other common organic solvents and, therefore, could not be purified by recrystallization. As a result, the elemental analysis of our product did not agree with the theoretical.

Melting points were recorded on a Hoover capillary melting point apparatus and were uncorrected. Elemental analyses were carried out by Robertson Laboratory, Inc., Madison, N. J. Melting point and analysis of the products (literature data and calculated values in parentheses) were

1. Benzotriazolatotriphenyltin(IV): 261 to 262°C; C, 61.35 (61.58); H, 3.92 (4.09); N, 8.87 (8.98)
2. Bis-adeninatodiphenyltin(IV): >355°C; C, 46.23 (48.83); H, 3.70 (3.35); N, 21.91 (25.88)

The techniques employed in our studies are based on the crown-gall potato disc bioassay outlined by Ferrigni and colleagues.[14] Upon further development and optimization of his technique, a modified bioassay was reached and employed for the remainder of the investigations. This modified bioassay is briefly described below.

Several moderate-sized, unpeeled red potatoes (*Solanum tuberosum*) were soaked for 20 min in a 20% vol/vol sodium aqueous hypochlorite (Clorox®) solution (i.e., 1% sodium hypochlorite, 0.13M). This effectively sterilized the surface of the tubers. After sterilization, the ends of the tubers were cut off and potato discs obtained by placing a sterilized #12 (15 mm) cork borer through the center of each tuber. The resulting core of each potato was cut into 0.5-cm-thick discs with a surface-sterilized scalpel. All work took place under aseptic conditions to prevent contamination.

Petri dishes containing 1.5% agar (w/v) were prepared and five potato discs placed in each dish. The discs were then inoculated with 0.10 mℓ of a 24-hr culture of *A. tumefaciens* containing about 5×10^9 cells per milliliter. The petri dishes were then incubated for 12 days at 27°C.

Four sets of eight plates each (each plate containing five potato discs) were assembled. The first set was inoculated with *A. tumefaciens*, but not treated with the organotin compounds and served as a control. The three remaining sets were inoculated with the bacterium and treated with a test compound. The three test compounds consisted of diphenyldiadeninatotin(IV), diphenyltin(IV) dichloride, and triphenylbenzotriazolatotin(IV).

Four plates from each set of test plates were treated with the test compound after 2 days of incubation postinfection. The remaining four plates were treated after 7 days of incubation.

Solutions of the test compounds were prepared by dissolving 2.0 mg of the compound in 0.25 mℓ ethanol. Sterile, distilled water was then added for a total volume of 10 mℓ. The final concentration of each compound, whether in solution or suspension, was 0.2 mg/mℓ.

After the appropriate incubation period, the discs in the test plates were treated with 0.1 mℓ of the prepared test compound (0.02 mg per disc). A flamed loop was used to spread the compound evenly over the disc surface. The plates were then reincubated at 27°C.

Following an incubation period of 12 days, the resulting macroscopic tumors were examined and counted with the aid of a binocular dissecting microscope. Tumor tissue was also weighed and recorded and these tumor weight values were used to determine and compare antitumor effects. Tumor counts, though useful and comparable, do not take into account the fact that tumors vary in size and mass. (See Table 1 where percent inhibition data from both weight and tumor count are displayed.)

V. RESULTS AND DISCUSSION

Our preliminary results, summarized in Table 1, indicate that all three of the organotin compounds exhibit significant inhibition of tumor growth at a concentration of 0.02 mg per disc in either solution or suspension when the discs were treated 2 days postinfection. Treatment on day 7 also showed significant reduction of growth with the exception of diphenyldiadeninatotin when administered in solution. The greatest reduction in tumor tissue was found when the test compounds were applied onto the potato discs 2 days after the discs were infected with *A. tumefaciens*. A plausible explanation for this effect is that not only could the compounds inhibit tumor cell growth and proliferation, but also prevent the early transformation or initiation process from taking place, i.e., initiation could be prevented by dispensing with the induction period altogether.

Table 1
PERCENT INHIBITION OF TUMOR GROWTH ON POTATO DISCS TREATED WITH ORGANOTIN COMPOUNDS IN SUSPENSION OR SOLUTION ON DAYS 2 AND 7[a]

Compound	Suspension		Solution	
	Day 2 (%)	Day 7 (%)	Day 2 (%)	Day 7 (%)
Ph_3SnBz	98(92)	78(70)	78(73)	75(62)
Ph_2SnCl_2	95(87)	66(61)	64(59)	28(22)
Ph_2SnAd_2	90(88)	52(53)	61(59)	7(11)[b]

[a] *A. tumefaciens* inoculated discs were treated with 0.02 mg per disc of the test compound on days 2 and 7 postinfection. On day 12 postinfection, the weight of the tumor tissue was determined both for the untreated controls and the experimental groups and percent inhibition calculated. Numbers in parentheses are percent inhibition based upon tumor-count data. The percent inhibition (growth assay, masses) =
$$\frac{\text{mass of tumor tissue of untreated control} - \text{mass of tumor tissue of treated experimentals}}{\text{mass of tumor tissue of untreated controls}} \times 100$$

[b] Not significant.

Attachment and penetration of the bacterial cells into the host plant cells and the subsequent release of the TI plasmid is believed to occur within the first 2 to 6 hr of infection. Thus, the observed effects are on the mechanism(s) of the tumorigenesis rather than on the bacterial cells themselves. It should also be pointed out that the concentration used (0.02 mg per disc) shows no toxicity in our system,[37] and further studies are underway. The bacteria apparently survive treatment with the organotin solutions/suspensions at the concentrations used.

Overall, each of the compounds exhibited maximum inhibition of tumor growth when used in suspension as opposed to solution. Solutions were made by dissolving the compounds in 95% ethanol, while suspensions resulted from using distilled water. Bond angles between the constituents of organotin molecules may be important in the binding of the compound to the active sites on enzymes or other macromolecules. The steric configuration of the organotin molecules and their binding ability might be different for each phase. This requires further investigation.

Galsky et al.[12,13] and Ferrigni et al.,[14,15] using known potent anticancer drugs (nonmetallic) and appropriate inactive controls, have shown clearly that there is a good correlation between the crown-gall potato disc assay and the in vivo P-388 mouse leukemia system. Potato disc actives were defined as those which inhibited about 20% or more of the tumors in two subsequent assays, using both the initiation assay (tumor counts) and growth assay (masses); this decision was made by considering the activity of a known P-388 active compound as a model.

Whether the crown-gall system will be effective in screening organotin compounds for their antitumor activity is not fully known. Our initial preliminary studies seem promising, but much remains to be done.

REFERENCES

1. **Smith, E. F. and Townsend, C. O.**, A plant tumor of bacterial origin, *Science*, 25, 671, 1907.
2. **White, P. R. and Braun, A. C.**, A cancerous neoplasm of plants: autonomous bacteria-free crown-gall tissue, *Cancer Res.*, 2, 597, 1942.

3. **Braun, A. C.**, *The Cancer Problem*, Columbia University Press, New York, 1969, 209.
4. **Dickinson, C. H. and Lucas, J. A.**, *Plant Pathology and Plant Pathogens*, John Wiley & Sons, New York, 1977, 161.
5. **Kiraly, Z., Klement, Z., Solymosy, F., and Voros, J.**, *Methods in Plant Pathology*, Akademia Kiado, Budapest, 1970, 509.
6. **Zaenen, I., Van Larebeke, N., Teuchy, H., Van Montagu, M., and Schell, J.**, Supercoiled DNA in crown-gall inducing *Agrobacterium* strains, *J. Mol. Biol.*, 86, 109, 1974.
7. **Schell, J.**, The role of plasmids in crown gall formation by *A. tumefaciens*, in *Genetic Manipulation with Plant Materials*, Ride, M., Ed., Plenum Press, New York, 1975, 163.
8. **Schell, J. and Van Montagu, M.**, The Ti plasmid as natural and as practical gene vectors for plants, *Biotechnology*, 1, 175, 1983.
9. **Chilton, M. D.**, A vector for introducing new genes into plants, *Sci. Am.*, 248, 50, 1983.
10. **Watson, B., Currier, T. C., Gordon, M. P., Chilton, M. D., and Nester, E. W.**, Plasmid required for virulence of *Agrobacterium tumefaciens*, *J. Bacteriol.*, 123, 255 1975.
11. **Braun, A. C.**, *The Story of Cancer*, Addison-Wesley, Reading, Mass., 1977.
12. **Galsky, A. G., Wisley, J. P., and Powell, R. G.**, Crown-gall tumor-disc bioassay, *Plant Physiol.*, 65, 184, 1980.
13. **Galsky, A. G., Kozimor, R., Piotrowski, D., and Powell, R. G.**, The crown-gall potato-disc bioassay as a primary screen for compounds with antitumor activity, *J. Am. Cancer Inst.*, 67, 689, 1981.
14. **Ferrigni, N. R., Putnam, J. E., Anderson, B., Jacobson, L. B., Nichols, D. E., Moore, D. S., McLaughlin, J. L., Powell, R. G., and Smith, C. R., Jr.**, Modification and evaluation of the potato disc assay and antitumor screening of *Euphorbiacea* seeds, *J. Nat. Prod.*, 45, 679, 1982.
15. **Ferrigni, N. R., McLaughlin, J. L., Powell, R. G., and Smith, C. R., Jr.**, Use of potato disc and brine shrimp to detect activity and isolate piceatannd as the antileukemic principle from the seeds of *Euphorbia-Lagascal*, *J. Nat. Prod.*, 47, 347, 1984.
16. **Braun, A. C.**, Thermal studies on the factors responsible for tumor initiation in crown gall, *Am. J. Bot.*, 34, 234, 1947.
17. **Morel, G.**, On some peculiarities of nitrate metabolism of tissues of *Agrobacterium tumefaciens*, *C. R. Soc. Biol.*, 160, 52, 1966.
18. **Kerr, A.**, Acquisition of virulence by non-pathogenic isolates of *Agrobacterium radiobacter*, *Physiol. Plant Pathol.*, 1, 241, 1971.
19. **Kerr, A.**, Transfer of virulence between strains of *Agrobacterium*, *Nature*, 223, 1175, 1969.
20. **Quetier, F., Huguet, T., and Guille, E.**, Induction of crown gall: partial homology between tumor-cell DNA, bacterial DNA, and the G + C-rich DNA of stressed normal cells, *Biochem. Biophys. Res. Commun.*, 34, 128, 1969.
21. **Srivastava, B. I. S.**, DNA-DNA hybridization studies between bacterial cell DNA, crown gall tumor cell DNA, and the normal cell DNA, *Life Sci.*, 9, 889, 1970.
22. **Lippincott, J. A. and Lippincott, B. B.**, Morphogenic determinants as exemplified by the crown gall disease, in *Physiological Plant Pathology*, Heitfuss, R. and Williams, P. H., Eds., Springer-Verlag, New York, 1976, 356.
23. **Ream, L. W. and Gordon, M. P.**, Crown-gall disease and prospects for genetic manipulation of plants, *Science*, 218, 854, 1982.
24. **Caplan, A., Herrera-Estrella, L., Inze, D., Van Haute, E., Van Montagu, M., Schell, J., and Zambryski, P.**, Introduction of genetic material into plant cells, *Science*, 222, 815, 1983.
25. **Braun, A. C. and Stonier, T.**, *Morphology and Physiology of Plant Tumors*, Springer-Verlag, New York, 1958, 93.
26. **Laetsch, W. M. and Cleland, R. E.**, *Papers on Plant Growth and Development*, Little, Brown, Boston, 1976, 479.
27. **Lippincott, B. B. and Lippincott, J. A.**, Bacterial attachment to a specific wound site as an essential stage in tumor initiation by *Agrobacterium tumefaciens*, *J. Bacteriol.*, 97, 620, 1969.
28. **Beardsley, R. E.**, The inception phase in the crown gall disease, *Prog. Exp. Tumor Res.*, 15, 1, 1972.
29. **Rosenberg, B., Van Camp, L., Troski, J. E., and Mansour, V. H.**, Platinum compounds: a new class of potent antitumor agents, *Nature*, 222, 385, 1969.
30. **Cleare, M. J.**, Some aspects of platinum complex chemistry and their reaction to anti-tumor activity, *J. Clin. Oncol.*, 7, 1, 1977.
31. **Crowe, A. J. and Smith, P. J.**, Dialkyltin dihalide complexes: a new class of metallic derivatives exhibiting anti-tumor activity, *Chem. Ind. (London)*, 23, 171, 1980.
32. **Haiduc, I., Silverstru, C., and Gielen, M.**, Organotin compounds: new organometallic derivatives exhibiting anti-tumor activity, *Bull. Soc. Chim. Belg.*, 92, 187, 1983.
33. **Barbieri, R., Pellirito, L., Ruisi, M., Lo Giudice, M. T., Huber, F., and Atassi, G.**, The antitumor activity of diorganotin (IV) complexes with adenine and glycylglycine, *Inorg. Chim. Acta*, 66, L39, 1982.

34. **Crowe, A. J., Smith, P. J., and Atassi, G.**, Investigations into the antitumor activity of organotin compounds. I. Diorganotin halide and di-pseudohalide complexes, *Chem. Biol. Interact.*, 32, 171, 1980.
35. **Gassend, R., Delmas, M., Maire, J. C., Richard, Y., and More, C.**, Etude par spectroscopie Mossbauer d'organstannylazoles, *J. Organomet. Chem.*, 42, C29, 1972.
36. **Pellerito, L., Ruisi, G., Bertazzi, M., Guidice, M. T., and Barbieri, R.**, Synthesis and Mossbauer spectroscopy of diorganotin(IV) complexes, *Inorg. Chim. Acta*, 17, L9, 1976.
37. **Mascio, A. A., Montelius, A. D., and King, B.**, unpublished data.

Chapter 16

ORGANOTINS AS INSECT CHEMOSTERILANTS

K. R. S. Ascher and J. Meisner

TABLE OF CONTENTS

I.	Sterilization of Insects	180
II.	Chemosterilization vs. Radiosterilization	180
III.	Chemosterilants and Antitumor Activity	181
IV.	Expressions of Chemosterilization	182
V.	Classes of Insect Chemosterilants	182
VI.	Organotins as Biocides	182
VII.	Organotins as Chemosterilants	183
	A. Effects on Egg Hatchability (Fertility)	183
	1. Diptera	183
	2. Coleoptera	187
	3. Lepidoptera	188
	4. Hemiptera	190
	5. Tetranychid Mites	190
	B. Effects on Fecundity	191
	1. Diptera	191
	2. Coleoptera	192
	3. Lepidoptera	192
	4. Orthoptera	194
	5. Hemiptera	194
	C. Other Properties of Organotins Relevant to Chemosterilization	195
	1. Absence of Significant Oviposition Repellence	195
	2. Effects of Organotins on Predation and Parasitism	195
	3. Chemosterilizing Effects in Mammals	195
Acknowledgment		196
References		196

I. STERILIZATION OF INSECTS

The sterility method to control insect pest populations comprises mass production and release into nature of sterilized insects, which however, are sexually both vigorous and fully competitive, or direct sterilization of natural insect populations. To bring about sterility* by either of these two means, several schemes have been used with varying degrees of success or have been considered seriously: radiosterilization using X-ray or gamma-radiation; high-intensity photoflash discharges; and chemosterilization and other genetic pathways, such as cytoplasmatic incompatibility, hybrid sterility, and translocation-induced sterility or semisterility.

Whereas the principles of genetic insect control were first formulated by Serebrovsky[1] in the U.S.S.R. as early as 1940, the theoretical aspects of chemically induced sterility for control programs were elaborated by Knipling[2,3] in the U.S. Earlier and contemporaneous findings on insect sterility achieved by mutagenic, carcinogenic, and carcinolytic chemicals (mostly as a by-product of genetic studies, mainly with *Drosophila melanogaster* Meig.) were published by von Gelei and Csik[4] (on colchicine), Auerbach and Robson,[5] Rapoport,[6-8] Battacharya,[9] Demerec et al.,[10] Bird,[11] Auerbach,[12] Wallace,[13] Auerbach and Moser,[14] Fahmy and Fahmy,[15-17] and others. In pioneering studies Goldsmith et al.,[18,19] Goldsmith and Harnly,[20] and Goldsmith and Frank[21] achieved a lowering or complete inhibition of oviposition in *D. melanogaster* by folic acid antagonists such as aminopterin (4-aminopteroylglutamic acid) and methotrexate (amethopterin; 4-amino-N^{10}-methyl-pteroylglutamic acid), both used then in the treatment of leukemia and other neoplastic diseases. However, the search for practical chemosterilants was initiated by the U.S.[22,23] Department of Agriculture (USDA) and independently in Israel[24,25] in 1955.

The subject of chemosterilants has been reviewed, inter alia, by Ascher,[26,27] Bertram,[28] Bořkovec,[29] Smith et al.,[30] Adolphi,[31] Campion,[32-34] Gruner,[35] Rukavishnikov,[36,37] Kilgore,[38] Bořkovec et al.,[39] Schumakow,[40] Proverbs,[41] Stüben,[42] Büchel,[43] and in the books on chemosterilants by Bořkovec[44] and LaBreque and Smith.[45] Bibliographies have been compiled by Sharma and Brooks[46] (includes 1294 references of works published up to June 1974) and by Fye and LaBreque[47] (includes 1475 references of works published through March 1974).

II. CHEMOSTERILIZATION VS. RADIOSTERILIZATON

Insect chemosterilization is evidently a natural consequence of the success in insect control with radiation-sterilized males. The most famous example of the latter, the successful eradication of the screwworm, *Cochlyomia hominivorax* Coquerel, first from the 170-mi^2 island Curaçao and subsequently from Florida and other states of the U.S. through the release of billions of radiation-sterilized males, is as a classic example of a successful economic entomology control project. Radiation sterilization, as used with the screwworm, seems to be adequate especially in situations in which only comparatively few sterile insects might be required to prevent establishment or to control or stamp out infestations or populations that have been reduced to a low level by conventional means. However, for most insects the rearing, sterilization, and release method alone would be impracticable for regulating well-established field populations, since it would require the mass release of sterilized males in numbers greater than the field population. Such a release may be often not only undesirable but also damaging, if not impossible, even if the damage and/or nuisance due to the released insects is only temporary. It cannot be applied, for instance, to insects that are mechanical vectors of pathogens. Very often the method is not feasible at all because many insects

---

* This specific type of "sterility" often constitutes not a change in the fertility of the treated insects, but rather of "reproduction," in that the embryos die at some stage of development.

cannot be obtained or reared in the laboratory, or the cost of rearing them may be prohibitive. It requires large, expensive, and highly specific plants; arrangements for rearing, transporting, and irradiating the insects (irradiation is usually most effective in the pupal stage); and demands a miniature airfleet to disperse the sterilized insects. In some species, e.g., the boll weevil, *Anthonomus grandis* Boheman; the gypsy moth, *Lymantria (Porthetria) dispar* (L.); the yellowfever mosquito, *Aedes aegypti* (L.) etc., the irradiation dose necessary to achieve sterility is so high that it drastically reduces the sexual competitiveness and vigor of the treated insects or even kills them. Satisfactory sexual competitivity, adequate sperm production, and tolerance to environmental hardships and stresses are essential for the sterilized insect to seek and reach its victim, namely, its mating partner in nature. The sterilized insect should be capable of penetrating all parts of the environment and of successfully competing sexually with fertile insects of the same sex, wherever they are, even in microniches. The shortcomings of sterilization by radiation mentioned above led naturally to the idea of *chemosterilization*.

III. CHEMOSTERILANTS AND ANTITUMOR ACTIVITY

Even before the start of the large and well-coordinated USDA research project in 1958, Mitlin et al.[23] had made valuable contributions to the chemical prevention of ovarian development and to subsequent sterility in the house fly. In the wake of Goldsmith's reports,[18-21] they too investigated folic acid antagonists such as aminopterin and other mitotic poisons, e.g., the nitrogen mustard mechlorethamine (methyl-bis-β-chlorethylamine) and colchicine, the classic compound interfering with the division of the cell nucleus. Mitlin and co-workers[23] showed that these and certain other mitotic poisons inhibit ovarian growth in the house fly, *Musca domestica* L. This was demonstrated both by complete prevention of oviposition and by inhibition of ovarian growth. Female house flies, unless fed proteins, have ovaries that can barely be seen with the naked eye. When the flies are fed with milk, the ovaries develop to about 2.5 mm in diameter each, and the females start to lay eggs. When mitotic poisons, e.g., 0.02% aminopterin or the nitrogen mustard at 0.2%, were added to the milk fed to female house flies, the latter laid no eggs and the ovaries remained undeveloped. On the other hand, oviposition was not affected when untreated females mated with males fed treated milk.

Since the materials found to be active were antitumor drugs, Mitlin and Baroody[48] proposed an idea that proved extremely fruitful for the subsequent development of the chemosterilant field. They reasoned that since some of the compounds found active in inhibiting the growth of the house fly ovary are also known to possess a certain antitumor activity, might not the house fly ovary serve as a screening site for potential tumor-inhibiting drugs? Indeed, this supposition proved to be reasonably accurate, as judged by testing the effect of 26 compounds of the most varied chemical groups on the housefly ovary. In a previous, comparative study edited by Gellhorn and Hirschberg[49] these 26 compounds, 12 of which had known antitumor activity, had been screened in 74 tumor and nontumor systems, including 15 experimental tumors, 21 microbiological systems of viruses, bacteriophages, bacteria, and fungi, 17 differentiation and developmental systems in a slime mold, in frog and chick embryos and *Drosophila,* and 21 biochemical indices of synthetic processes in tumors and rat spleen. Mitlin and Baroody[48] found that 15 substances inhibited ovarian growth in the house fly. Of the 12 known antitumor compounds, 8 were detected on feeding to house fly females in milk, through growth inhibition of the house fly ovary. A relationship was thus established between insect chemosterilants and antitumor compounds. It is quite conceivable that a compound effective in one system could also affect the other. The reproductive tissues always contain components with rapidly dividing cells, which at least in some respects are similar to those in a growing tumor. One must beware of oversimplification or of drawing mechanical conclusions. However, in accordance with a simple reversal of Mitlin's reasoning,[48] most of the chemosterilants found in the U.S. since 1960 belong to classes of compounds which are generally recognized as carcinostatic or potentially carcinostatic, that is, cancer chemotherapeutic agents or closely related compounds. In brief, the American school of thought argues that interference with the fertility of an organism at the cellular level is similar to interference with the reproduction of cells in a tumor.

IV. EXPRESSIONS OF CHEMOSTERILIZATION

The most frequent form of sterility induced in insects by chemosterilants has been dominant lethality in the mature ova and sperm; other effects related to sperm inactivation or endocrine misfunction may also occur. The dominant lethal mutation is a nuclear change in a germ cell, which does not prevent the zygote from reaching maturity. Death usually occurs before blastoderm formation, but may occur as late as the larval or pupal stage. It is generally agreed that dominant lethality induced by radiation or chemosterilants is associated with chromosome breakage. If breaks are not restored, the degree of dominant lethality is likely to be high. Apart from this, chemosterilants can, as noted above, also lower the fecundity of the females and cause aspermia or sperm inactivation in the males.

V. CLASSES OF INSECT CHEMOSTERILANTS

Among the chemosterilants are found the alkylating agents, the ethyleneimins or aziridines, e.g., tepa and thiotepa, which have been used as palliatives in certain neoplastic diseases and in containing adenocarcinoma of the breast and ovary; their methyl derivatives metepa and methiotepa; and apholate, also considered promising in cancer research. Incidentally, all these compounds are cross-linking agents used in the textile industry to strengthen synthetic fibers and to flameproof and confer crease resistance in fabrics made from natural fibers. Another aziridine chemosterilant is the well-known anticancer compound triethylenemelamine or tretamine (TEM) and its methyl derivative, methyl tretamine. There is also the sulfonic acid-type of alkylating-agent chemosterilants, such as busulfan (also called myleran), 1,3-propanediol dimethanesulfonate, which is used in the treatment of the chronic blood disease, myeloid leukemia.

Other chemosterilants belong to the compounds grouped together under the name of antimetabolites, e.g., the folic acid antagonists and anticancer drugs already mentioned, aminopterin and amethopterin. Numerous folic acid, purine, and pyrimidine antagonists and other antimetabolites, e.g., 5-fluorouracil, 5-fluoro-orotic acid, 6-azauridine, 6-methylmercapto 3 deazapurine, etc., inhibit ovarian development and affect maturing eggs.

It is fascinating to note in this context that organotins have rather distinct chemosterilant properties.

VI. ORGANOTINS AS BIOCIDES

The organotins offer an outstanding example of versatile, multipurpose biocides. This is true for the triphenyltins or *fentins*, e.g., fentin acetate (FA), which is the active ingredient of Hoechst's "Brestan"; fentin hydroxide (FH), the basis of Duphar's "Duter"; and the less-known fentin chloride (FCl), Hoechst's "Brestanol". These fentins, originally developed as highly effective agricultural fungicides and as marine antifoulants, were soon found to be also bactericides, potent molluscicides, and even effective algicides. Some closely related compounds which, except for Shell's "Vendex", hexabutatin oxide, are tricyclohexyltins (e.g., Dow's "Plictran", cyhexatin; or Bayer's "Peropal", azocyclotin), are widely used acaricides. The biocidal properties of organotins were recently reviewed by Davies and

Table 1
FENTINS IN THE DIET AS HOUSE FLY REPRODUCTION INHIBITORS

Compound	Conc. for 95% reduction of reproduction (ppm)	Approx. LC_{95} (ppm)
Fentin		
Acetate (FA)	125	250
Hydroxide (FH)	62	1000
Chloride (FCl)	62	250
Fluoride	62	1000
Benzyl	250	1000
Cyclopentadienyl	250	1000
Stearate	250	>1000
Bis(fentin)		
Sulfide	62	1000
Ethylene	<125	1000
Tris(fentin)		
Borate	62	250

From Kenaga, E. E., *J. Econ. Entomol.*, 58, 4, 1965.

Smith[50,51] and in the books of Bock[52] (fentins only), Thayer,[53] Blunden et al.,[54] and Evans and Karpel.[55]

Most of these organotin biocides have aroused interest also in insect pest control. In fact, apart from toxic effects on insects in the strict sense, fentins and related organotins are both antifeedants[56,57] and *chemosterilants*.

VII. ORGANOTINS AS CHEMOSTERILANTS

The effect of organotins, both aryl and alkyltins, on the reproduction of insects is reviewed hereunder. Section VII.A covers the effects on egg fertility (hatchability and egg viability) following treatment of adults, pupae, and larvae; Section VII.B deals with effects on fecundity, i.e., on number of eggs laid, ootheca produced, etc.

A. Effects on Egg Hatchability (Fertility)
1. Diptera

Kenaga[58] at the Dow Chemical Company, U.S.A. was the first to discover that organotins, in particular fentins, are chemosterilants for the house fly, *M. domestica* L., on ingestion. Kenaga's screening included 30 fentin derivatives, of which the most active ones are listed in Table 1. Kenaga[59] was also the first to demonstrate that feeding of only one sex with fentins almost always caused an only moderate rate of sterility. Mating of treated females with untreated males was more effective than vice versa, and females could be sterilized by lower concentrations than males. At 0.05% FH fed continuously to males had no effect during the first days of life on sperm motility in either testes or spermathecae. After 3 days the sperm in the testes was no longer motile, and after 4 days sperm in the testes was scarce. The ovaries in females fed with this concentration did not develop fully, and the flies could not lay eggs; 0.025% delayed the development of the ovary, and all the eggs were sterile. At 0.0125% the treated ovary was of approximately normal size, but egg laying was delayed and the eggs were sterile. At 0.0062 and 0.0031% egg laying was not delayed, but nearly

Table 2
THE INFLUENCE OF FENTINS AT 100 PPM IN THE DIET ON HOUSE FLY EGG HATCHABILITY

Compound	Hatch compared with control (%)
Fentin	
Acetate (FA)	7
Hydroxide (FH)	12
Benzoate	6
Thiocyanate	5
Phthalate	0
Hydrogenphthalate	0
Methoxy	1
Ethoxy	8
Bis(fentin)	
Oxide	21

From Byrdy, S., Ejmocki, Z., and Eckstein, Z., *Bull. Acad. Pol. Sci. Ser. Chim.*, 13, 683, 1965.

all eggs were sterile. There was no difference in the size of eggs of treated and untreated insects. To achieve effective rates of sterility (100% or very near to it) in the house fly with various fentins at concentrations not producing mortality in the treated adults, Kenaga had to feed both sexes simultaneously. This finding was confirmed by Polish researchers, Byrdy et al.,[60] who tested nine fentins including FA and FH, on an adult house fly population containing both sexes (Table 2).

Kenaga[59] found that the fentins on topical application did not penetrate the cuticle of the adult house fly in amounts sufficient to control reproduction without causing high mortality in the treated flies.

Similar results were obtained in the U.S. by Fye et al.[61] (cf. also page 328 of Reference 62 and Tables 21 and 23 [*vide* substances CS-43 and 44] of Reference 63), with the five fentins FA, FH, FCl, allylfentin, and bis(fentin)sulfide, which were effective house fly sterilants at low concentrations when fed to both sexes simultaneously. When fed to males only, FA, FCl, and allylfentin did not sterilize at a concentration of 0.25% in the fly food made up of sugar, milk powder, and powdered egg yolk. FH and bis(fentin)sulfide sterilized males, when fed at 0.01 and 1.0%, respectively, in a sugar-only diet, but not in the fly food.

Kissam and Hays[64] in the U.S. fed both sexes of the house fly with 0.00425% FA or 0.00375% FCl for 10 days; fertility based on the weight of larvae per female per day was reduced to 2 and 5%, respectively, of the control. However, there was considerable mortality of the adults (males somewhat more than females) during the protracted feeding period.

A more differentiated analysis was conducted by Hays[65] in 1968: (1) feeding 1-day-old house-fly females for 48 hr with FA or FCl at a rate of 0.025% in the diet reduced the average percentage of egg hatch during a 14-day observation to 22 and 29%, respectively (control = 99% hatch). Similar treatment of 1-day-old males was much less effective, with eclosion rates of 71 and 50% for FA and FCl, respectively (control = 95%). (2) Feeding

7-day-old ovipositing females with the same concentration and again for 48 hr, Hays obtained only 15 and 13% hatch for FA and FCl, respectively (control = 91%). (3) In a further test series male and female flies were allowed to feed together on an untreated diet in two groups, namely, for either 5 or 8 days, to ensure mating. The females were then separated from the males and a diet of 0.0125% fentin was offered to the first group for 8 days and to the second group for 5 days. Then (i.e., after 13 days for both groups) the females were transferred to untreated food for an additional 5 days. Percent egg hatch was zero as from the second day of treatment in females fed FA after 5 or 8 days of life and in females fed FCl for 8 days after 5 days of life; egg hatch remained zero until the end of the experiment. The females fed with FCl for only 5 days produced a few viable eggs (3% eclosion) when an untreated diet was fed after the treatment.

In the experiments of Ascher et al.[66] in Israel, virgin females of the Oriental house fly, *M. domestica vicina* Macquart, were mated with virgin males that had been fed 0.05% FA or FH in milk for 3 days. Egg fertility gradually deteriorated over the following 2 weeks. Life span was not affected in the FA and only slightly in the FH treatment. To determine whether all or only some of a batch of females was affected, single-pair tests were conducted with FA. Normal egg fertility was found in some females and gradually increasing, or even complete egg sterility from the start of oviposition, in others. Dissections showed some of spermatozoa in the spermathecae to be weakly motile or nonmotile. This was ascribed to the slow-poisoning effect of fentin on the sperm of the treated male in the spermathecae of the female ("stored sperm" effect in the sense of Bořkovec, see pages 26 and 51 of Reference 44).

Koula and Rajchartová[67] in the C.S.S.R. fed organotins (*n*-trialkyltins, fentins, and tri-benzyltins) in the food to males or females of the house fly, *M. domestica*. A 74% reduction in hatching was produced by tri-*n*-butyltin laurate fed to males, whereas none of the substances tested reduced hatching when fed to female house flies.

Byrdy's group[68] investigated 32 organotins — 11 trialkyltins, 2 diphenyltins, and 19 fentins — as chemosterilants for the house fly. A mixture of milk and sugar containing 0.01% of the organotin was offered to equal numbers of 1-day-old male and female flies. The females were allowed to oviposit on an uncontaminated larval medium 3 days later; the hatched larvae were counted after 6 days. At least 11 out of the 19 fentins tested inhibited reproduction by more than 90%, e.g., FCl (100%) and FA (94%); FH was somewhat less effective (87% reproduction inhibition). When some of the active compounds were fed only to females which then mated with untreated males, the results obtained with most of the fentins at this low concentration were practically identical to those of the both-sexes treatment. A notable exception in this respect was fentin propionate (females treated = 56% sterility; both sexes treated = 99.5%) and, to a lesser extent, fentin 2-methyl-4-chlorophenoxyacetate. The conclusion drawn by the authors was that at 0.01% the investigated compounds affected the females, whereas they were inactive against the males.

Among the trialkyltins assayed by Brydy et al.,[68] some gave an only moderate sterility rate, e.g., *n*-propyltin propionate (71%), *n*-butyltin fluoride (66%), *n*-butyltin acetate (68%), and n-$C_4H_9SnOCOCH_2SC_6Cl_5$ (66%). Of the two diphenyltins tested, only diphenyltin dichloride was quite active (91%).

When only virgin females of *M. domestica vicina* were fed 0.025 to 0.045% FA or FH in milk for 3 days and then mated with untreated males,[69] egg viability was initially nearly zero, but then gradually recovered during the 14-day observation period. The ultimate level of egg hatchability reached depended on the fentin concentration administered; with 0.025% FA or FH it was practically normal. Female longevity was reduced by treatment with 0.035% FA to 9.3 days on the average (14.9 in control), with 0.04% to 10.5 days (15.1), and with 0.045% to 7.6 days (15.0). No corresponding shortened life span occurred with FH-treated females or with fentin-treated males. Similar curves of gradual recovery of egg hatchability were obtained when females were fed 0.06 to 0.08% FA or 0.07% FH for 1 day only, but these treatments did not reduce the life span. When both sexes were fed FA in milk for 3 days and then mated, the egg hatchability remained very low (between 2 and 20%) throughout the observation period. This was ascribed to the fentins acting at first on the females by depressing egg viability early in the experiment, and later, in the second half of the 14-day experiment, by slowly poisoning sperm from treated males stored in the spermathecae. This was probably the reason that Kenaga[59] had to feed both sexes of the house fly to achieve high egg sterility.

Pausch[70] in the U.S. exposed adult house flies (*M. domestica*) to an FH-treated cord baited with a light corn syrup, hung from the roof in the center of a cage for 3 days. There was no hatch at an FH concentration of 1%, 5% hatch at 0.5%, 38% at 0.25%, and between 50 and 60% for concentrations between 0.125 and 0.015%. When the flies were exposed to the baited chemosterilant for 7 instead of 3 days, mortality at 1% FH was 64% and at 0.5% was 42%, whereas at the concentrations between 0.25 and 0.015% mortality was negligible. This shows that the two concentrations which caused high sterility, 1 and 0.5% FH, were very toxic at the 7-day exposure.

Krzemińska[71] in Poland investigated the effect of FH and "Decafentin" (decyltriphenylphosphonium bromochlorotriphenylstannate) on the reproduction of *M. domestica*. Adults of both sexes, separately and together, were fed on diets containing the compounds for 3 days, starting approximately 24 hr after emergence. At 0.00625 to 0.2%, FH caused 38 to 94% sterility in the T♂ × T♀ experiments and 29 to 92% sterility in the U♂ × T♀ experiments. "Decafentin" at 0.0625 to 1% caused 46 to 97% sterility in T♂ × T♀ and 9 to 91% in U♂ × T♀. The higher dosages of both organotins resulted in high mortality among the treated flies. Females were sterilized by a lower concentration than males.

Krzemińska[72] extended these experiments to FA and repeated them with FH at 0.00625 to 0.2% and "Decafentin" at ten times these concentrations, again fed in the diet to adults of *M. domestica* for 3 days from about 24 hr after emergence. The highest concentration of each material reduced the reproductive capacity of both sexes by about 90%.

In Diptera other than the house fly, the following results were obtained.

Pausch[73] offered 2, 1, 0.5, 0.25, and 0.015% FA-, FH-, and FCl-treated food for 24 hr separately to male and female adults of the little house fly, *Fannia canicularis* (L.), which then mated with untreated individuals of the opposite sex. The experiments with FA and FCl were soon discontinued, as these compounds were far too toxic to this species even at low concentrations. FH was efficient in producing sterility only at concentrations causing an appreciable level of mortality already after 3 days; it was more active at lower concentrations in females than in males. High sterility rates were also attained, again only at concentrations causing high mortality, when syrup-baited FH was offered, together with untreated fly food and water, to unsexed flies for an unlimited time in free-choice experiments.

Mulla[74] in the U.S. exposed adult males and females of the eye gnat *Hippelatus collusor* (Townsend) to organotins in sugar baits at 0.05, 0.1, and 1% concentrations and allowed the insects to feed on them for 24 and 48 hr. Egg hatch was practically normal.

Some work was conducted also with trypetid flies.

Orphanidis and Patsakos[75-77] in Greece tested FH in the form of a 60% wettable powder (WP) of Du-Ter Extra against two species of Trypetidae: the olive fly, *Dacus oleae* (Gmelin), and the Mediterranean fruit fly, *Ceratitis capitata* Wiedemann. The compound was supplied for 48 hr in the adults' food. Egg fertility was not substantially reduced in *D. oleae* when either males or females were offered food containing 0.5 or 1% FH. In *C. capitata*, on the other hand, eclosion (egg hatch) at 1% was lowered to an average of approximately 20% in both the male and the female treatment (controls = 75 and 74%, respectively). At 2%, there was no hatch in either treatment. A strong effect of FA on fecundity was obtained in both species (see below) when females were fed with the substance, but FA fed at 0.1 or 2% to *C. capitata* had no effect on egg fertility.[76]

Abdel-Megeed et al.[78] in Egypt showed that by rearing larvae of *C. capitata* on artificial diets treated with different FH concentrations, apart from toxic effects on larvae and pupae (males being more susceptible than females), weight reduction of fully grown larvae, pupae, and adults, and reduced emergence of adults and egg hatch were obtained. Biochemical studies showed that such larval treatment with FH caused a slight reduction in free amino acid, protein amino acid and lipid content of larvae and pupae, a significant reduction of reducing sugars, and an increase in organic acid content.[79,80] FH had little apparent effect on the morphology of the ovaries and the testes.[79]

Singh and Teotja[81] in India fed 1% FH in a treated sugar medium to pairs of both sexes of newly emerged melon flies (*Dacus cucurbitae* Coquerel) for 1, 4, and 5 days. The treatment proved quite toxic, with mortality within 17 days ranging from 52 to 76%. With the 1- and 4-day treatments, egg hatch was normal; 5-day ingestion was toxic.

White[82] in England demonstrated that at 0.5 ppm FH and two other fentins were strongly larvicidal for the yellowfever mosquito, *A. aegypti*. Treatment of aquatic stages, 5-hr tarsal (insect foot) exposure to fentin residues, and feeding females and/or males for 6 days with aqueous fentin solutions which the author considered as being saturated, had no effect on fertility.

2. Coleoptera

Byrdy et al.[60] (see also Byrdy[83]) investigated the fertility and the fecundity (see below) of the Colorado potato beetle, *Leptinotarsa decemlineata* (Say), placed on potato plants sprayed with 0.002% FH or bis(fentin)oxide. Their results showed that the average egg fertility was only slightly reduced by FH (53% hatch; control = 79% hatch). Only eggs laid on the first day of oviposition in the FH treatment had a low (7%) hatching rate; 0.002% bis(fentin)oxide affected the hatching rate only slightly (68%). Byrdy et al.[68] used the same technique to carry out experiments on the effect of three other fentins on the egg fertility of the Colorado potato beetle: fentin cyanide, propionate, and 2-methyl-4-chlorophenoxy acetate, in 0.1 and 0.01% suspensions. It is doubtful whether the sparse data presented lend themselves to unequivocal interpretation.

Koula and Rajchartová[67] fed organotins (trialkyltins, fentins, and tribenzyltins) to males of the first generation of *L. decemlineata* and to overwintering males under field conditions. In the first generation males the greatest reduction in hatching was brought about by tri-*n*-propyltin acetate, tri-*n*-butyltin laurate, and FA, whereas in overwintering males the best results were obtained with tri-*n*-propyltin laurate, followed by the corresponding acetate.

Klassen et al.[84] in the U.S. showed that FA at concentrations ranging from 0.2 to 0.05% and FH ranging from 0.1 to 0.001% incorporated into a synthetic diet were toxic when offered to males of the boll weevil, *A. grandis*, for 3 days. Eggs laid after the 0.005% FA treatment showed an egg hatch of >30%. These fentins are, therefore, not suitable for sterilization of the boll weevil.

Hayes et al.[85] in the U.S. tested five fentins (including FA, FH, and FCl) against the boll weevil by dipping the adults (mixed sexes) and by feeding them with the substances in a 10% sucrose solution. The compounds were generally very toxic to the weevils, but at lower, slightly less toxic or nontoxic dosages there was no sterility.

Ladd[86] in the U.S. applied FA, FH, and FCl topically to both sexes of the Japanese beetle, *Popillia japonica* Newman, simultaneously, prior to mating. Only at a dosage which markedly reduced longevity, 6.25 µg per insect, were high rates of egg sterility achieved, with FA being more effective (100% sterility) than FH (78%) and FCl (73%). The results obtained with this dosage may not be reliable due to the very low fecundity (0.1, 0.6, and 0.3 eggs per female for FA, FH, and FC1, respectively, vs. 6.0 in control; see also below), but also at two lower topical application dosages, 3.13 and 1.56 μg per insect, the order of the (insufficient) sterility rates produced by the substances was FA > FH > FCl.

Kenaga[59] incorporated 0.1, 0.05, 0.025, and 0.01% FH or allylfentin into the diet of the confused flour beetle, *Tribolium confusum* Duval, at concentrations not appreciably toxic of the adults (mixed sexes), and infested the diet with pupae. With the exception of allylfentin at 0.1% concentration in the diet, there was low adult mortality 14 days after the treatment. At the observation 45 days after treatment, allylfentin totally inhibited reproduction at all concentrations tested, whereas FH was much less effective (100% inhibition of reproduction only at 0.1% concentration). Adult mortality rose to 100% in the three highest concentrations of allylfentin and in the highest concentration of FH. This left little margin between adult-killing and adult-sterilizing concentrations.

Findlay[87] in South Africa found that the reproduction potential of adults of the yellow mealworm, *Tenebrio molitor* L., feeding on a 0.1% FH-treated diet, was reduced markedly (to 7% of the control), whereas on an 0.1% FA-treated diet it was moderately diminished (to 42% of control.)

Nagasawa et al.[88] in Japan established that topical application of FH to females of the Azuki bean weevil (southern cowpea weevil), *Callosobruchus chinensis* L., caused them to lay sterile eggs. Males were not sterilized by a similar treatment. The median sterilizing dose was 0.29 μg per female, which is close to the figure of 0.20 μg when both females and males were treated in an earlier work.[89] Males treated with 0.0025 μg FH were fully competitive sexually with untreated males, when paired with untreated females.[88]

3. Lepidoptera

Findlay[87] fed freshly emerged paired adults of both sexes of the Egyptian cotton leafworm, *Spodoptera littoralis* (Boisduval), with honeywater containing either FA or FH. He used a concentration gradient which expressed itself in a gradually descending percentage hatch of the eggs laid. FH had a slightly more pronounced effect than FA, but even at the highest concentration tested (0.5%), percentage eclosion was not reduced below 15% (control = 79% hatch). Dipping fresh (younger than 24 hr old) pupae of *S. littoralis* in suspensions of the two fentins resulted in both pupal mortality and reduced egg viability. Some of the data presented by Findlay[87] in his M.Sc. thesis can also be found in a later publication.[90]

Elbadry et al.[91] in Egypt studied larval and pupal mortality and chemosterilization by feeding third-instar *S. littoralis* larvae a castor bean (*Ricinus communis*) leaf disk "sandwich", of which one disk had been treated with FH in acetone. Concentrations of FH between 0.5 and 0.1% caused 100% mortality within 3 to 8 days. Surviving adults deriving from larvae fed 0.05, 0.01, and 0.005% FH (viz., both sexes treated), laid eggs with 16, 17, and 26% hatch, respectively (control = 98%). A much lower egg hatch rate was achieved when treated males were mated with untreated females, than vice versa.

The effect of FH on reproduction in *S. littoralis* by treatment of larvae was investigated intensively in Egypt.[92,93] Third-instar *S. littoralis* larvae were fed for 48 hr leaves of castor bean sprayed with FH at concentrations between 0.00025 and 0.5%, and then transferred to clean leaves. The moths obtained were mated as follows:

- Males from treated larvae × untreated females (T♂ × U♀)
- Untreated males × females from treated larvae (U♂ × T♀)
- Males × females, both reared from treated larvae (T♂ × T♀)
- Males × females, both reared from untreated larvae (U♂ × U♀) (control)

The egg hatchability due to these larval treatments ranged from 52% at 0.00025% to 16% at 0.025% FH with T♂ × T♀, surprisingly, was somewhat lower with T♂ × U♀ (45 and 0%, respectively), and was much higher in U♂ × T♀ (86 and 37%, respectively). These results indicate that males were affected more strongly than females by larval FH treatment.

Further experiments involved treatment of adults. Separate sexes of newly emerged *S. littoralis* adults were allowed for 24 hr to drink dispersions of different concentrations (0.05, 0.15, and 0.25% active ingredient (AI) prepared from a 50% FH WP [Du-Ter]) in a 10% sugar solution and then paired in small vials according to the scheme outlined in the larval feeding tests. In some of these combinations, egg viability of adults fed 0.25 or 0.15% FH was zero or nearly zero: with T♂ × U♀, egg viability reached 62, 4, and 0%, respectively, for 0.05, 0.15, and 0.25% AI; with U♂ × T♀, 72, 64, and 32%, respectively; and with T♂ × T♀, 50, 0, and 0%, respectively.

For contact application to *S. littoralis* adults, glass jars were coated internally with dilutions of the 50% FH WP at different AI concentrations, and cotton leaves sprayed with the same concentrations were introduced into the jars. Newly emerged moths were transferred, each sex separately, to the treated jars, left there for 24 hr, and then transferred in pairs to clean jars as follows: T♂ × T♀, T♂ × U♀, U♂ × T♀, and U♂ × U♀ (control).

In contrast with the results obtained on feeding, the degree of reduction of egg viability upon exposure to FH residues was much less pronounced (34% egg fertility at 0.25% with T♂ × T♀ vs. 100% in control).

FH treatments reduced moth longevity by feeding more than by contact;[93] this effect was especially pronounced in females. For example, females fed on 0.05, 0.15, and 0.25% FH lived for 6.5, 5, and 5 days, respectively, vs. 9.5 days in the untreated control.

Mitri and Kamel[94] in Egypt fed pairs of *S. littoralis* with FA, FH, cyhexatin ("Plictran"), and "Decafentin" at 0.25 and 0.5% AI dispersed in 10% aqueous sugar solutions, from emergence throughout their lives. Egg fertility was 1.5, 61, 62, and 75% with 0.25% FH, FA, "Decafentin", and cyhexatin, respectively, and 0.5, 40, 0.3, and 0%, respectively, with 0.5% of these materials, vs. 98% hatchability in the untreated control. These results (Mitri and Kamel[94]) for FH were in agreement with those obtained by Abo-Elghar and Radwan[92] and Elbadry et al.[93] When Mitri and Kamel[94] fed the adults with the organotins for 48 hr only and then with untreated sugar solutions, hatchability on 0.25% of the four substances was, in contrast to the findings of the previously mentioned Egyptian authors, practically normal. With 0.5% FH, FA, cyhexatin, and "Decafentin" it was 10, 3, 39, and 80%, respectively (99% in the control). In further studies Mitri and Kamel[95] exposed pairs of freshly emerged moths throughout their lives to cotton shoots sprayed with 0.25, 0.5, and 1.0% FH, FA, and FCl; an untreated 10% sugar solution served as nutrient for the moths. With most concentrations there was no pronounced effect on egg fertility: hatchability was 54% with 1% FCl and, paradoxically, 37, 58, and 81% with 0.25, 0.5, and 1% FH, respectively.

Joshi et al.[96] in India dipped fresh pupae of the tobacco caterpillar, *Spodoptera litura* (F.), for 10 min in 0.075% FA dilution. Adult emergence was reduced to 40 vs. 79% in the untreated control. The average longevity of adults of both sexes was shortened to approximately 3 days, vs. 7.4 and 9.2 in untreated females and males, respectively. Fecundity was reduced markedly (see below). None of the eggs laid by the females in T♂ × T♀ hatched, and only very few of those laid by U♂ × T♀ or T♂ × U♀.

Campion and Outram[97] in England realized that FA and FH were nearly inactive as sterilants when topically applied to or injected into adult males of the red bollworm, *Diparopsis castanea* Hmps. The only exception was in injection of 15 μg FH per male which reduced hatch to 40 vs. 75 to 85% in the control. Subsequently, Campion and Lewis[98] demonstrated that the LD_{50} of FA, 8.5 μg per male injected into *D. castanea*, was considerably lower than the calculated 50% sterilizing dose (SD_{50}), 16.1 μg per male. This implied that without strongly enhanced mortality, complete sterility could not be achieved by FA in a population of this insect.

When FH was administered by Salem et al.[99,100] in Egypt for 24 hr to adults of the spiny bollworm, *Earias insulana* (Boisduval), orally in honey at concentrations between 0.062

and 0.5%, the numbers of eggs laid (see below) on okra pods and their viability were reduced. Egg viability for 0.5% was 24 vs. 90% in the control. The percentage of hatched eggs on different days was subject to fluctuations, with the intensity of the sterilizing effect decreasing as time elapsed after the treatment. There was no significant difference between the diameter of testes in treated and untreated males, whereas the length of ovarioles was reduced by the FH treatment.

Shaaban et al.[101] in Egypt applied 0.5, 1, and 2 μg FH per larva topically to fourth-instar larvae of the greasy cutworm, *Agrotis ipsilon* Rott., or fed them castor bean leaves which had been dipped in 0.005, 0.01, or 0.02% FH. Both modes of application reduced percent pupation and moth emergence only slightly, but curtailed adult longevity markedly in both males and females obtained from treated larvae, to between 20 and 45% of the control; also, the preoviposition period was prolonged considerably. Fecundity was reduced (see below) and egg fertility at the highest dosage and by treatment of both sexes contemporaneously was lower than 10% with both modes of application.

Wolfenbarger et al.[102] in the U.S. obtained efficient sterilization by topical application of relatively massive doses of FH to larvae (both sexes) of the tobacco budworm, *Heliothis virescens* (F.), (with 3.8 μg/g larva, female moths laid 100% sterile eggs) and the bollworm, *Heliothis zea* (Boddie), (3.5 μg/g larva, 99.7% sterile eggs). Printing errors in the names of compounds in Table 2 of the paper by Wolfenbarger et al.[102] and the fact that the first sentence of the discussion of the data of this Table does not, therefore, correspond to the Table do not allow one to draw conclusions on the sterilizing capacity of FA from this article (see footnote 5 in Ascher et al.[69]). Compounds active at much higher dosages were FCl in *H. virescens* and trioctyltin chloride in *H. zea*.

Bonnemaison[103] in France fed third-instar larvae of the diamondback moth, *Plutella maculipennis* Curtis, for 24 hr with leaves painted with 0.025% FH or brought them into a 4-hr contact with FH residues on glass. In addition, male adults were fed for 24 hr on 0.05% FH in a 30% sucrose solution and then mated with untreated females. In none of these treatments did sterility exceed 21%. Tarsal contact of adults of *P. maculipennis* and of the cabbage moth, *Mamestra brassicae* L., with massive residues of FH, 6.25 mg/cm^2 (= 62.5 g/m^2), for 30 min brought about 100% sterility[104] and also influenced fecundity (see below). Such high concentrations had to be used since at lower ones the sterilizing effect due to tarsal contact was either very weak or nil.[105]

4. Hemiptera

Ansari and Khan[106] in India exposed adult females of the cotton stainer, *Dysdercus cingulatus* (F.), to residues (films) of FA (0.35, 0.7, and 1.4 mg/in.^{2}, i.e., approximately 0.5, 1, and 2 g/m^2) for periods of 0.5, 1, 4, and 12 hr. At the lowest concentration and shortest exposure no mortality was encountered, but with the longer exposure times with this concentration mortality reached 25% before mating. The two highest concentrations caused 40 and 50% female mortality, respectively. Egg hatch was reduced from 95% in the control to between 54 and 71% for the various exposure times and concentrations. When males were exposed similarly to FA,[107] mortality and significant reduction in fertility were observed only with 12 hr exposure to 1.4 mg/in.^{2}; FA was thus less effective in sterilizing males than females of *D. cingulatus*.

5. Tetranychid Mites

Redfern[108] in the U.S. reported that 2% FA and FH had no effect on the fertility or fecundity of the twospotted spider mite, *Tetranychus urticae* Koch, when the compounds were sprayed directly on mite-infested lima bean plants (postinfestation treatment) or when gravid females were exposed to residues of the compounds on lima bean leaf disks (preinfestation treatment). On the other hand, Boykin and Campbell[109] in the U.S. found that FH tends to decrease the average female longevity and slightly reduces the reproductive potential of this mite.

B. Effects of Fecundity
1. Diptera

Kenaga[59] found that by feeding a mixed population of male and female house flies (*M. domestica*) with 0.05% FH for 3 days, oviposition was totally inhibited during the 8 days of the experiment; the ovaries developed to only two thirds of the normal size.

Kissam and Hays[64] fed 0.00425% FA and 0.00375% FCl in milk to mixed populations containing equal numbers of 1-day-old male and female house flies. During the 10-day feeding and test period, fecundity in FA was 51% and in FCl 42% of the control, but female mortality was significantly higher in the treated flies than in the control.

Fye et al.[61] reported that no oviposition occurred when adult house flies of both sexes were offered fly food (a mixture of sugar, milk powder, and powdered egg yolk) containing 0.0025% FA, 0.01% FH, or 0.05% FCl, or granulated sugar containing 0.25% FA, 0.5% FH, or 0.25% FCl; FH caused high mortality of females during the preoviposition period. For allylfentin the values with fly food and granulated sugar were >0.025 and 0.5%, respectively. Bis(fentin)sulfide was much less active than the other fentins.

Hays[65] found that feeding 1-day-old females of the house fly for 48 hr with 0.025% FCl in their diet reduced fecundity to approximately one-third of the control, whereas FA had no effect on fecundity under these conditions. A similar treatment of 1-day-old males with either compound was claimed to reduce fecundity. When 6- to 7-day-old ovipositing females were fed for the same length of time on 0.025% FA or FCl, the number of eggs produced was 53 and 58% of the control.

The effect of feeding nonlethal fentin concentrations, 0.025 to 0.045%, for 3 days (see above), on the fecundity of female *M. domestica vicina*[69] was either slight (FH) or not very pronounced (FA). In the 1-day feeding of females with high fentin concentrations (0.06 to 0.08%, see above), fecundity was practically normal. Dissections showed that immediately after starting to feed females with undeveloped ovaries with 0.04% FA in milk, ovarian growth and the development of oocytes were slower than in the controls and that the two first ovarian cycles were longer in treated than in untreated females. Fecundity during the period when the fentin effect on egg viability in treated females was waning (see above) was equal to that in controls.

When FA and FH were administered to 0 to 4-hr-old females of *M. domestica* as 0.1% of the food and "Decafentin" at 1%, Krzemińska[110] found that, apart from inhibition of vitellogenesis (yolk production), the ovaries in treated females were only at the second stage of development at the age of 5 and 10 days. Very few granules of vitelline substance were visible around the oocyte (a female gamete before maturation), whereas in the ovaries of untreated females mature eggs were present. Fecundity was reduced to zero by the FH treatment.[72]

Wang et al.[111] in Malaysia treated 12-to-24-hr-old sexed adults of *M. domestica vicina* by topical application with tri-*n*-propyltin and tri-*n*-butyltin acetate at the LD_{50} level and found no reduction vs. control in the fecundity of the survivors and in subsequent egg hatchability. However, when they treated third-instar larvae by topical application with concentrations causing 10 to 15% mortality, the fecundity of adult flies surviving the treatment was reduced to 43 and 42% of the control in tri-*n*-propyltin acetate and tri-*n*-butyltin acetate, respectively.

In sugar baits, 1% (but not lower concentrations) of FA and FCl (but not FH) somewhat reduced fecundity of *H. collusor* following a 48-hr exposure.[74]

By incorporating FH in an artificial diet of *C. capitata* (see above), the preoviposition period was prolonged[78] and the oviposition and postoviposition periods were shortened.

Fecundity was lower,[78] with a negative correlation between daily number of eggs and FH concentration,[79] although the compound had no apparent effect on the number of oocytes in the ovaries of newly emerged and old females.[80]

Orphanidis and Patsakos[75,77] fed FH, as described above, to adults of *D. oleae* and *C. capitata* for 48 hr. Administration of FH to females of *D. oleae* reduced fecundity markedly: with 0.5%, the number of eggs laid was only about 1.5% of that of the controls, whereas with 1.0% the figure was about 11%. Fed to males, 0.5% FH had no appreciable effect on the fecundity of the females which mated with them; 1.0% FH fed to males inhibited oviposition in the females to 25% of the control. In *C. capitata* 0.5, 1.0, and 2.0% FH fed to females reduced fecundity to 3.6, 4.6, and 1.5%, respectively, of the control values. No clear-cut effect on fecundity was obtained when males of this species were fed FH.

Singh and Teotja,[81] on feeding pairs of *D. cucurbitae* adults for 1, 4, and 5 days with 1% FH (see above), found that fecundity was normal with the 1-day feeding; with the 4-day feeding there were two normal egg layings, after which oviposition stopped; and after the 5-day ingestion, no eggs were laid.

White[82] was unable to demonstrate any detrimental influence of the fentins on the fecundity of *A. aegypti*.

2. Coleoptera

In a field trial conducted in Switzerland in 1960 by Murbach and Corbaz[112] on potato plots which were artificially and uniformly contaminated with pairs of adults of the Colorado potato beetle, *L. decemlineata*, FA treatment induced, in an unknown way, a strong reduction in the number of egg batches and larvae. In further field trials in 1962 Murbach[113] found that the adults were as numerous on treated as on untreated plots, but gnawed potato leaflets only slightly (antifeedant effect) and soon stopped feeding entirely. The consequence of this fasting was a decline in the female fecundity, as expressed in few egg batches (122) as compared with check plots (296).

Byrdy et al.[60] (see also Byrdy[83]) found that on placing adults of *L. decemlineata* on potato plants (five males and five females per plant) sprayed with 0.02% FH or bis(fentin)oxide, only a few eggs were laid, and those exclusively on the first day. Oviposition then stopped completely, whereas in the control it continued normally for about 2 weeks, after which the experiment was discontinued. The authors reported that in the same sort of trial, but with a tenfold lower concentration, 0.002%, the two fentins brought about oviposition on the second day of the experiment, whereas in the control it started only on the tenth day. The total number of eggs laid in the FH treatment (471) was of the same order of magnitude as in the control (380), but bis(fentin)oxide seemed to reduce fecundity at this low concentration (162 eggs).

Haynes et al.[85] found that no eggs were laid when boll weevil (*A. grandis*) populations of mixed sexes were dipped into or fed with FA, FH, FCl, and allylfentin at most of the concentrations tested; however, the concentrations inhibiting oviposition caused a 100% mortality of the weevils 7 to 14 days after the treatment. Bis(fentin)sulfide had no effect on fecundity.

Ladd,[86] in his investigation with the Japanese beetle, *P. japonica*, found a dosage-related decline in the number of eggs per female-days after topical application of FA, FH, and FCl to pairs of adult beetles (Table 3). The decrease in fecundity could thus not be attributed solely to the severely reduced female longevity induced by increasing dosages of the fentins.

3. Lepidoptera

Findlay,[87,90] in his study of *S. littoralis*, demonstrated that fecundity is reduced by dipping the pupae of both sexes for 30 sec in FA or FH dilutions. With FA at 0.01%, the number of eggs was 38% of the control; 0.05% FA, 17%; and 0.1% FA, 8% of the control. No

Table 3
EFFECT OF THREE FENTINS APPLIED TOPICALLY TO PAIRS OF *POPILLIA JAPONICA* NEWMAN ON THE FECUNDITY OF THE FEMALES

Dose (μg/insect)	Mean number of eggs per female per day		
	FA	FH	FCl
1.56	0.37	0.19	0.18
3.13	0.16	0.14	0.15
6.25	0.01	0.04	0.03
12.5	0.03	0	0
0.0 (control)	0.25		

From Ladd, T. L., Jr., *J. Econ. Entomol.*, 61, 577, 1968.

eggs were laid at 0.5% FA, but at this concentration in only 50% of the treated pairs of female and male pupae did both partners emerge normally. With 0.01% FH, the number of eggs was 27% of the control; with 0.05% FH, 17%; and with 0.1% FH, 4%. Here, too, no eggs were laid at 0.5%, and again, in only 30% of the pairs did both partners emerge normally. There was a highly significant difference between the number of eggs laid per treatment, and this trend was closely correlated with the concentration gradient. Pairs of adults of both sexes fed continuously on fentin-treated honey-water showed the following fecundity values: FA, 0.01% - 17%; 0.1% - 25%; 0.5% - 5% of the control; and FH, 0.01% - 18%; 0.1% - 25%; 0.5% - 4% of the control. These treated adults had an estimated mean life span of only 7 days; untreated control adults survived up to a maximum of 12 days longer.

Elbadry et al.[91] and Abo-Elghar and Radwan[92] stated that when third-instar larvae of *S. littoralis* were fed 0.025, 0.005, and 0.0025% FH in leaf "sandwiches" (as described above), fecundity of the resulting females was 18, 26, and 26%, respectively, of the control, when both sexes were derived from treated larvae. When only one of the sexes was derived from treated larvae, fecundity was only slightly higher, with reduction in fecundity being the least in U♂ × T♀. This seemed to indicate that with this mode of administration the male *S. littoralis* was more sensitive to FH than the female. In the adult feeding tests (drinking FH in sugar solutions, see above), Abo-Elghar and Radwan[92] and Elbadry et al.[93] found that there was a strong reduction in fecundity: at 0.25% FH, with T♂ × U♀ to 19%, U♂ × T♀ to 15%, and T♂ × T♀ to 4% of the control, respectively. At two lower concentrations, 0.15 and 0.05%, reduction of fecundity was the same in T♂ × T♀ and U♂ × T♀, whereas in the T♂ × U♀ treatment it was lower. The males of *S. littoralis* were more easily affected by contact (see above) than the females: with T♂ × U♀ at 0.05, 0.15, and 0.25% FH fecundity was 18, 17, and 9% of the control, respectively; about the same results were obtained with T♂ × T♀. With U♂ × T♀, fecundity was 35, 31, and 21% of control at the three concentrations, respectively.

Mitri and Kamel,[94] on feeding FA, FH, cyhexatin, and "Decafentin" at 0.25 and 0.5% AI in a 10% sugar solution to pairs of *S. littoralis* adults (see above), found the following rates of fecundity (expressed as percent of control): 0.25% FH, FA, cyhexatin, and "Decafentin" — 12, 53, 90, and 37% fecundity; 0.5% FH, FA, cyhexatin, and "Decafentin" — 7, 28, 20, and 16%, respectively. Contact of adults with FH-treated cotton shoots (see above) had a slight and paradoxical effect on fecundity: only at 0.25%, but not at the higher concentrations, was the fecundity significantly lower (52% of control). The number of eggs laid on all FA and FCl concentrations was consistently higher in the contact tests than in the control.

When Joshi et al.[96] dipped fresh pupae of *S. litura* in 0.075% FA for 10 min, the number of eggs per female from adult pairs derived from treated pupae of both sexes (T♂ × T♀) was 9, for U♂ × T♀, 54, for T♂ × U♀, 296, and for the untreated control, 2149. FA treatment in the pupal stage of *S. litura* had thus a very strong effect on adult fecundity.

Salem et al.[99,100] fed *E. insulana* adults with FH in honey (see above). Fecundity was reduced, e.g., to 65 and 68% of control by 0.25 and 0.125% FH, respectively.

When *A. ipsilon* fourth-instar larvae were treated with FH topically or by feeding on treated castor bean leaves,[101] fecundity was strongly reduced, e.g., to 20% of the control by 2 μg FH/larva topically applied or to 23% by feeding 0.02% FH. The number of eggs produced increased when treated adults of only one sex were used or with a reduction of concentration.

According to the paper of Wolfenbarger et al.,[102] FH applied topically to larvae of *H. zea* and *H. virescens*, did not seem to reduce fecundity (untreated control fecundity data are lacking). FCl at 25 μg/g larva inhibited oviposition completely in an experiment with *H. zea*. For FA no conclusion can be reached from the data of these authors for the reasons advanced above.

Bonnemaison[104] stated that the sterilizing tarsal contact of adults of both *P. maculipennis* and *M. brassicae* with 6.25 mg/cm^2 FH for 30 min (see above) also reduced fecundity very strongly.

Dale and Saradamma[114] in India confined first-instar larvae of the Indian mealworm, *Corcyra cephalonica* (Staint.) to FA-treated wheat flour. At 0.02, 0.01, and 0.0025% mortality of larvae and pupae was 100, 80, and 20%, respectively. The fecundity for 0.01, 0.0025%, and untreated control was 63, 311, and 386 eggs per female, respectively; practically all the eggs laid by treated and untreated females hatched.

4. Orthoptera

Kenaga[59] performed some experiments on the German cockroach, *Blattella germanica* (L.) When fourth-instar nymphs were fed 0.1% FH in their diets, the resulting adults displayed a considerable but incomplete "reproduction inhibition", based on reduced ootheca and nymphal offspring counts.

Krzemińska[72] stated that FH fed to nymphs of *B. germanica* at a concentration of 1% in the food reduced the reproductive capacity of females about fourfold in comparison with the controls.

5. Hemiptera

Ansari and Khan[106] found that contact of females of *D. cingulatus* with 0.7 and 1.4 mg/in.^{2} FH for 12 hr reduced the fecundity to approximately 45% of the control. Shorter exposure times and a weaker concentration (0.35 mg/in.^{2}) were still, though considerably less, active.

Bonnemaison[115] showed that a 30-min exposure of second-stage nymphs of the rosy apple aphid, *Dysaphis plantaginea* (Passerini sensu Bonnemaison), to 2 mg/cm^2 (= 20 g/m^2) FH in petri dishes did not affect mortality rates or fecundity of the adults. Subsequently, he found[104] that mean fecundity is reduced by 50 to more than 60% by a 3-hr contact with 1.3 mg/cm^2 (= 13 g/m^2) FH in *S. plantaginea* or by 1.5-hr contact in the cabbage aphid, *Brevicoryne brassicae* L. It is not clear whether contact in this case was effected with nymphs or with wingless apterous adults.

Bhalla and Robinson[116] in Canada allowed third-instar nymphs of the pea aphid, *Acyrthosiphon pisum* (Harris), to feed through a membrane on an artificial liquid diet containing 0.01 or 0.05% FH. Reduced fecundity was obtained with both concentrations, but the higher one was toxic.

Chawla et al.[117] in Canada showed that by topical application of fentins on the potato aphid, *Macrosiphum euphorbiae* (Thomas), FH was a more effective sterilant than fentin fluoride, but both affected the fecundity of the offspring as well as that of the treated aphids themselves.

When the statements about reduced fecundity are evaluated, those which deal with toxic concentrations shortening female longevity considerably should be viewed with extreme caution. A female weakened by any toxic agent to such an extent as to have a drastically shortened life span, may well be incapable of producing an adequate number of eggs, even if egg production is calculated on the basis of eggs per female-days. A similar criterion as regards longevity should be applied, apropos, to chemosterilant activity in male insects. We certainly agree with the statement of Kissam and Hays[64] that the fentins "are fairly good chemosterilants, but their apparent toxicity at the sterility threshold may be a problem."

C. Other Properties of Organotins Relevant to Chemosterilization

1. Absence of Significant Oviposition Repellence

Our search of the literature did not include oviposition-repelling effects of organotins. However, Sáringer[118] found that residues from 1% solutions of FA and FH on the garden poppy (*Papaver somniferum* L.) had no antioviposition effect on the poppy weevil *Ceutorhynchus macula-alba* Herbst.

Cyhexatin was slightly oviposition-repellent[119] for females of the European grape-berry moth, *Lobesia* (*Polychrosis*) *botrana* (Den. & Schiff.), on grapes treated with 0.0375% AI. No such effect was found with the codling moth, *Cydia pomonella* L.

2. Effects of Organotins on Predation and Parasitism

Abdul Kareem et al.[120] conducted experiments in which FA, FH, and FCl at concentrations of 0.025 to 0.1% were sprayed on apterous female adults of the cowpea aphid, *Aphis craccivora* Koch, which were then fed to adult lady beetles, *Menochilus sexmaculatus* (F.). The fentins affected normal predation only very slightly or not at all; for instance, the percent predation at 0.1% (and in control) was FA, 71 (83); FH, 94 (94); and FCl, 77 (88).

Abdul Kareem et al.[121] also evaluated FA, FH, and FCl at 0.1 and 0.05% for their effects on egg hatchability of the Mealworm, *C. cephalonica* , and on parasitism by its egg parasite, *Trichogramma australicum* Gin., by direct spray on the eggs of the host. The effect on eggs was in the order FCl > FH > FA, and the maximum reduction of egg hatch was to 23% of the control, with 0.1% FCl. Although the organotins thus reduced egg hatch of the host considerably, they did not hamper parasite emergence: parasitism (with both 0.05 and 0.1% FH) ranged from 72 to 93%, with 95% recorded for the control treatment. In the remaining two compounds, FA and FCl, the level of parasitism at 0.05% was similar to the untreated control.

3. Chemosterilizing Effects in Mammals

The fentins have a strong effect on the fertility of rats. In males[122] FA and FCl at 10 mg/kg daily administered in the food produced several degenerative changes in testicular tissue, including a decrease in the number of cell layers per seminiferous tubule, a decrease in tubule diameter, an overall decrease of testicular size to one half to one quarter of normal, a depletion of the more advanced cell forms from the tubules, and a 99% closure of the tubule lumina. Within a 19-day treatment 100 and 60 to 70% sterility was achieved by FA and FCl, respectively. In similarly treated females[123] there was a decreased number of mature follicles, an increased incidence of atresia in early follicle growth, and a pronounced decrease in the number of corpora lutea (yellow secretory cells in the cavity of a ruptured Graffian follicle) present. All these changes and especially the last indicated a decreased ovulation potential and, therefore, a significant decrease in fertility. The gross size of ovaries of the treated animals was about half that of the ovaries of control animals. The effects produced by FA and FCl in females were similar. Some further studies on the effect of FA, FH, and cyhexatin on fertility in the rat were reviewed by McCollister and Schober.[124]

ACKNOWLEDGMENT

This article is a contribution from the Agricultural Research Organization, the Volcani Center, Bet Dagan, Israel (No. 1727-E, 1986 series).

REFERENCES

1. **Serebrovsky, A. S.**, On the possibility of a new method for the control of insect pests (in Russian), *Zool. Zh.*, 19, 618, 1940; (in English) Proc. panel organized by the joint FAO/IAEA Division of Atomic Energy in Food and Agriculture, Panel Proc. Ser. STI/PUB/224, 1969, 123.
2. **Knipling, E. F.**, Possibilities of insect control or eradication through the use of sexually sterile males, *J. Econ. Entomol.*, 48, 459, 1955.
3. **Knipling, E. F.**, Potentialities and progress in the development of chemosterilants for insect control, *J. Econ. Entomol.*, 55, 782, 1962.
4. **von Gelei, G. V. and Csik, L.**, Die Wirkung des Colchicins auf *Drosophila melanogaster*, *Biol. Zbl.*, 60, 275, 1940.
5. **Auerbach, C. and Robson, J. M.**, Experiments on the Action of Mustard Gas in *Drosophila*. Production of Sterility and of Mutation, Report No. W3979, Ministry of Supply of Great Britain, London, 1942.
6. **Rapoport, I. A.**, Inheritance changes taking place under the influence of diethyl sulphate and dimethyl sulphate, *Dokl. Akad. Sel.-Khoz, Nauk*, 12, 12, 1947.
7. **Rapoport, I. A.**, Derivatives of carbamic acid and mutations, *Byull. Eksp. Biol. Med.*, 23, 198, 1947.
8. **Rapoport, I. A.**, A selective sterile modification induced by dimethyl phosphate and other compounds, *Dokl. Akad. Nauk SSSR*, 147, 943, 1962.
9. **Battacharya, S.**, Tests for a possible action of ethylene glycol on the chromosomes of *Drosophila melanogaster*, *Proc. R. Soc. Edinburgh* 63, B, (17), 242, 1949.
10. **Demerec, M., Wallace, B., Witkin, E. M., and Bertani, G.**, The gene, *Carnegie Inst. Washington Yearb.*, 48, 154, 1949.
11. **Bird, M. J.**, Production of mutations in *Drosophila* using four aryl-2-halogenoalkylamines, *Nature (London)*, 165, 491, 1950.
12. **Auerbach, C.**, Problems in chemical mutagenesis, *Cold Spring Harbor Symp. Quant. Biol.*, 16, 199, 1951.
13. **Wallace, B.**, Dominant lethals and sex-linked lethals induced by nitrogen mustard, *Genetics (Princeton)*, 36, 364, 1951.
14. **Auerbach, C. and Moser, H.**, Analysis of the mutagenic action of formaldehyde food. II. The mutagenic potentialities of the treatment, *Z. Indukt. Abstamm. Vererbungsl.*, 85, 547, 1953.
15. **Fahmy, O. G. and Fahmy, M. J.**, Cytogenetic analysis of the action of carcinogens and tumour inhibitors in *Drosophila melanogaster*. II. The mechanism of induction of dominant lethals by 2:4:6-tri(ethyleneimino)-1:3:5-triazine, *J. Genet.*, 52, 603, 1954.
16. **Fahmy, O. G. and Fahmy, M. J.**, Cytogenetic analysis of the action of carcinogens and tumour inhibitors in *Drosophila melanogaster*. The cell stage response of the male germ line to the mesyloxy resins, *Genetics (Princeton)*, 46, 361, 1961.
17. **Fahmy, O. G. and Fahmy, M. J.**, Cytogenetic analysis of the action of carcinogens and tumour inhibitors in *Drosophila melanogaster*. Mutagenetic efficiency of the mesyloxy esters on the sperm in relation to molecular structure, *Genetics (Princeton)*, 46, 1111, 1961.
18. **Goldsmith, E. D., Tobias, E. B., and Harnly, M. H.**, Folic acid antagonists and the development of *Drosophila melanogaster*, *Anat. Rec.*, 101, 743, 1948.

19. **Goldsmith, E. D., Harnly, M. H., and Tobias, E. B.,** Folic acid analogs in lower animals. I. The insects: *Drosophila melanogaster, Ann. N.Y. Acad. Sci.,* 52, 1342, 1950.
20. **Goldsmith, E. D. and Harnly, M. H.,** Reversal of folic acid antagonist 4-aminopteroylglutamic acid in *Drosophila melanogaster, Cancer Res.,* 10, 220, 1950.
21. **Goldsmith, E. D. and Frank, I.,** Sterility in the female fruit fly, *Drosophila melanogaster,* produced by the feeding of a folic acid antagonist, *Am. J. Physiol.,* 171, 726, 1952.
22. **Mitlin, N.,** Inhibition of development in the house fly by 3,4-methylenedioxyphenyl compounds, *J. Econ. Entomol.,* 49, 683, 1956.
23. **Mitlin, N., Butt, B. A., and Shortino, T. J.,** Effect of mitotic poisons on house fly oviposition, *Physiol. Zool.,* 30, 133, 1957.
24. **Ascher, K. R. S.,** Prevention of oviposition in the housefly through tarsal contact agents, *Science (N.Y.),* 125, 938, 1957.
25. **Ascher, K. R. S.,** Investigations on a fluorocarbon as "O.I.T.C.-agent" (oviposition-inhibiting tarsal contact agent) in mosquitoes, *Riv. Malariol.,* 36, 209, 1957.
26. **Ascher, K. R. S.,** A review of chemosterilants and oviposition-inhibitors in insects, *World Rev. Pest Control,* 3, 7, 1964.
27. **Ascher, K. R. S.,** Insect pest control by chemosterilants and antifeedants — Magdeburg 1966 to Milan 1969, *World Rev. Pest Control,* 9, 140, 1970/1971.
28. **Bertram, S. D.,** A symposium on chemosterilants in pest and vector control. I. Entomological and parasitological aspects of vector chemosterilisation, *Trans. R. Soc. Trop. Med. Hyg.,* 57, 296, 1964.
29. **Bořkovec, A. B.,** Insect chemosterilants, *Residue Rev.,* 6, 87, 1964.
30. **Smith, C. N., LaBreque, G. C., and Bořkovec, A. B.,** Insect chemosterilants, *Annu. Rev. Entomol.,* 9, 269, 1964.
31. **Adolphi, H.,** Chemosterilantien in der Schädlingsbekämpfung, *Z. Angew. Zool.,* 52, 133, 1965.
32. **Campion, D. G.,** The present status of research on chemosterilants in the United States and Central America for the control of insect pests, *Pest Artic. News Summ. (PANS),* 11A, 467, 1965.
33. **Campion, D. G.,** The sterilisation of lepidopterous pests by radiation and chemosterilants, *Pest Artic. News Summ. (PANS),* 13A, 392, 1965.
34. **Campion, D. G.,** Insect chemosterilants: a review, *Bull. Entomol. Res.,* 61, 577, 1972.
35. **Gruner, L.,** Les chimiostérilisants des insectes, *Rev. Zool. Agric. Appl.,* 65, 1, 1966.
36. **Rukavishnikov, B. I.,** Sexual Sterilization as a Method of Combatting Harmful Insects, *Lit. Rev. (Moscow),* 2, 14, 1966.
37. **Rukavishnikov, B. I.,** Radiation and Chemical Sterilization of Harmful Insects, *Itogi Nauki Zool. (Moscow),* 6, 1966.
38. **Kilgore, W. W.,** Chemosterilants, in *Pest Control: Biological, Physical and Selected Chemical Methods,* Kilgore, W. W. and Doutt, R. L., Eds., Academic Press, New York, 1967, 197.
39. **Bořkovec, A. B., Fye, R. L., and LaBreque, G. C.,** Aziridinyl chemosterilants for house flies, Agric. Res. Serv., Publ. No. ARS 33-129, U.S. Department of Agriculture, Washington, D. C., 1968.
40. **Schumakow, E. M.,** Hauptrichtungen in der Erforschung der Sterilisationsmethoden bei Insekten, *Pflanzenschutzberichte,* 38, 157, 1968.
41. **Proverbs, M. D.,** Induced sterilization and control of insects, *Annu. Rev. Entomol.,* 14, 81, 1969.
42. **Stüben, M.,** Chemosterilantien, *Mitt. Biol. Bundesanst. Land- Forstwirtsch.,* 133, 1, 1969.
43. **Büchel, K. H.,** Chemosterilantien, in *Chemie der Pflanzenschutz- und Schädlingsbekämpfungsmittel,* Wegler, R., Ed., Band 1, Springer-Verlag, Berlin, 1970, 475.
44. **Bořkovec, A. B.,** Insect Chemosterilants, *Adv. Pest Control Res.,* 7, 1966.
45. **LaBreque, G. C. and Smith, C. N., Eds.,** *Principles of Insect Chemosterilization,* Appleton-Century-Crofts, New York, 1968.
46. **Sharma, V. P. and Brooks, G. D.,** Insect Chemosterilant Bibliography, Doc. WHO/VBC/75.526, World Health Organization, Geneva, 1975.
47. **Fye, R. L. and LaBreque, G. C.,** Bibliography of Arthropod Chemosterilants, Doc. ARS-S-93, U.S. Department of Agriculture, Washington, D. C., 1976.
48. **Mitlin, N. and Baroody, A. M.,** Use of the housefly as a screening agent for tumor-inhibiting agents, *Cancer Res.,* 18, 708, 1958.
49. **Gellhorn, A. and Hirschberg, E.,** Investigation of diverse systems for cancer chemotherapy screening, *Cancer Res.,* Suppl. 3, 1, 1955.
50. **Davies, A. G. and Smith, P. J.,** Recent advances in organotin chemistry, *Adv. Inorg. Chem. Radiochem.,* 23, 1, 1980.
51. **Davies, A. G. and Smith, P. J.,** Tin, in *Comprehensive Organometallic Chemistry,* Wilkinson, G., Stone, F. G. A., and Abel, E. W., Eds., Pergamon Press, Oxford, 1982, 519.
52. **Bock, R.,** Triphenyltin compounds and their degradation products, *Residue Rev.,* 79, 1, 1981.
53. **Thayer, J. S.,** *Organometallic Compounds and Living Organisms,* Academic Press, New York, 1984.

54. **Blunden, S. J., Cusack, P. A., and Hill, R.,** *The Industrial Uses of Tin Chemicals,* The Royal Society of Chemistry, London, 1985.
55. **Evans, C. J. and Karpel, S.,** *Organotin Compounds in Modern Technology,* Elsevier, Amsterdam, 1985.
56. **Ascher, K. R. S. and Rones, G.,** Fungicide has residual effect on larval feeding, *Int. Pest Control,* 6(3), 6, 1964.
57. **Ascher, K. R. S.,** Organotin insect antifeedants: an overview, in *Tin as a Vital Nutrient: Implications in Cancer Prophylaxis and Other Physiological Processes,* Cardarelli, N. F., Ed., CRC Press, Boca Raton, 1968, 211.
58. **Kenaga, E. E.,** Triphenyl tin compounds as insect reproduction inhibitors, Proc. 12th Int. Congr. Entomology, London, July 8 to 16, 1965, 517.
59. **Kenaga, E. E.,** Triphenyl tin compounds as insect reproduction inhibitors, *J. Econ. Entomol.,* 58, 4, 1965.
60. **Byrdy, S., Ejmocki, Z., and Eckstein, Z.,** Organotin compounds as insect chemosterilants. Evaluation of the activity of some triphenyltin derivatives on the Colorado potato beetle (*Leptinotarsa decemlineata* Say) and house fly (*Musca domestica* L.), *Bull. Acad. Pol. Sci. Ser. Sci. Chim.,* 13, 683, 1965.
61. **Fye, R. L., LaBreque, G. C., and Gouck, H. K.,** Screening tests of chemicals for sterilization of adult house flies, *J. Econ. Entomol.,* 59, 485, 1966.
62. **USDA/ARS,** Materials evaluated as insecticides, repellents and chemosterilants at Orlando and Gainesville, Fla., 1952—1964, Handbook No. 340, U.S. Department of Agriculture, Washington, D.C., 1967.
63. **WHO,** Evaluation of insecticides for vector control. A collaborative programme conducted by the World Health Organization. I. Compounds evaluated in 1960—67, Doc. WHO/VBC/68.66, World Health Organization, Geneva, 1968.
64. **Kissam, J. B. and Hays, S. B.,** Mortality and fertility response of *Musca domestica* adults to certain known mutagenic or antitumor agents, *J. Econ. Entomol.,* 59, 748, 1966.
65. **Hays, S. B.,** Reproduction inhibition in house flies with triphenyl tin acetate and triphenyl tin chloride and in combination with other compounds, *J. Econ. Entomol.,* 61, 1154, 1968.
66. **Ascher, K. R. S., Meisner, J., and Nissim, S.,** The effect of fentins on the fertility of the male housefly, *World Rev. Pest Control,* 7, 84, 1968.
67. **Koula, V. and Rajchartová, O.,** Some organic tin compounds as chemosterilants of insects, *Ochr. Rostl. (Praha),* 5, 265, 1969.
68. **Byrdy, S., Ejmocki, Z., and Eckstein, Z.,** Insect chemosterilizing activity and chemical structure of some organotin derivatives, *Bull. Acad. Pol. Sci. Ser. Sci. Biol.,* 18, 15, 1970.
69. **Ascher, K. R. S., Avdat, N., Meisner, J., and Moscowitz, J.,** The effect of fentins on the fertility of the female housefly — incorporating a review of their influence on insect fertility and fecundity in general, *Z. Angew. Entomol.,* 69, 285, 1971.
70. **Pausch, R. D.,** Local house fly control with baited chemosterilants. I. Preliminary laboratory studies, *J. Econ. Entomol.,* 64, 1462, 1971.
71. **Krzemińska, A.,** The sterilizing effect of some organotin compounds on the house fly *Musca domestica* L., *Roczn. Nauk Roln.* 139, 1973; *Rev. Appl. Entomol.,* 64B, 359, No. 1260, 1976.
72. **Krzemińska, A.,** Effect of organotin fungicides on insect reproductive capacity, *Wiadomaści Parazytologiezne,* 23(1/3), 269, 1977; *Rev. Appl. Entomol.,* 67B, 267, No. 2082, 1979.
73. **Pausch, R. D.,** A laboratory evaluation of baits and chemosterilants on the little house fly, *J. Econ. Entomol.,* 62, 25, 1969.
74. **Mulla, M. S.,** Chemosterilants for control of reproduction in the eye gnat and the mosquito, *Hilgardia,* 39, 297, 1968.
75. **Orphanidis, P. S. and Patsakos, P. G.,** Chimiostérilisation des *Dacus oleae* (Gmel.) et *Ceratitis capitata* Wied. au moyen de substances chimiques avec ou sans propriétés d'alkylation, *Ann. Inst. Phytopathol. Benaki,* 9, 134, 1970.
76. **Orphanidis, P. S.,** Stérilisation en laboratoire de *"Ceratitis capitata"* Wied., et de *"Dacus oleae"* Gmel. au moyen d'aziridines, acaricides et de sels minéraux, Repr. Lect. II-19, 2ème Congr. Int. Antiparasitaires, Naples, Italy, March 15 to 17, 1965.
77. **Orphanidis, P. S. and Patsakos, P. G.,** Nouvelles expériences sur la stérilisation de deux espèces de Tripetidae (*Dacus oleae* (Gmel.) et *Ceratitis capitata* Wied.) au moyen de substances chimiques, avec ou sans propriétés d'alkylation, Repr. Lect. No. 27, 3ème Congr. Int. Antiparasitaires, Milan, Italy, October 6 to 8, 1969.
78. **Abdel-Megeed, M. I., Zidan, Z. H., Awadallah, A. M., and El-Abbassi, T. S.,** Latent effects of Du-Ter on the Mediterranean fruit fly *Ceratitis capitata* Wied., *Bull. Entomol. Soc. Egypt,* 12, 119, 1980/81; *Rev. Appl. Entomol.,* 73A, 605, No. 5396, 1985.
79. **Abdel-Megeed, M. I., Zidan, Z. H., Awadallah, A. M., and El-Abbassi, T. S.,** Effect of triphenyltin hydroxide, Du-Ter, on gonads, reproductive potential and certain biochemical constituents of larvae and pupae of the Mediterranean fruit fly, *Ceratitis capitata, Agric. Res. Rev.,* 58, 181, 1980; *Rev. Appl. Entomol.,* 71A, 288, No. 2435, 1983.

80. **Abdel-Megeed, M. I., Zidan, Z. H., Awadallah, A., and El-Abbassi, T. S.**, The action of Du-Ter on the biochemical constituents and ovaries of the Mediterranean fruit fly, *Ceratitis capitata* Wied., *Bull. Entomol. Soc. Egypt*, 12, 107, 1980/81; *Rev. Appl. Entomol. Ser.*, 73A, 673, No. 5998, 1985.
81. **Singh, O. P. and Teotja, P. S.**, Effect of triphenyltin hydroxide on the mortality and reproduction of the melon fly, *Dacus cucurbitae* Coq., Inf. Circ. Radiation Techniques and Their Application to Insect Pests (FAO/IAEA), 17, Abstr. No. 24, 1974.
82. **White, G. B.**, The Effects of Sterilizing Chemicals on the Reproduction of *Aedes aegypti* (L), Ph.D. thesis, London School of Hygiene and Tropical Medicine, London, 1966.
83. **Byrdy, S.**, Chemical methods as one of the factors of integrated pests and diseases control, *Roczn. Nauk Roln. Ser. A*, 93, 789, 1968.
84. **Klassen, W., Norland, J. F., and Bořkovec, A. B.**, Potential chemosterilants for boll weevils, *J. Econ. Entomol.*, 61, 401, 1968.
85. **Haynes, J. W., Mitlin, N., Davich, T. B., and Sloan, C. E.**, Evaluation of candidate chemosterilants for the boll weevil, ARS/USDA Prod. Res. Rep. No. 120, U.S. Department of Agriculture, Washington, D.C., 1971.
86. **Ladd, T. L., Jr.**, Some effects of three triphenyltin compounds on the fertility and longevity of Japanese beetles, *J. Econ. Entomol.*, 61, 577, 1968.
87. **Findlay, J. B. R.**, The use of anti-feeding compounds as protectants against insect damage to plants, M.Sc. thesis, University of Pretoria, Pretoria, Republic of South Africa, 1968.
88. **Nagasawa, S., Shinohara, H., and Shiba, M.**, Differential susceptibilities in sexes of *Callosobruchus chinensis* L. (Coleoptera, Bruchidae) to the sterilizing effects of triphenyltin hydroxide, *J. Stored Pro. Res.*, 3, 177, 1967.
89. **Nagasawa, S., Shinohara, H., and Shiba, M.**, Sterilizing effect of Dowco-186 on the Azuki bean weevil, *Callosobruchus chinensis* L., with special reference to the hatchability of the eggs deposited by treated weevils. Studies on chemosterilants of insects. VI., *Botyu Kagaku*, 30, 91, 1965.
90. **Findlay, J. B. R.**, Laboratory studies on the effects of triphenyltin acetate and triphenyltin hydroxide on the stages in the life-cycle of *Spodoptera littoralis* (Bois.), *Phytophylactica (South Africa)*, 2, 91, 1970.
91. **Elbadry, E. A., Abo Elghar, M. R., and Radwan, H. S.**, Chemosterilization of larvae of the cotton leafworm, *Spodoptera littoralis* (Boisd.) by Du-Ter, *Z. Pflanzenkr. Pflanzenschutz*, 78, 700, 1971.
92. **Abo-Elghar, M. R. and Radwan, H.**, Toxicological, chemosterilant and histopathological effects of triphenyl-tin-hydroxide on *Spodoptera littoralis* Boisd., *Acta Phytopathol. Acad. Sci. Hung.*, 6, 261, 1971.
93. **Elbadry, E. A., Abo Elghar, M. R., and Radwan, H. S.**, Chemosterilant effects of Du-Ter on adults of the Egyptian cotton leafworm, *Spodoptera littoralis* (Boisd.), *Z. Angew. Entomol.*, 71, 140, 1972.
94. **Mitri, S. H. and Kamel, A. A. M.**, The sterilant effect of certain antifeedants on the moth of *Spodoptera littoralis*, *Bull. Entomol. Soc. Egypt, Econ. Ser.*, 6, 79, 1972.
95. **Mitri, S. H. and Kamel, A. A. M.**, Further studies on the sterilant effect of certain antifeedants on the adult stages of *Spodoptera littoralis* (Boisd.) (Lepidoptera: Noctuidae), *Bull. Ent. Soc. Egypt, Econ. Ser.*, 7, 143, 1973.
96. **Joshi, B. G., Ramaprasad, G., and Narasimhayya, G.**, Note on fentin acetate as a reproduction-inhibitor of the tobacco caterpillar, *Spodoptera litura* (Fabricius), *Indian J. Agric. Sci.*, 43, 324, 1973.
97. **Campion, D. G. and Outram, I.**, Insecticidal and possible chemosterilant effects of certain organo-metal compounds against red bollworm, *Int. Pest Control*, 10(2), 21, 1968.
98. **Campion, D. G. and Lewis, C. T.**, Studies of competitiveness, chemosterilant persistence and sperm structure in treated red bollworms, *Diparopsis castanea* (Hmps.), in Sterility Principle for Insect Control or Eradication, Publ. STI/PUB/265, IAEA, Vienna, Austria, 1971, 183.
99. **Salem, Y. S., Abdel-Megeed, M. I., and Zidan, Z. H.**, Triphenyl-tin-hydroxide "Du-Ter" as inhibitor of the spiny bollworm *Earias insulana* (Boisd.) (Lepidoptera: Noctuidae), *Bull. Entomol. Soc. Egypt, Econ. Ser.*, 9, 293, 1975.
100. **Salem, Y. S., Abdel-Megeed, M. I., and Zidan, Z. H.**, Du-Ter as inhibitor to the reproduction of the spring bollworm, *Earias insulana* (Boisd.) (Lep., Noctuidae), *Z. Angew. Entomol.*, 81, 187, 1976.
101. **Shaaban, A. M., Youssef, H. J., Kamel, A. A., and Abulghar, M. R.**, Effect of certain chemosterilants on the larvae of the greasy cutworm, *Agrotis ipsilon* Rott., *Z. Angew. Entomol.*, 78, 386, 1975.
102. **Wolfenbarger, D. A., Guerra, A. A., and Lowry, W. L.**, Effects of organometallic compounds on Lepidoptera, *J. Econ. Entomol.*, 61, 78, 1968.
103. **Bonnemaison, L.**, Essais de substances chimiostérilisantes. II. Action sur divers lépidoptères, *Phytia. Phytopharm.*, 15, 79, 1966.
104. **Bonnemaison, L.**, Essais de chimiostérilisantes sur quelques homoptères, coléoptères et lépidoptères, Repr. Lect. No. 5, 3ème Congr. Int. Antiparasitaires, Milan, Italy, October 6 to 8, 1969.
105. **Bonnemaison, L.**, personal communication, 1971.
106. **Ansari, H. J. and Khan, M. A.**, Effect of triphenyltin acetate on the fecundity and fertility of *Dysdercus cingulatus* F. (Heteroptera: Pyrrhocoridae), *Curr. Sci.*, 42, 280, 1973.

107. **Ansari, H. J. and Khan, A.**, Effect of triphenyltin acetate on the fertility of (the) male red cotton bug, *Dysdercus cingulatus* F. (Heteroptera: Pyrrhocoridae), *Comp. Physiol. Ecol.*, 4, 121, 1979; *Entomol. Abstr.*, 11, 35, No. 2421-E11, 1980.
108. **Redfern, R. E.**, Evaluations of candidate chemosterilants for control of two-spotted spider mites, *J. Econ. Entomol.*, 63, 357, 1970.
109. **Boykin, L. S. and Campbell, W. V.**, Rate of population increase of the twospotted spider mite (Acari: Tetranychidae) on peanut leaves treated with pesticides, *J. Econ. Entomol.*, 75, 966, 1982.
110. **Krzemińska, A.**, The effect of triphenylstannous compounds on ovarian development in the house fly (*Musca domestica* L.)., *Roczniki Państwowego Zakładu Higieny*, 31, 79, 1980; *Rev. Appl. Entomol. Ser.*, 69B, 64, No. 473, 1981.
111. **Wang, C.-Y., Sudderuddin, K. I., and Kumar Das, V. G.**, Insecticidal evaluation of triorganotin (IV) compounds against the housefly *Musca domestica* L., *Malays. Appl. Biol.*, 11, 117, 1982.
112. **Murbach, R. and Corbaz, R.**, Influence de trois types de fongicides utilisés en Suisse contre le mildiou de la pomme de terre [*Phytophthora infestans* (Mont.) de Bary] sur la densité de population du doryphore (*Leptinotarsa decemlineata* Say), *Phytopathol. Z.*, 43, 182, 1963.
113. **Murbach, R.**, Effect en plein champ de fongicides à base de fentin-acétate, de manèbe et d'oxychlorure de cuivre sur la densité de population du doryphore de la pomme de terre (*Leptinotarsa decemlineata* Say), *Rech. Agron. (Suisse)*, 6, 345, 1967.
114. **Dale, D. and Saradamma, K.**, Effect of continuous feeding of fentin acetate on the biology of the Indian mealworm, *Corcyra cephalonica* S. (Pyralidae: Lepidoptera), *Bull. Grain Technol.*, 12, 66, 1974; Rev. Appl. Entomol, 64A, 346, No. 1157, 1976.
115. **Bonnemaison, L.**, Action stérilisante du tépa et du D.M.S.O. sur divers insectes, *Phytia. Phytopharm.*, 17, 105, 1968.
116. **Bhalla, O. P. and Robinson, A. G.**, Effects of chemosterilants and growth regulators on the pea aphid fed an artificial diet, *J. Econ. Entomol.*, 61, 552, 1968.
117. **Chawla, S. S., Perron, J. M., and Cloutier, M.**, Topical application effects of three chemosterilants on the potato aphid, *Macrosiphum euphorbiae* (Thomas) (Homoptera: Aphididae), *Phytoprotection*, 55, 43, 1974; *Rev. Appl. Entomol.*, 63A, 757, No. 2813, 1975.
118. **Sáringer, Gy.**, Oviposition behaviour of *Ceutorrhynchus macula-alba* Herbst. (Col.: Curculionidae), *Symp. Biol. Hung.*, 16, 241, 1976.
119. **Deseö, K. V.**, Influence of cyhexatin on the oviposition preference of *Lobesia botrana* Den. & Schiff. (Lepidoptera, Tortricidae), Abstr., Regulation of Insect Reproduction, Bechyně, CSSR, June 14 to 18, 1982.
120. **Abdul Kareem, A., Thangavel, P., Balasubramaniam, G., and Balasubramanian, M.**, Studies on the predatism of the lady bird beetle, *Menochilus sexmaculatus* (F.) on (the) bean aphid, *Aphis craccivora* Koch, treated with antifeeding compounds, *Z. Angew. Entomol.*, 83, 406, 1977.
121. **Abdul Kareem, A., Jayaraj, P., Thangavel, P., and Navarajan Paul, A. V.**, Studies on the effects of three antifeedants on the egg hatchability of *Corcyra cephalonica* Staint. (Galleriidae: Lepidoptera) and parasitism by *Trichogramma australicum* Gin. (Trichogrammatidae: Hymenoptera), *Z. Angew. Entomol.*, 83, 141, 1977.
122. **Pate, B. D. and Hays, R. L.**, Histological studies of testes in rats treated with certain insect chemosterilants, *J. Econ. Entomol.*, 61, 32, 1968.
123. **Newton, D. W. and Hays, R. L.**, Histological studies of ovaries in rats treated with hydroxyurea, triphenyltin acetate and triphenyltin chloride, *J. Econ. Entomol.*, 61, 1668, 1968.
124. **McCollister, D. D. and Schober, A. E.**, Assessing toxicological properties of organotin compounds, in *Environmental Quality and Safety—Global Aspects of Chemistry, Toxicology and Technology as Applies to the Environment*, Vol. 4, Georg Thieme, Stuttgrt, 1975, 80.

Chapter 17

BIOACTIVITY OF SOME ORGANOTIN COMPOUNDS ON INSECTS

R. N. Sharma, Vrushali Tare, and S. B. Bhonde

TABLE OF CONTENTS

I.	Introduction	202
II.	Materials and Methods	202
III.	Results and Discussion	203
References		209

I. INTRODUCTION

Organotin compounds have long been known to possess unique bioactivity toward different classes of organisms. Ascher and Nissim[1] have comprehensively reviewed the action of various tin compounds on insects. Apart from their insecticidal properties, the organotins are also known for potent biolgoical activity on such different taxa as fungi, mollusks, and mammals.[1,2] The role of tin as a trace element of possibly vital significance in complex and intricate endocrine and developmental processes has also been hinted.[1,3] The property of many organotin compounds as insect antifeedants has been highlighted especially by Ascher and his group at the Volcani Insitute in Israel.[1,4] Any group of compounds possessing this broad array of biological effects on such a diverse range of organisms must be investigated more comprehensively in the hope of elucidating their true role and significance in biological processes. We have earlier reported[5] on the comprehensive screening of two organotin compounds against a number of species for a broad range of bioactivities. We describe here results of a recent investigation on more compounds belonging to the same series of organotins.

II. MATERIALS AND METHODS

The compounds used in the present investigations are listed in Table 1. In the following text, the compounds shall be referred to by their corresponding numbers in this table. It may be added that tri-*n*-butyltin deoxycholate and trimethyltin cholate are also listed in Table 1, even though most of the work done with them has been reported earlier.[5] With minor variations, the procedures and insect species as reported in the earlier investigations[5] have been used. These are, nevertheless, recounted here in brief.

Insecticidal action was studied on 2- to 5-day-old adult houseflies, *Musca domestica*, and the rice weevil, *Sitophilus oryzae*. Larvicidal activity was assessed for the 5th instar larvae of the tobacco leaf-eating caterpillar, *Spodoptera litura*, and the army worm, *Mythimna separata*. In addition, insecticidal activity against the fourth-instar larvae of three mosquito species viz., the yellow fever mosquito, *Aedes aegypti*; the malaria vector, *Anopheles stephensi*; and the filaria vector, *Culex fatigans*.

The compounds were topically applied in different concentrations in suitable solvents to the houseflies. In the case of the rice weevil, the latter was exposed to residual films of different strength on glass surfaces for 24 hr. For the lepidopteran larvae the topical application technique was also used. Finally, for the mosquito larvae, an aqueous suspension of the test compounds was applied to the holding waters in various doses, as detailed in the relevant tables.

Juvenile hormone (JH) activity of the test organotin compounds was assessed by using the red cotton bug, *Dysdercus koenigii*, as indicator species. The compounds were applied on freshly emerged fifth-instar nymphs kept on water and metamorphosis inhibition if any was recorded at the time of larval adult molt.

Antifeedant action of the test organotins was studied against *M. domestica* adults and *S. litura* larvae. In the former case the compounds were mixed with the vital dye Light Green (Centron Research Labs, Bombay, India) and offered in 0.05 *M* sucrose solution to the test fly. The effect on feeding activity was gauged by dissections of the test flies 24 hr later. In case of *S. litura*, early fourth-instar larvae were starved for 1 hr before being offered castor leaves treated with selected doses of the test compounds. Observations on the area of the leaf eaten/protected were made 24 and 48 hr later.

The effect of a few compounds on the total body protein contents of *S. litura* larvae was also examined using the standard Lowry's method[6] of protein estimation. The fourth instar larvae were exposed to treated castor leaves for 48 hr, whereafter they were removed and kept on untreated leaves for another 48 hr before being sacrificed for body protein estimation.

Table 1
ORGANOTIN COMPOUNDS INVESTIGATED[a]

No.	Compound	
1	Triphenyltin cholate	
2	Cholesteryl-n-butylstannate	
3	Triphenyltin testosterone	
4	Tri-n-butyltin deoxycholate	
5	Triphenyltin cholesterol ether	
6	Triphenyltin cholesterol ether	isomers
7	Tri-n-butyltin deoxycholate	
8	Tri-n-butyltin deoxycholate	isomers (or fractions) of no. 4
9	Tri-n-butyltin deoxycholate	
10	Cholesteryl tri-n-butyltin ether	
11	Cholesteryl tri-n-butyltin ether	isomers
12	Cholesteryl tri-n-butyltin adipate	
13	Cholesteryl tri-n-butyltin adipate	isomers
14	Tri-n-butyltin cholate	
15	Testosteronyl-n-butylstannate	
16	Triphenyltin testosteronyl ether	
17	Triphenyltin dehydroisoandrosterone	
18.	Estronyl-n-butyl stannate	
19	Trimethyltin cholate	
20	Di-n-butyltin dicholate	
21	Cortisonyl n-butylstannate	

[a] Used as received from N. F. Cardarelli and S. V. Kanakkanatt of Unique Technologies, Inc., Akron, Ohio. Names are based upon stoichiastic considerations. See References 7 to 9.

Two compounds showing distinct antifeedant action and two others inactive thus were also used to compare developmental inhibition and effects on total body proteins, if any, on younger *S. litura* larvae. In this case, second-instar larvae were used. These larvae were exposed as before to treated leaves for 48 hr, whereafter they were kept on untreated leaves, and some of them were sacrificed at the fifth-instar stage for body protein estimation while the remaining ones were allowed to complete development.

Barring only compounds **7**, for which 70% ethanol had to be used and **2** and **21** which were soluble in tetrahydrofuran (THF), all other compounds were soluble in acetone which was used as the delivery solvent.

In all cases, insecticidal action was examined at an appropriate high dose for a given insect species. Relevant lower doses were applied against the latter only if >95% toxicity was obtained at the high dose.

In our earlier investigation[5] we had used the pulse beetle, *Callosobruchus maculatus*, as one of the test insect species. In the present work, we have replaced this with the rice weevil, *S. oryzae*. In this report we have included the result of the application of tri-n-butyltin deoxycholate and trimethyltin cholate on the rice weevil, also.

Different doses used for assessing biological activities are given in the appropriate tables of results. All results are based on an average of a minimum of three replicates. Further details of procedures and calcuations are given in our earlier work.[5]

III. RESULTS AND DISCUSSION

For the sake of convenience of comparison we are including here results obtained earlier[5]

Table 2
ADULTICIDAL ACTIVITY OF SOME TIN COMPOUNDS AGAINST INSECTS

	Mortality (%)					
	Musca domestica			Sitophilus oryzae		
Compound	1.0 μg/insect	5.0 μg/insect	10.0 μg/insect	1.0 μg/cm²	5.0 μg/cm²	10.0 μg/cm²
1	—	—	10	—	—	0
2	—	—	10	—	—	0
3	—	—	75	—	—	0
*4	—	—	0	—	—	10
6	10	30	100	—	—	0
7	—	—	0	—	—	0
8	0	5	96.7	—	—	0
9	—	—	90	—	—	0
10	—	—	90	—	—	0
11	0	20	100	—	—	0
12	—	—	85	—	—	0
13	0	20	100	—	—	0
14	—	—	10	—	—	0
15	—	—	0	—	—	0
16	—	—	75	—	—	0
17	5	40	100	—	—	0
18	—	—	0	—	—	0
*19	0	100	100	95	100	100
20	—	—	0	—	—	0
21	—	—	65	—	—	0

Note: — not tested.

with compounds 4 and 19 wherever these fit into the present series of investigations. These have been specially indicated with asterisks in the different tables.

A perusal of the data depicted in Tables 2 to 6 permits certain broad inferences. Thus, it is quite apparent that in an overall context, compound **19** remains the most toxic compound even in the enlarged list of total organotins examined so far. The toxicity of compound **19** to *M. domestica*, *S. litura*, and the newly introduced *S. oryzae* is the highest (Tables 2 and 3). On the other hand, this compound shows relatively less toxicity to mosquito larvae in comparison with some of the other newer compounds introduced, e.g., **3, 6, 10, 12 to 14**, and **17** (Table 3).

A second general observation was that a knock-down effect such as was obtained with compound **19** for the house flies[5] was not obtained with any of the compounds tested in the present work. Likewise, the phenomenon of hemolymph exudation[5] from the bodies of lepidopteran larvae was also not elicited by any other compound. However, in general, many compounds did show high toxicity to the housefly adults and also to mosquito larvae. Curiously, only compound **19** exhibited notable toxicity to the rice weevil adults and the lepidopteran larvae (Tables 2 and 3). These observations established compound **19**'s high- and broad-spectrum toxicity as well as possible neurotoxic mode of action. On the other hand, the toxicity of the other tin compounds is comparatively lesser and is probably of a different nature.

It may also be stressed that values of >90% mortality at the low dose of 1 μg/cm² for *S. oryzae* and 100% at 5 μg per insect for housefly adults and lepidopteran larvae by compound **19** are decidedly of interest from an applied viewpoint. Similarly, 100% toxicity of mosquito larvae by a number of compounds at 5 ppm are also encouraging.

Table 3
LARVICIDAL ACTIVITY OF SOME TIN COMPOUNDS AGAINST INSECT PESTS/VECTORS

Compound	Aedes aegypti			Culex fatigans			Anopheles stephensi			Spodoptera litura			Mythimna separata		
	1.0 (ppm)	5.0 (ppm)	10.0 (ppm)	1.0 (ppm)	5.0 (ppm)	10.0 (ppm)	1.0 (ppm)	5.0 (ppm)	10.0 (ppm)	1.0 (μg/insect)	5.0 (μg/insect)	10.0 (μg/insect)	1.0 (μg/insect)	5.0 (μg/insect)	10.0 (μg/insect)
1	70.0	76.7	100	46.7	100	100	—	100	100	—	—	0	—	—	0
2	—	—	0	—	—	0	—	—	—	—	—	—	—	—	—
3	60.0	100	100	0	100	100	—	100	100	—	—	0	—	—	0
4	—	—	93	66	100	100	—	—	96.7	—	—	0	—	—	0
6	36.7	100	100	93	100	100	—	100	100	—	—	0	—	—	0
7	—	—	0	—	—	0	—	—	—	—	—	—	—	—	—
8	—	—	60	80	100	100	—	—	0	—	—	30	—	—	0
10	43.0	100	100	87.5	100	100	—	—	100	—	—	0	—	—	30
11	0	80	100	—	100	100	—	—	96.7	—	—	10	—	—	0
12	10	100	100	10	100	100	—	100	100	—	—	0	—	—	0
13	40	100	100	—	100	100	—	100	100	—	—	0	—	—	0
14	25	100	100	50	100	100	—	100	100	—	—	0	—	—	0
15	—	—	0	—	—	0	—	—	0	—	—	—	—	—	—
16	—	—	93	80	100	100	—	100	100	—	—	0	—	—	0
17	0	100	100	5	100	100	—	—	20	—	—	0	—	—	0
18	—	—	0	—	—	15	—	—	0	—	—	0	—	—	0
*19	—	—	63	0	73.3	100	—	—	23.3	20	100	100	65	100	100
20	—	—	0	—	—	0	—	—	0	—	—	0	—	—	0
21	—	—	40	—	—	83	—	—	—	—	—	—	—	—	0

Note: — = Not tested.

Table 4
JUVENILE HORMONE (JH) ACTIVITY OF SOME TIN COMPOUNDS AGAINST *DYSDERCUS KOENIGII*

Compound	% Inhibition at 10.0 μg per insect
1	0.66
2	—
3	0.6
*4	0
6	0
7	0
8	1.65
10	7.102
11	0.83
12	2.5
13	15.77
14	7.25
15	0
16	0
17	5.625
18	1.0
*19	0
20	0
21	—

Note: — = not tested.

Juvenile hormone (JH) activity as measured on red cotton bug was present but very low for some compounds. Highest JH activity was shown by compound **13** (Table 4). This compound also exhibited high toxicity to some other insects and induced ecdysial failures, albeit of a very low percentage, in the case of treatments of mosquito larvae when exposed from second instar onward. Work on this aspect is incomplete but still continuing.

In keeping with the known insect antifeedant properties of organotin compounds, many of the present series also exhibited high-feeding deterrance against *S. litura* larvae. However, none of the compounds showed any feeding deterrance against houseflies, suggesting that this action may be limited to lepidopteran larvae. Compounds **3**, **6**, **8**, and **11** to **14**, **16**, and **17** gave >90% leaf protection against *S. litura* larvae, which can be treated as synonymous with antifeedant action. These values compare very well with the ones obtained especially for compound **19**.[5] Compounds **12** to **14** showed some toxicity to the lepidopteran larvae in these antifeedant bioassays. Other compounds did not exhibit such effects. The mortality induced by compounds **12** to **14** cannot be due to oral toxicity since there was no feeding at all. It can only be adduced that these toxic effects may be because of the high intrinsic toxicity of these specific compounds which became manifest only as a consequence of their continued contact with test insects which were under additional duress of forced starvation due to the high feeding deterrance of these organotin compounds. In any case, as we had observed earlier,[5] >90% antifeedant action at doses as low as 0.1% for so many compounds is highly encouraging and promises to afford opportunities for selection of a few less toxic ones for insect management by behavior manipulation.

We have limited our investigations into fluctuations of total body protein contents to a few randomly chosen compounds only. Some of these exhibited antifeedant action while others did not. Again, some were exposed to the test compounds in the second-instar stage

Table 5
ANTIFEEDANT ACTIVITY OF SOME TIN COMPOUNDS AGAINST *SPODOPTERA LITURA*

Compound	% Protection at 0.1%[a]	
	24 hr	48 hr
1	75.99	80.93
2	9.4	2.89
3	100	100
*4	84	—
6	94.99	95.98
7	31.81	0
8	100	100
10	72.37	28.79
11	100	100
12	100	100
13	100	100
14	100	100
15	3.9	0
16	100	95.27
17	100	98.04
18	0	0
19	96.84	—
20	0	0
21	75.0	37.24

Note: — = not tested.

[a] Calculated as $\dfrac{X - Y}{XR} \times 100$ where X = area consumed in control and Y = area consumed in the test.

while others were exposed in the fourth instar. Overall results (Table 6) show that of the seven compounds so assessed, five did not affect the protein contents. However, two (compounds **11** and **21**) apparently induced an increase in the latter. Curiously, the five inactive compounds were those manifesting little or no feeding deterrance. These results are again similar to the ones we obtained earlier,[5] where compound **19** had exhibited both antifeedant action and the effects of inducing an increase in total body protein content as well as hemolymph exudation. As mentioned earier, **11** and **21** did not, however, induce the latter phenomenon. It is also interesting to note that exposure of the larvae to the active compounds, whether during second or fourth instar, had similar effects in terms of inducing elevated protein levels. It may also be recalled that these compounds deter feeding in lepidopteran larvae, but not in the house flies. Thus, both the phenomena of feeding deterrance and elevation of body proteins seem to occur in the case of lepidopterans. Whether the two are coextant or correlated cannot be assessed on the basis of the present preliminary data. It may be pointed out here that we[10] have observed such phenomena, e.g., elevation of total body protein content and exudation of hemolymph with physiologically potent doses of some known antifeedants and growth regulators such as azadirachtin and some synthetic JH mimics. It would be premature to draw inferences from such apparent similarities in selective biochemical effects, but the latter do suggest possible connection of the tin moiety with the growth, hormonal, metabolic, and/or developmental processes of insects.

Table 6
EFFECT OF SOME TIN COMPOUNDS ON TOTAL BODY PROTEIN CONTENTS OF *SPODOPTERA LITURA*

Compound	Total body protein content mg/g body weight	
	Second instar exposed to 0.01% treated leaf[a]	Fourth instar exposed to 0.1% treated leaf[a]
Control (acetone)	39.57	37.32
15	—	29.04
Control (tetrahydrofuran [THF])	—	35.57
2	—	40.11
21	—	59.26
7	—	34.87
11	47.52	—
18	36.87	—
20	37.09	—

Note: — = not tested.

[a] Explanation in text.

In conclusion, attention is drawn once again to the high antifeedant action and toxicity of some tin compounds assessed in the present investigations. These definitely have applied potential, and further developmental work on them is obviously indicated. Of importance also are the interesting and possibly highly significant aspects of the mode of action of these compounds and their role in the various vital functions of insects. Understanding of these latter aspects may lead to important insights into the significance of this element in the biological processes of organisms in general.

REFERENCES

1. **Ascher, K. R. S. and Nissim, S.,** Organotin compounds and their potential use in insect control, *World Rev. Pest Control.,* 3, 188, 1964.
2. **Cardarelli, N. F.,** Controlled release organotins as mosquito larvicides, *Mosq. News,* 38, 328, 1978.
3. **Cardarelli, N. F.,** personal communication, 1984.
4. **Ascher, K. R. S. and Moscowitz, J.,** Pennsalt TD-5032, an experimental organotin insecticide with antifeedant properties, *Int. Pest Control,* 11, 1969.
5. **Sharma, R. N., Tare, V., and Bhonde, S. B.,** Toxicity and chosen behavioural and physiological effects of some tin compounds on selected insect species, in *Tin as a Vital Nutrient: Implications in Cancer Prophylaxis and Other Physiological Processes,* Cardarelli, N. F., Ed., CRC Press, Boca Raton, 1986, 221.
6. **Lowry, O. H., Rosebrough, N. J., Farr, A. L., and Randall, R. J.,** Protein measurements with Folin phenol reagent, *J. Biol. Chem.,* 193, 265, 1951.
7. **Kanakkanatt, S.,** Synthesis of tin steroids and the relation between structure and anticancer activity, in *Tin As a Vital Nutrient: Implications in Cancer Prophylaxis and Other Physiological Processes,* Cardarelli, N. F., Ed., CRC Press, Boca Raton, 1986, 189.
8. **Cardarelli, N. F.,** Tin steroids, in *Tin As a Vital Nutrient: Implications in Cancer Prophylaxis and Other Physiological Processes,* Cardarelli, N. F., Ed., CRC Press, Boca Raton, 1986, 197.

9. **Cardarelli, N. F. and Kanakkanatt, S. V.,** Tin steroids and their use as antineoplastic agents, U.S. Patent 4,541,956, 1985.
10. **Sharma, R. N., Tare, V., and Bhode, S. B.,** unpublished data.

Chapter 18

COMPUTER-ASSISTED STRUCTURE — ANTICANCER ACTIVITY CORRELATIONS OF ORGANOTIN COMPOUNDS

Mohamed Nasr, Kenneth D. Paull, and V. L. Narayanan

I.	Introduction		212
II.	Results and Discussion		213
	A.	4-Coordinated Tin Compounds	213
		1. Diorganotins $R_2Sn\text{-}(HT)_2$	213
		2. Triorganotin Compounds R_3 Sn-HT	224
		3. Monoorganotin Compounds $RSn\text{-}(HT)_3$	224
		4. Tetraorganotin Compounds R_4Sn	224
		5. Tetraheterotin Compounds $Sn\text{-}(HT)_4$	224
	B.	5-Coordinated Tin Compounds	224
	C.	6-Coordinated Tin Compounds	224
		1. Diorganotin Compounds $R_2Sn\text{-}(HT)_4$	224
		2. Triorganotin Compounds $R_3Sn\text{-}(HT)_3$	224
		3. Hexaheterotin Compounds $Sn\text{-}(HT)_6$	224
	D.	Miscellaneous Types	224
		1. Diorganotin Compounds R_2 Sn	224
		2. Diorganotin Compounds $[(R_2Sn)HT]_x$	224
		3. Monoorganotin Compounds $RSn\text{-}(HT)_2$	225
		4. Tin Amino Acids	225
		5. Tin Sulfinates	225
		6. Compounds with Tin Bonded to Tin or to a Different Metal	225
III.	Conclusions		226
References			226

I. INTRODUCTION

The National Cancer Institute (NCI) and others have a continuing interest in exploring the anticancer potential of metal and metalloidal compounds.[1-6] The number of metal-containing compounds in the NCI collection is given in Table 1. Table 2 gives the number of compounds tested against the in vivo murine P388 and L1210 lymphocytic leukemia anticancer screens and the percentage of actives found for each test system.

Although metals and metalloidal compounds represent only a small fraction of the total NCI file (3.5%), organotin compounds are the largest class among metals as represented by more than 1800 compounds. This emphasis is the natural consequence of the wide biological use[7-9] of tin compounds and their subsequent availability for anticancer screening by the NCI. A good deal of work has been done on the chemistry,[10,11] toxicology,[12-14] and metabolism[15,16] of tin compounds. This study focuses on the structure-anticancer activity of tin-containing compounds evaluated by the NCI.

We report here an analysis of the various structural types of tin compounds tested by the NCI and the performance of these types as a group against the two in vivo murine leukemias P388 and L1210. This study seeks to utilize the computer's ability to group compounds according to precise structural definitions and to manipulate these groups using Boolean logic to create additional interesting subgroups. This technique has been used by us previously to analyze other classes of compounds.[17-19]

Many tin compounds are active against the standard P388 leukemia test system routinely used by the NCI, but only one of 700 tested showed confirmed activity* against the standard L1210 leukemia system. Thus, tin compounds as a group exhibit a high frequency of activity against P388 and low frequency of activity against L1210, although individual compounds may not be highly active against either system. This usage of "high activity", meaning a high frequency of actives instead of a high level of activity, is used throughout this study.

Approximately 29% of all tin compounds have demonstrated confirmed activity against P388, but only 1% against L1210. These percentages are slightly higher than calculated based on the numbers of confirmed actives in Table 3. The reason for the difference has been described.[17,18] The percentages used throughout Tables 2 and 3 are computed using a projection technique. This technique uses historical data to estimate the expected outcome of partially completed testing on a set of compounds.

To understand the relevance of these findings, it is essential to compare these results with NCI's total screening experience against both P388 and L1210 systems comprising approximately 150,000 compounds in each category. Using the projection technique described above, we find the overall percentage of actives for P388 and L1210 to be 7.6 and 1.8%, respectively. For each test system, the total percentage represents a composite of primary (first time a compound is tested) and secondary testing (compound already known to be active in another test system). Because there is a correlation among most tumor systems, the yield of actives from secondary testing is much higher than from primary testing. Thus, the composite values of 7.6 and 1.8 for P388 and L1210, respectively, are distinctly higher than the primary testing values which we estimate as 5 and 1% for P388 and L1210, respectively. Using these overall percentages, tin compounds seem to have been active against P388 almost six times as frequently as the overall percentage would predict and about the same frquency of activity against L1210 as would have been expected. Thus, P388 is far more sensitive than expected to tin compounds, while L1210 is not especially sensitive. The reason for this differential sensitivity is not known. As will be noted below,

---

* Because of biological variations, it is customary to retest compounds showing initial activity in a secondary test, and confirmed activity refers to the accepted NCI criteria (20% increase in survival time for P388 and 25% for L1210).

Table 1
METAL AND METALLOID COMPOUNDS TESTED BY THE NATIONAL CANCER INSTITUTE[a]

Transition elements										3A Al 89	4A	5A	6A
Sc	Ti	V	Cr	Mn	Fe	Co	Ni	Cu	Zn	Ga	Ge	As	Se
8	77	75	248	251	848	820	734	1218	838	51	206	1246	710
Y	Zr	Nb	Mo	Tc	Ru	Rh	Pd	Ag	Cd	In	**Sn**	Sb	Te
10	55	28	162	0	127	238	418	139	123	18	**1888**	349	51
La[b]	Hf	Ta	W	Re	Os	Ir	Pt	Au	Hg	Tl	Pb	Bi	Po
27	15	15	86	19	25	22	1455	111	811	37	287	81	0
Ce	Pr	Nd	Pm	Sm	Eu	Gd	Tb	Dy	Ho	Er	Tm	Yb	Lu
30	22	27	0	20	76	18	38	22	12	18	12	13	11

[a] Number tested as of March 1987.
[b] Lanthanides (bottom row).

this unpredicted sensitivity of P388 to tin compounds becomes far more evident once the structural details of the tin compounds are considered.

II. RESULTS AND DISCUSSION

The results of the analysis are summarized in Table 3. This table shows the basic structural types of tin compounds and shows the effect of structural modifications of antitumor activity. The total number of compounds containing the indicated substructure that have been tested in any in vivo or in vitro test system is shown. In addition, Table 3 depicts the number of compounds that have been tested against P388 and/or L1210 leukemia, the number of confirmed actives (CA) and the percentage of activity.[17,18] For each substructure type, an example of an active compound is given except in cases where no active was found.

The information generated in Table 3 is indicative rather than definitive. The presence of relatively many active compounds within an analyzed group is considered a reasonable basis for additional, more thorough studies on the group. It should be noted that a high percentage of actives cannot be considered proof that the subject substructure is required for the antitumor activity or even relevant to it. On the other hand, if few active compounds are found among a relatively large group having a given substructure, it is safe to assume that the particular substructure is not particularly relevant to that type of anticancer activity.

The results of our analysis are discussed below.

A. 4-Coordinated Tin compounds
1. Diorganotins $R_2Sn\text{-}(HT)_2$*

This represents a highly active class against P388. The activity varies somewhat with the nature of the organic substituent, R, and the electronegative substituent, HT. In general, the diorganotin compounds (Z2)** showed 54% activity against P388; 60% with HT = O (Z3), 46% with HT = S (Z12), 48% with HT = N (Z16), and 39% with HT = halogen (Z18). Excellent activity of 94% against P388 was obtained with R = Et, HT = O (Z5), and 89% with R = Ph and HT = O (Z8). All the three bis-diorganotin compounds (Z10) tested against P388 demonstrated confirmed activity. When R = Ph and HT = S (Z15), the four compounds tested against P388 are all confirmed actives. The diorganotin nitrogen

* HT is used to indicate electronegative substituents.
** "Z" code is a serial number used for computer programming purposes.

Table 2
METAL AND METALLOID COMPOUNDS TESTED BY THE NATIONAL CANCER INSTITUTE[a] — PERCENTAGE OF ACTIVES AGAINST P388 AND L1210

Transition elements

Sc	Ti	V	Cr	Mn	Fe	Co	Ni	Cu	Zn
1[b] 6[c]	43 13	34 24	86 117	88 97	219 422	252 380	270 387	408 442	250 405
0[d] 0[e]	2 0	1 1	6 1	27 2	10	15 2	9 3	6 1	14 2

Y	Zr	Nb	Mo	Tc	Ru	Rh	Pd	Ag	Cd
6 5	21 21	22 24	81 78	0 0	64 33	126 136	145 216	34 63	27 54
0 0	5 1	7 0	4 1		40 7	20 2	6 3	2 1	4 0

La[f]	Hf	Ta	W	Re	Os	Ir	Pt	Au	Hg
12 15	3 8	10 12	30 40	5 6	11 11	8 12	429 982	74 37	179 345
0 0	0 0	0 0	3 0	13 0	12 0	23 6	52 23	33 1	10 6

							3A	4A	5A	6A
							B 3			
							Al 40 32 / 8 0			
							Ga 28 16 / 14 6	Ge 94 60 / 10 0	As 217 305 / 40 1	Se 308 185 / 9 7
							In 2 12 / 0 0	**Sn 973 700 / 29 1**	Sb 83 147 / 23 1	Te 21 9 / 5 0
							Tl 43 13 / 2 0	Pb 76 192 / 32 0	Bi 41 20 / 18 5	Po 0 0 / 0 0
							Er 9 10 / 0 0	Tm 6 6 / 0 0	Yb 8 5 / 0 0	Lu 5 6 / 0 0

Lanthanides:

Ce	Pr	Nd	Pm	Sm	Eu	Gd	Tb	Dy	Ho
15 5	13 5	16 10	0 0	12 7	65 11	12 5	33 5	16 5	8 3
6 0	0 0	0 0		0 0	6 0	0 0	2 0	0 0	3 0

[a] Data as of October 1984.
[b] Number tested against P388.
[c] Number tested against L1210.
[d] Percentage activities against P388 (see discussion).
[e] Percentage activities against L1210.
[f] Lanthanides (bottom row).

Table 3

Z code no.	Substructure[a]	No. of compounds	P388			L1210			Examples	
			No. tested	No. CA[b]	% Activity	No. tested	No. CA	% Activity[c]	NSC[d]	Structure
1	All Sn	1888	973	259	29	700	1	1	329882	$H_2N-CH_2-CH_2-CH_2-S-Sn(Cl)(Me)_2$
2	4-Coordinate $R_2Sn(HT)_2$	450	228	118	54	147	1	1	8786	Bu_2SnOAc_2
3	R_2SnO_2	200	90	52	60	83	1	2	345311	$Ph_2Sn-O-SnPh_2$ with ONO_2 groups
4	Me_2SnO_2	31	21	7	33	8	0	0	348067	$Me_2Sn-O-SnMe_2$ with OCOEt groups
5	Et_2SnO_2	25	17	16	94	10	1	10	221283	$(M_3\text{ Me O CH}_2\text{-SO}_3)_2\text{Sn-Et}_2$; Active P388 & L1210
6	Pr_2SnO_2	2	0			1	0	0	221191	$Pr_2Sn(OSO_2Me)_2$
7	Bu_2SnO_2	93	35	19	59	37	0	1	146118	Ph-substituted cyclic $SnBu_2$ peroxide

Table 3 (continued)

Z code no.	Substructure[a]	No. of compounds	P388 No. tested	P388 No. CA[b]	P388 % Activity	L1210 No. tested	L1210 No. CA	L1210 % Activity[c]	NSC[d]	Examples Structure
8	Ph_2SnO_2	23	9	8	89	15	0	0	356206	$Ph_2Sn(OCOPh)_2$
9	$R_2Sn(OCO)_2$	56	26	10	40	19	0	0	306914	$\begin{array}{c} C(O)O \\ \diamond\ SnEt_2 \\ C(O)O \end{array}$
10	$(R_2Sn)_2\text{-}O$	73	3	100	1	0	0	294263		MeOCO-Sn-O-Sn-OCOMe (Et, Et, Et, Et)
11	$R_2Sn(OSO_2C)_2$	9	4	3	75	6	1	17	306907	$Et_2Sn(OSO_2Me)_2$
12	R_2SnS_2	85	42	18	46	17	0	0	202858	$Me(CH_2)_3\text{-}Sn(SCN)_2(CH_2)_3Me$
13	Me_2SnS_2	31	18	7	39	6	0	0	351601	$Me_2Sn(SP(S)Me_2)_2$
14	Bu_2SnS_2	28	13	4	41	6	0	0	202886	$Bu_2Sn(SBu)_2$
15	Ph_2SnS_2	12	4	4	100	4	0	0	351602	$Ph_2Sn(SP(S)Ph_2)_2$

#	Type								Structure
16	R$_2$SnN$_2$	28	25	11	48	4	0	292415	Me$_2$Sn(NCS)$_2$
17	R$_2$SnN$_2$ (N$_2$ are ring nitrogens)	18	15	9	61	3	0	342927	imidazole-Sn(Me)$_2$-imidazole
18	R$_2$SnX$_2$	74	38	14	39	20	0	302600	Et$_2$SnCl$_2$
19	R$_3$Sn-HT	415	171	16	14	222	0	358324	1,4-C$_6$H$_4$(SnEt$_2$Cl)(SnEt$_2$Cl)
20	R$_3$Sn-O	196	80	3	10	96	0	173032	(CH$_2$=CH)$_3$-Sn-OAc
21	R$_3$Sn-S	76	34	3	11	43	0	161513	Ph$_3$Sn-S-C(S)-N(morpholine)
22	R$_3$Sn-N	44	23	0	3	22	0	142120	4-MeC$_6$H$_4$SO$_2$NHSnEt$_3$
23	R$_3$Sn-X	78	29	10	39	43	0	202912	Et$_3$SnF
24	R$_3$Sn-X (two moieties in same molecule)	5	4	2	50	3	0	341996	1,4-C$_6$H$_4$(SnMe$_2$Cl)(SnMe$_2$Cl)
25	RSn – (HT)$_3$	38	15	3	20	11	0	294232	Ph-Sn-O-(CH$_2$)$_2$-NH-CH$_2$-CH$_2$-O (cyclic)

Table 3 (continued)

Z code no.	Substructure[a]	No. of compounds	P388			L1210			Examples	
			No. tested	No. CA[b]	% Activity	No. tested	No. CA	% Activity[c]	NSC[d]	Structure
26	$RSnO_2Cl$	6	6	3	50	0			294232	
27	$Sn(HT)_4$	142	56	1	5	72	0	1	229572	
28	N_2SnX_2	3	3	0	0	0			325297	
29	N_2SnO_2	3	3	0	0	0			346400	
30	R_4Sn	368	188	8	5	149	0	0	348111	$(H_2C=HC-CH_2)_2SnEt_2$
31	$R_2Sn(CH_2COOMe)_2$	5	5	4	80	1	0	0	323991	$Et_2Sn(CH_2COOMe)_2$

#	Description									Structure
32	Ph—SnR₃ (fusion allowed on phenyl)	89	28	3	16	58	0	1	351184	Ph-Sn(CH₂COOMe)₂ | Et | Cl
33	All 5-coordinate Sn compounds	137	73	11	19	68	0	1	162794	(Ph₂Sn complex with 8-hydroxyquinoline, Cl, O, N)
34	R₂Sn(HT)₃	18	16	10	68	4	0	0	162794	
35	All 6-coordinate Sn compounds	326	230	83	39	104	0	1	303784	
36	R₂Sn(HT)₄	172	163	79	50	26	0	0	303784	Et₂Sn(bipy)Br,I complex
37	R₂SnX₂N₂	116	113	55	49	12	0	0	292424	
38	R₂SnO₂N₂	10	10	6	80	3	0	0	292424	Me₂Sn(O-C₆H₄-CH=N-(CH₂)₂-N=CH-C₆H₄-O)

Table 3 (continued)

Z code no.	Substructure[a]	No. of compounds	P388			L1210			NSC[d]	Examples Structure
			No. tested	No. CA[b]	% Activity	No. tested	No. CA	% Activity[c]		
39	R_2SnN_4	14	14	8	58	4	0	0	326390	
40	$R_2SnN_2S_2$	5	5	2	40	0			334724	
41	R_2SnO_4	12	12	4	41	1	0		254041	

#	Structure	Name						ID
42		$R_2SnO_2S_2$	4	4	1	25	0	0	0	297324
43		Y_2SnX_4 (Y = any atom)	36	14	2	15	12	0	0	157846
44		N_2SnX_4	8	8	2	26	1	0	0	7890
45		$R_3Sn(HT)_3$	6	4	0	5	0	0	0	297500
46		$Sn(HT)_6$	132	47	3	12	76	0	1	320529

Table 3 (continued)

Z code no.	Substructure[a]	No. of compounds	P388 No. tested	P388 No. CA[b]	P388 % Activity	L1210 No. tested	L1210 No. CA	L1210 % Activity[c]	NSC[d]	Examples Structure
47	SnX_6	19	3	0	3	0			43602	$\overset{+4}{Sn}\overline{Cl}_6 \; 2\,NH_4^+$
48	$[R_2Sn]x$	6	4	2	50	1	0	0	162819	$[Ph-Sn-Ph]_x$
49	$[(R_2Sn)O]x$	27	15	6	44	8	0	9	323987	$[(PhBuSn)O]x$
50	$[(R_2Sn)S]x$	8	4	1	25	2	0	29	92620	$[(Bu_2Sn)S]x$
51	$(HT)_2Sn-R$	10	4	2	50	5	0	0	96391	$Me(CH_2)_3SnO_2H$
52	SnO_3	3	0			3	0	0	221193	$ROSnO_2R$ R = Bi–O–Sn=O
53	Sn-N-CCOO (amino acids)	23	21	7	37	3	0	0	346395	amino acid tin complex (PhCH₂, CH₂Ph substituents with NH₂/COO coordination to Sn)

54	![structure with Sn, N, O ring]	17	16	7	48	2	0	0	358913 ![Me, Me, S, Bu₂Sn-NH₂, O structure]
55	![bicyclic structure with H₂N, N, Sn, O]	4	4	4	100	1	0	0	326392 ![Bu, Bu, Sn⁺², H₂C-NH₂, N, C=O structure]
56	Sn–O-S(O)R	15	14	0	5	1	0	0	251424 Bu₂Sn(OS(O)Ph)₂
57	Sn – Sn	18	3	0	7	14	0	0	92633 n-Bu₃Sn–SnBu₃₋ₙ
58	Sn – M M = any metal other than Sn	16	8	3	38	10	0	0	294516 (Ph₃Ge – Sn(OEt)₃
59	Sn – P	1	0			1	0	0	209801 Ph₂P – SnCl₄

a HT = any atom except C or H; X = halogen.
b Confirmed actives, i.e., compound showed activity in two separate tests.
c Percentages of actives are rounded to the nearest whole number.
d The NSC identify each compound in the NCI collection, and upon request antitumor data and other information can be retrieved for each NSC number.

compounds with the nitrogens as part of a ring system (Z17) showed 61% activity against P388.

2. Triorganotin Compounds R_3Sn-HT

The class (Z19) showed 14% activity against P388 and no activity against L1210. A very advantageous electronegative substituent in this class appears to be halogen (Z23); and within that class, the subclass (Z24) having two moieties of R_3SnX in the same molecule is even better.

3. Monoorganotin Compounds RSn-$(HT)_3$

The overall activity, 20%, for this category (Z25), is derived from the activity, 50% of the subtype $RSnO_2Cl$ (Z26). No other compound of the RSn-$(HT)_3$ class showed any activity against either P388 or L1210.

4. Tetraorganotin Compounds R_4Sn

The class (Z30) in general showed poor activity, but the subclass (Z31) showed 80% activity. The active compounds possess two carboxyalkyl ligands. It has been postulated that the cleavage of a carboxyalkyl ligand to tin is enhanced by the ability of the carboxy group to stabilize the carbanion $^-CH_2COOR$ in the transition state.[11] The antileukemic activity of these compounds might be related to the ease of cleavage of such ligands.

5. Tetraheterotin Compounds Sn-$(HT)_4$

This class showed 5% activity against P388 (Z27) and, as such, represents the least active class of tetracoordinated tin compounds. Compounds with two nitrogen ligands and either two halogen (Z28) or two oxygen ligands (Z29) were devoid of any P388 activity.

B. 5-Coordinated Tin Compounds

As a class, 5-coordinated tin compounds have good P388 activity, 19% (Z33); the diorganotin type (Z34) is the only significantly active subclass (68%).

C. 6-Coordinated Tin Compounds

1. Diorganotin Compounds R_2Sn-$(HT)_4$

Most of these show good activity against P388. The best subclass (Z38) has two oxygen and two nitrogen ligands. No diorganotin compound with four halogen ligands has been tested.

2. Triorganotin Compounds R_3Sn-$(HT)_3$

Only four compounds (Z45) were tested against P388, and they are inactive.

3. Hexaheterotin Compounds Sn-$(HT)_6$

This class showed 12% activity against P388 (Z46). Compounds with two nitrogens and four halogens (Z44) showed 26% activity against P388.

D. Miscellaneous Types

1. Diorganotin Compounds R_2Sn

Of the four compounds (Z48) tested against P388, two are active.

2. Diorganotin Compounds $[(R_2Sn)HT]_x$

Compounds of type $[(R_2Sn)O]_x$ (Z49) showed 44% activity against P388 and 9% activity against L1210. (Among the eight tested, one compound showed initial activity against L1210.) Of the four compounds of type $[(R_2Sn)S]_x$ (Z50) that were tested against P388, one showed confirmed activity. Of the two compounds tested against L1210, one showed initial activity.

3. Monoorganotin Compounds RSn-(HT)$_2$

Of the four monoorgano compounds (Z51) tested against P388, two have shown confirmed activity.

4. Tin Amino Acids

Tin amino acids showed 37% activity against P388 (Z53). All four cyclic tin amino acids (Z55) are active against P388.

5. Tin Sulfinates

Of the 14 compounds that were tested against P388, only 5% are active (Z56).

6. Compounds with Tin Bonded to Tin or to a Different Metal

The three compounds with the tin bonded to another tin (Z57) were all inactive against P388. In contrast, compounds with tin bonded to different metals (Z58) showed good activity against P388.

III. CONCLUSIONS

Many organotin compounds have demonstrated anticancer activity against the murine P388 leukemia routinely used as the primary screen by the NCI. The diorganotin compounds, regardless of their overall coordination number, constitute the most frequently active subclass. In contrast, organotin compounds are generally inactive against The L1210 leukemia. Also, it should be noted that a selected group of 24 P388-active tin compounds was further tested in the five murine and three human tumor xenograft test systems of the NCI tumor panel.[22] None of them showed any activity to warrant further development.

REFERENCES

1. **Rosenberg, B.**, Clinical aspects of platinum anticancer drugs, *Met. Ions Biol. Syst.*, 11, 168, 1980.
2. **Narayanan, V. L.**, Strategy for the discovery and development of novel anticancer agents, in *Developments in Pharmacology*, Vol. 3, Reinhoudt, D. N., Connors, T. A., Pinedo, H. M., and van dePall, K. W., Eds., Martinus Nijhoff, Boston, 1983, 5.
3. **Wolpert-DeFillipps, M. K.**, Strategy for the discovery and development of novel anticancer agents, in *Cis-Platin: Current Status and New Developments*, Prestayko, A. W., Crooke, S. T. and Carter, S. K., Eds., Academic Press, New York, 1980, 183.
4. **Cleare, M. J. and Hydes, P. C.**, Antitumor properties of metal complexes, *Met. Ions Biol. Syst.*, 11, 1, 1980.
5. **Crowe, A. J., Smith, P. J., and Atassi, G.**, Investigations into the antitumor activity of organotin compounds, *Chem. Biol. Interact.*, 32, 171, 1980.
6. **Lippard, S. J., Ed.**, *Platinum, Gold and Other Chemotherapeutic Agents*, ACS Symp. Ser. 209, American Chemical Society, Washington, D.C., 1983.
7. **Cardarelli, N. F.**, Slow release pesticides utilizing organotins, *Tin Its Uses*, 93, 16, 1972.
8. **van der Kerk, G. J. M. and Luijten, J. G. A.**, Organotin compounds, preparation and antifungal properties, *J. Appl. Chem.*, 6, 56, 1956.
9. **Hof, T. and Luijten, J. G. A.**, Organotin compounds as wood preservatives, *Timber Technol.*, 67, 83, 1959.
10. **Davis, A. G. and Smith, P. J.**, Recent advances in organotin chemistry, *Adv. Inorg. Chem. Radiochem.*, 23, 41, 1980.

11. **Wardell, J. L.**, Reactions of electrophilic reagents with tin compounds containing organofunctional groups, in *Organotin Compounds: New Chemistry and Applications*, Zuckerman, J. J., Ed., ACS Adv. Chem. Ser. No. 157, American Chemical Society, Washington, D.C., 1967, 113.
12. **Barnes, J. M. and Stoner, H. B.**, Toxic properties of dialkyl and trialkyl Sn salts, *Pharmacol. Rev.*, 11, 211, 1959.
13. **Cardarelli, N. F., Ed.**, *Tin as a Vital Nutrient: Implications in Cancer Prophylaxis and Other Physiological Processes*, CRC Press, Boca Raton, 1986.
14. **Smith, P. J. and Smith, L.**, Organotin compounds and applications, *Chem. Br.*, 11, 208, 1975.
15. **Thayer, J. S.**, Organometallic compounds and living organisms, *J. Organomet. Chem.*, 76, 265, 1974.
16. **Kimmel, E. C., Fish, R. H., and Casida, J. E.**, Metabolism of organotin compounds in microsomal monooxygenase systems and in mammals, *J. Agric. Food Chem.*, 25, 1, 1977.
17. **Nasr, M., Paull, K. D., and Narayanan, V. L.**, Computer structure activity correlations, *Adv. Pharmacol. Chemother.*, 20, 123, 1984.
18. **Paull, K. D., Nasr, M., and Narayanan, V. L.**, Computer assisted structure activity correlations of benzo[de]isoquinoline-1,diones, *Arzneim. Forsch. Drug Res.*, 34(2), 1243, 1984.
19. **Sadler, P. J., Nasr, M., and Narayanan, V. L.**, The design of metal complexes as anticancer drugs, *Dev. Oncol.*, 17, 290, 1984.
20. *In Vivo Cancer Models*, NIH Publ. No. 84-2635, Developmental Therapeutic Program, Division of Cancer Treatment, National Cancer Institute, 1984.
21. **Paull, K. D., Hodes, L., and Simon, R. M.**, Efficiency of antitumor screening relative to activity criteria, *J. Natl. Cancer Inst.*, 76, 1137, 1986.
22. **Venditti, J. M., Wesley, R. A., and Plowman, J.**, Current NCI preclinical antitumor screening in vivo, *Adv. Pharmacol. Chemother.*, 20, 1, 1984.

INDEX

A

A11 chain, 114
αβ dimers, 115
Acac-carbonyl carbons, 75
Acac ligands, 76
Acac-methyl carbons, 75—76
Accessory cells, 147, 148
Acetyl CoA, 120, 122
ACTH, 157
Activator T cells, 147
Acyrthosiphon pisum, 195
Adenocarcinoma, 3, 54—57
Adenosine derivatives, 44—45
Adrenal-thymus interactions, 157
Adrenocorticosteroid levels, 149
Aged, diseases of, 30
Age-related thymus involution, 149
Agglutinin, peanut, 142
Agrobacterium tumefaciens, 172—173, 175
Agrotis ipsilon, 190
A helix, 111, 114
Alanine, 114
ALA synthase, 126, 130
Alcohol conversion, 60—64
Aldopyranose sugars, 62
Algae, tin in, 9
Algicides, 69—70, 182
Alkoxide derivatives
  dialkyltin, 64—67
  trialkyltin, 60—64
Alkoxide method, 47
Alkylating agents, 182
Alkyltin compounds, 6, 71, 81
Alkyltin-soil systems, 7
Allograft rejection, 151
Alloimmune memory responses, 138
Allosteric equilibrium, 114
Alluvial deposits, 5
Allylfentin, 188
Amethopterin, 150, 182
Amino acids, 108—112, 145, 162—165, 225
Aminopterin, 182
Analytical procedures, 8—9
Animals, , 10, 13—15, see also Mammals
Anthropogenic inputs, 7—8
Anthropomorphic input, 8
Antibodies, 148, 149
Anticancer agents, 54—57, 80—81, 212—225
Anticancer hormone, 57
Anticancer screening, 47
Antifecundity agents, 191—195
Antifeedants, 183, 202, 207—209
Antifertility agents, 183—191
Antifoulants, 7
Antifouling paints, 6, 70
Antigens
  blood-borne, 141
  differentiation of, 146
  histocompatibility, 142
  HLA, 144
  Lyt, 142
  thymocyte surface, 141—142
Antihistone antibodies, 167
Antimetabolites, 182
Antiproliferative bovine thymus substances, 54
Antiproliferative thymic steroid hormone, 3
Anti-T-cell tumor agents, 84
Antitumor-active organotins, 40, 45
  covalent targeting of, 41
  cyclodextrin inclusion compounds, 42
  1,3-dioxa-2-stannacyclo-pentanes and hexanes, 42—44
  water-soluble, 41—42
Antitumor agents, 84—85, 174—176, see also Antitumor-active organotins
  activity of, 3
  chemosterilants as, 181—182
  effects of, 87—98
  metal-based, 40
  screening agent for, 172—173
  screening of, 175—176
Apholate, 182
Arachidonate release, 96—99, 104
Ariridines, 182
Ascorbate ligand, 40
Ascorbic acid complexes, 43, see also Vitamin C
Atmosphere, 7, 9
Atomic absorption techniques, 8
ATP, 94, 95, 99
Atropine sulfate derivatives, 43—44
Autoimmune disease, 150
Autoimmunity, 146
Autophosphorylation, 120—121
Autoradiography, 118
Azadirachtin, 208
Azathioprine, 150
Azeotropic dehydration, 64
Azeotropic removal, 62

B

Bacterial tests, 72
B cells, 147, 150
Benzo(a)pyrene hydroxylase activity, 126—127, 130
Benzotriazolatotrophenyltin(IV), 174—175
Benzotriazole, 174
Benzoylation, 61
Benzoyl groups, 60
Bezssonoff-Comsa extract, 156—158
Bile pigment, 127
Biocides, 69, 182—183
Biosphere, tin in, 9—12
2,2'-Bipyridyl complexes, 40—41
Birds, tin in, 13
Bis(fentin)oxide, 187, 192

Bis (trialkyltin) carbonates, 79, 80
Bis(trimethyltin) carbonate, 77, 80
Bis-pyridyl complex, 40
Blast cells, 139
Blatella germanica, 194
Blood-thymus barrier, 141
Bracken, 10
Brain protein phosphorylation, 119—123
Breast cancer, mummified, 30
Busulfan, 182
n-Butyltin, 6, 43, 47

C

Cadmium, 151
Calcium, 98—101
Callosobruchus
   chinensis, 188
   maculatus, 203
Cancers, 29—31, see also Carcinoma(s); Sarcoma; Tumors
Canned foods, 10
Carbohydrates, see also Sugars
   alkoxide derivatives of, 60—67
   indirect methods of linking tin atoms to, 69—72
   synthesis of organotin derivatives of, 60—72
   thiolate derivatives of, 68—69
   tin-carbon bond-containing compounds of, 67—68
Carbonates, oceanic, 5
Carboxyalkyl ligand, cleavage of, 224
Carboxy group, 224
Carboxypeptidases, 113
Carcinomas, 29—30, see also Cancer
Cassiterite, 5, 6, 9—10
Catechol violet method, 8
Cell proliferation suppression, 84—104
Ceratitis capitata, 186—187, 192
Chemical shift, 74
Chemoattractants, 144
Chemosterilants, insect, 180—196
Chemosterilization, 180—182, 195—196
Chemotherapeutic agents, 174, see also Antitumor agents
Chloride-hydroxide exchange, 13
Chlorinate oil stabilization, 7
Chlorophyll, 13
Chloroplasts, 13
Cholesterol, synthesis of, 54
Chromatin, 165, 167
Chromatography, 8
Cis-platin, 40
Cl-M-Cl bond angle, 40
CoA, 120
Coal-burning plants, 9
Colchicine, 181
Coleoptera, 187—188, 192
Color development, 8
Con A, 94, 96—99, 103
Continental shield sediment, 5
Copper, 151
Corticosteroid-hormone production, 149

Covalent targeting, 41
Cows, tin in, 13
CPMAS ^{13}C-nuclear magnetic resonance, 74—81
CPMAS nuclear magnetic resonance, 75—81
Creatine, 157
Cretinism, 2
Crown-ether products, 33, 34
Crown-Gall disease, 172—173
Crown-Gall tumor disc bioassay, 172—176
C-Sn-C bond angles, 78, 81
C-terminal regions, 162—163, 165
C/T × 100 index, 55
Cyclic AMP, 120, 122, 146
Cyclic anhydride, 70
Cyclic di-n-butylstannylene derivatives, 64
Cyclic GMP, 146
Cyclic organotin compounds, 42—44
Cyclodextrin organotin inclusion compounds, 42
Cyclophosphamide, 150
Cyhexatin, 195
Cysteine, thiol groups of, 108—111
Cysteine 13α, 108—111, 114
Cytochrome P-450, 126—127
   depletion of, 129—130
   depression of, 133
   organotin effects on, 128—129, 131—132
Cytotoxic drugs, 150

D

Dacus oleae, 186, 192
DAG, 96
DBDC, see D-n-butyltin dichloride
Decafentin, 186, 189, 191, 193—194
DEDC, see Diethyltin dichloride
Deficiency diseases, 2
Degradation processes, 7
Delayed hypersensitivity (DTH), 146, 151
Deoxyhemoglobin, 113
Dephosphorylation, 119
Diacylglycerolkinase, 96
Dialkyltins, 64—67, 84, 129, 133
cis-1,2-Diaminocyclohexane compound, 40
Dibasic acid monosucrose esters, 69
Dibromide, 40
Dibutylstannylene derivatives, 66
Di-butyltin complexes, 43
Dichloride, 40
Dicyclohexano crown-ether molecules, 33
Diethylboron groups, 64
Diethyltin dichloride (DEDC), 126—129, 133
Diethyltin diiodide, 40
Dimenthyltin(IV) bis(dithiocarbamates), 76
Dimeric dibutylstannyl derivatives, 65
1,2-Dimethylformamide (DMF), 66
Dimethyl organotin compounds, 41
Dimethylsulfoxide (DMSO), 54
Dimethyltin(IV) dichloride, 34
Dimethyltin compounds, 34, 47
2,2-Di-n-butyl-1,3,2-dioxastannolan, 43
Di-n-butylstannyl derivatives, 65

Di-*n*-butylstannylene derivative, 67
Di-*n*-butylstannylene-pyranosides, 44
Di-*n*-butyltin compounds, 43—45, 99, 102
  antitumor activity of, 88
  cytotoxic effects of, 88—92
  effect of, 93
Di-*n*-butyltin oxide, 43, 64, 66
cis-Diol pair, 62
Diorganotin(IV) compounds, 78, 172
Diorganotin compounds, 84, 129, 151, 174—176, 213, 224, 225
Diorganotin dichloride, 41
Diorganotin dihalides, 40, 42
1,3-Dioxa-2-stannacyclo-hexanes, 42—44
1,3-Dioxa-2-stannacyclo-pentanes, 42—44
Diparopsis castanea, 189
Diphenyldiadeninatotin(IV), 175
Diphenyltin(IV) dichloride, 174—175
cis-Diphenyltin(IV)s, 78
Diphenyltin chloride hydroxide, 40
Diphenyltin compounds, 40, 47, 78
Diphenyltin dibromide complex, 40
Diphenyltin dichloride, 40
Diptera, 183—187, 191—192
Dithiol method, 55
DMF, see 1,2-Dimethylformamide
DMSO, see Dimethylsulfoxide
DNA
  hybridization, 173
  plasmid, 172
  synthesis of, 85—87, 90
    acceleration of, 95
    inhibition of, 92, 99
    suppression of, 88—89
D-*n*-butyltin dichloride (DBDC), 126—129, 133
Dysaphis plantaginea, 194
Dysdercus
  cingulatus, 190, 194
  koenigii, 202, 207

E

Earias insulana, 189—190
ED_{50} inhibition index, 55
Effector T cells, 143, 147—148
Ehrlich-ascites tumor, 84, 87
Electrophilic attack, 60
Electrophilic substitution, 66
Emission control devices, 9
Endocrine system, 15, 138
Environmental contamination, 7—8
Epithelial cells, thymic, 139
Epoxy sugar, 67
Estradiol, 157
Ethyleneimins, 182

F

Fat tumor, 29
Fentins, 182, 183
  acetate, 182
  as antifecundity agents, 191—195
  antifertility effects of, 184—191
  chemosterilization in mammals with, 195—196
  chloride, 182
  house fly egg hatchability and, 184
  hydroxide, 182
Fertilizers, 10
Fetal life, trace metal supply in, 2
Flame spectroscopy, 8
Flies, 181, 183, 202—209, see also Diptera; *Musca domestica*
Flours, 10
Fluorine, excessive ingestion of, 29
fMet-Leu-Phe, 99, 101
Folic acid antagonists, 182
Food plants, tin in, 10—12
Foods, tin in, 10
Forest fires, 7
Fossil fuels, 9
Fraction V thymosins, 145
Fresh water inorganic tin, 6
Freundlich isotherms, 7
Fructose residues, 67
FTS, see Thymic serum factor
Fungicidal tests, 69, 70, 72

G

Galsky's bioassay technique, 172
Gas chromatography, 8
Genetic insect control, 180, see also Insect chemosterilization
Geosphere, tin in, 3—6
Germanium, 41
GH1 chain, 114
G helix, 114
Glucofuranose derivatives, 67
α-D-Glucopyranoside, 63
Glucose, 62, 67—69, 121
β-Glucuronidase release, 99
α-Glycosides, 62
Gonad-thymus interactions, 157
Graft-vs.-host (GvH) reactivity, 145—146, 151
Grand Haven Harbor, 6
Group-IV element compounds, 33
Growth factors, thymic, 147
Growth regulators, 208
GvH, see Graft-vs.-host reactivity

H

H2A:H2B complex, 161
H2A histones, 165, 167
H2A polypeptide chain, 160—161
H2B histones, 165, 167
H2B polypeptide chain, 160—161
H_4chol derivatives, 47
Halogen, 224
Halogenated hydrocarbons, 150—151
Hcholest derivatives, 47
Heavy metals, 151

HeLa cells, 84, 87
Heliothis species, 190, 194
Helper T cells, 143, 145, 147
Hematopoietic stem cells, 143
Heme, 113—114, 126—135
Heme oxygenase, 126, 127
   activity of, 127, 129, 130
   organotin effects on, 128, 131—132
   prolonged elevation of, 129
Hemeprotein synthesis, 129, 130
Hemipelagic sediment, 5
Hemiptera, 190, 194—195
Hemoglobins
   alpha chain sequences of, 109
   beta chain sequences of, 110
   binding to alpha subunit of, 112
   deoxy- and carbonyl-derivatives of, 113
   liganded, 113
   mutant, 115
   oxygen equilibria of, 112
   triethyltin binding to, 108—115
Hemolymph exudation, 204, 208
Herbicides, 70—71
Hexanes, 174
H helix, 114
Hibernation, 149
High performance liquid chromatography, 159—160
Hippocampus, protein phosphorylation in, 123
Histidine 113α, 108, 111, 114
Histiocytoma, fibrous, 29
Histocompatibility antigens, 142
Histone-HTH, 162, 167
Histone polypeptide chains, 160—161
Histones
   alignment of C-terminal segments of, 163
   amino acid sequences of, 162—165
   binding regions of, 167
   novel functions of, 160—162
   tryptic digestion of, 165
HLA antigens, 144
Hodgkin's disease, 29
Homeostasis, 2
Homeostatic thymus hormone (HTH), 156
   binding regions of, 167
   biological interactions of, 156—158
   chemical modifications of, 165
   chemical properties of, 159—167
   correlations of with binding region, 167
   endocrine function of, 157
   functional implications of, 165—167
   histone functions and, 160—162
   -histone-ubiquitin interactions, 167
   prohormone analogies of, 165
   properties of, 156
   purification and sequence determination of, 159—160
   sequence comparison with other thymic hormones and related proteins, 162—165
   substitute therapy with, 156
   thymus-thyroid interactions and, 157
HPLC, see High performance liquid chromatography

HTH, see Homeostatic thymus hormone
Human body, tin in, 15—18
Humus, 9
Hydrate formation, 33
Hydrogen, hydroxylic, 64
Hydrogen bonding, 33—36
Hydrolysis, 43
Hydrolytic cleavage, 7
Hydrosphere, tin in, 6—7
Hydroxyl groups, 60, 61
Hydroxylic sites, 61
cis-Hydroxyls, 62
Hydroxyls, 62—64, 66

I

IHP, see Inositol hexaphosphate
I-J gene locus, 148
IMC-carcinoma, 84, 87
Imidazole groups, 108, 111
Immune network, 149
Immune response, 149, 151, 157, 158
Immune system, 147—149, 152
Immunity, cell-mediated, 148
Immunocompetence, 142—143, 150—151
Immunocompetent cells, 143—144, 149
Immunodeficiency diseases, 143, 145—146
Immunoglobulin-fold domain structure, 167
Immunosuppressive drugs, 150
Inhibition indices, 55—56
Inorganic tin, 6—7, 12, 18—19
Inositol hexaphosphate (IHP), 113, 114
Insect chemosterilants, 180—186
   antitumor activity of, 181—182
   classes of, 182
   organotins as, 182—186
Insect chemosterilization, 180—182, see also Insect chemosterilants
Insecticides, 7
Insects, 180, 195, 202—209
Interleukin 2, 147
Iron production emissions, 7
Isotopes, stable, 8—9

J

$|J|$/angle correlation, 80—81
J couplings, 79
Juvenile hormone (JH), 202, 207, 208
$|J|$ values, 78—79, 81

K

KB epidermoid tumors, 3, 54, 55, 57
α-Keto acid oxidation, 84

L

L1210 lymphocytic leukemia, 212—214
Lakes, 6, 9
Lake trout, 13

Laminaria digitata, 9
Land plants, tin in, 9—10
Larvicides, 205—209
Lead compounds, 41
Lectins, T-cell, 145
Leiomyoma, calcified, 29
Lepidoptera, 188—190, 192—194, 202, 204, 207, 208
Leptinotarsa decemlineata, 187, 192
Leucine, 114
Leukemias, 142, 152
Ligands, 40, 76
Lipoma, 29
Lipomodulin, 99, 101
Liquid chromatography, high-performance, 159—160
Lost River tin district, 10
Lung cancer, mummified, 30
Ly1+, 143
Ly23+, 143
Ly123+, 143
Lymphatic system, tin in, 18, 54
Lymphocytes, 138—141, 147—149
Lymphocyte transformation
  biochemical events in, 92—98
  induction of, 99
Lymphocytosis, 144
Lymphoid cells, 138, 139
Lymphokine release, 148
Lys-Arg-Lys-Arg region, 165
Lys-Arg region, 165
Lyt, 142, 143, 146—148

M

Macrosiphum euphorbiae, 195
Magic-angle spinning cross-polarized solid state nuclear magnetic resonance, see CPMAS nuclear magnetic resonance
Malignant cells, organotin effects on, 87—88
Mammals, 13, 195—196
Mannose derivatives, 62, 63, 66
Marine animals, 13—15
Marine biomaterials, 9
Marine harbors, 6
Marine paint antifoulants, 7
Marine phosphates, 5
Marine plants, tin in, 9
Marine sources, 6—7
Meat products, tin in, 13
Melanoma, metastatic malignant, 29
Membrane-related biochemical changes, 84
Mercury, 151
Me-Sn-Me bond angles, 74—76, 78—79
Metal compounds, see also Organotins; specific compounds
  active against lymphocytic leukemias, 213—214
  immunocompetence and, 151
  structures of, 215—223
Metallic tin production emissions, 7
Metalocene dichlorides, 40

Metals, 2, 4, 18—19, 151, see also Metal compounds; specific metals
Meteoritic tin, 4
Metepa, 182
Methemoglobin complex, 114
Met-hemoglobins, 113
Methiotepa, 182
Methyl 4,6-di-*O*-benzylidine-α-D-glucopyranoside, 65
Methylmercury, 151
Methylstannonic acid polymers, 77
Methyltin, 6
Methyltin(IV) compounds
  amorphous polymers, 77—80
  noncrystalline, 76
  solids, NMR of, 75
  structure of, 77, 79—81
  studies of, 74
Methyl tretamine, 182
MHC, 143, 144, 148
Microbiol degradation, 7
Migration inhibition factor (MIF), 145
Milk, tin in, 15, 17
Mineral waters, tin in, 7
Miticides, 7
Mitochondria, 118—120, 127, 130—133
Mitogens, 84, 95, 151
Mitotic poisons, 181
MLC reactivity, 146
Mobile-belt shelf sediment, 5
Molecular structure, 74—81
Molluscicides, 182
Monoclonal antibodies, 144
Monooxygenase system, 130
Monorganotin compounds, 224, 225
Monosaccharide derivatives, 44
Mosquito larvae, 207
Mössbauer spectroscopy, 47, 49—51, 79
Mosses, 10
Mummification, tumors in, 29—30
Musca domestica, 181, 183, 185—186, 191, 202, 204
Muscle tumor, 29
Myoid cells, 139
Myositis ossificans, 29

N

NAD, 120
NADH, 120
National Cancer Institute anticancer agent screening, 212—225
Neoplasm, 29, see also Tumors
Neuroactive agents, 118
Neurotransmitters, release of, 122
Neutron activation analysis, 9
Nitrogen ligands, 224
Nitrogen mustard mechlorethamine, 181
NMR, see Nuclear magnetic resonance
Nopaline synthesis, 173
N-terminal regions, 162, 165

Nuclear magnetic resonance (NMR), 47, 74
  data from, 49—51
  in structural organotin chemistry, 74—81
Nucleophilic displacement, 67
Nucleosides, 44
Nutrient, vital, 2
Nutrition, trace metals in, 2

O

O-2, 65—66
O-3, 66
Oceanic carbonates, 5
Octastannylsucrose, 64
Octopine synthesis, 172—173
Oil burning emissions, 7
Oil-burning plants, 9
Oligosaccharides, perstannylated, 64
Organic tin, 7
Organometallics, 33—36, see also Organotins
Organotin-biomolecule complex structures, 81
Organotins, 3, 6
  active against lymphocytic leukemias, 213—214
  adulticidal activity of in insects, 204
  in algae, 9
  alterations in heme metabolism with, 126—135
  anticancer activity of
    computer analysis of, 212—225
    structural analysis of, 80—81
  antifeedant action of, 202, 207—209
  antitumor activity of, 40—45, 85
  bioactivity of on insects, 202—209
  biocidal, 69—72, 182—183
  ^{13}C-labeled, 81
  carbohydrate derivatives of
    alkoxide, 60—67
    containing tin-carbon bonds, 67—68
    indirect linking of tin and sugar atoms in, 69—72
    synthetic methods of, 60—72
    thiolate, 68—69
  chemosterilizing effects in mammals of, 195—196
  cytotoxic effects of on thymocytes, 88—92
  di substituted, 84
  effects of on predation and parasitism of insects, 195
  hydrogen bonding of in water, 33—36
  insect body protein effects of, 202, 209
  as insect chemosterilants, 180—196
  (IV) compounds, 33
  juvenile hormone activity in, 202, 207
  larvicidal activity of, 205—206
  linking of to sugars, 62
  molecular structure of, 74—81
  neurotoxicity of, 204
  oviposition-repelling effects of, 195
  plant growth and, 12—13
  solid state NMR in structural chemistry of, 74—81
  sources of, 7
  structures of, 215—223
  suppression of cell proliferation by, 84—104
  water-soluble, 41—42

Organotin steroids, 47—51
Organs, 13, 150
Orthoptera, antifecundity agents for, 194
O-Sn-O bonds, 51
O-Sn-O bridges, 51
O-Sn-O fragments, 42
O-Sn-S bonds, 43
Osteophyte, 29
Oviposition repellence, 195
Oxidation of hemes, 114
Oxygen, 111—113, 224
Oxyhemoglobin, oxidation of, 114

P

P_{50} change, 111—112
P388 lymphocytic leukemia, 3, 40, 54, 84, 87
  agents for, 212—225
  antitumor activity against, 41
  ED_{50} inhibition index for, 55
  organotins active against, 213—214
  suppression of, 57
Paleopathologic studies, 29—31
Papilloma, squamous, 29
Parasitism, 195
PDH, see Pyruvate dehydrogenase
Peanut agglutinin (PNA), 142
Peat ash, 9
Pelagic deposits, 5, 13
Peptide hormones, 145—146
Perfluoro-chemicals, 41
Perstannylation, 64
Pesticides, organotin, 12—13
$Ph_3Sn(cholest)$, 50—51
Phagolysosomes, 147
ortho-Phenanthroline complexes, 40—41
Phenylfluorene, 8
Phosphates, 5, 13
Phosphatidyl inositol (PI) turnover, 84, 96—99
Phospholipase activation system, 91, 97—98
Phospholipase C, 84, 99
Phospholipases, 99, 101
Phospholipids, 13, 84, 91—92, 94—96, 99, 102—103
Phosphoproteins, 119—121
Phosphorus uptake, inhibition of, 91
Phosphorylation, 118—123, 165
Photometric detection, 8
PI, see Phosphatidyl inositol
Pituitary-thymus interaction, 157
Plankton, 9
Plants, 9—13
Plasmids, tumor-inducing, 176
Platinum coordination compounds, 40
Plutella maculipennis, 190
PNA, see Peanut agglutinin
Polarographic methods, 8
Poly(vinylchloride) plastics, 7
Polybrominated biphenyls, 150
Polychlorinated biphenyls, 150
Polycrystalline organotin(IV)s, 75—76

Polymers, 76, 78—80
Polypeptide chains, histone, 160—161
Polyurethanes, 60
Popillia japonica, 187, 192, 193
Prethymic progenitor cells, 141
Prohormones, 165
Propane-1,3-diol, 43
1,3-Propanediol dimethanesulfonate, 182
Protein kinase, cyclic AMP-dependent, 122
Proteins
   allosteric equilibrium of, 114
   amino acid sequences of, 162—164, 166
   catabolism of, 167
   conformational and functional changes in, 112—115
   nonhistone, 145
   phosphorylation of in subcellular fraction, 118—123
   quarternary structure of, 113
Prothymocytes, 145
Psammoma bodies, 30
Pyridoxine complexes, 43
Pyrimidine antagonists, 182
Pyruvate dehydrogenage (PDH), 118—121
Pyruvate oxidation, 122

Q

Quarternary conformation, 112—114
Quercetin spectrophotometric method, 8

R

$R_2Sn(H_2chol)$ structures, 51
Radiation, 150, 158
Radiomimetic drugs, 150
Radiosterilization, 180—181
Rain water, 7
Reduction of hemes, 114
Regulatory T cells, 148—149
Reservoir waters, 6
Rhabdomyosarcoma, 29
Riboflavin derivatives, 43
Ribonucleosides, 64
River water, 6
RNA polymerase activities, 90, 92
RNA synthesis, 85—86, 89—90, 95, 100
Rock, tin content of, 4—5
R quaternary conformation, 112, 114
R-T equilibrium shifts, 113

S

Sarcomas, 29, 84, 87
SDS-PAGE, 118—119, 159, 161
Sea spray, 7
Sea water, tin in, 6
Second messenger phenomenon, 146
Sedges, 10
Sedimentary domains, 5
Sediments, tin in, 9
Selenium deficiency, 151
Serine phosphorylation/dephosphorylation, 165
Sex hormone, 149
S fraction, 54
Silicon, antitumor activity of, 41
Sitophilus oryzae, 202
Skeletal fish debris, 13
Skin tag, 29
Skin tumors, 29
^{113}Sn, 3
Sn-N bond lengths, 40
Sn-O bonds, 43
Soil tin, 3—6
Spectrochemical analysis, 4
Spectrophotometric quantization, 8
Spectroscopy, 8, 47—51, see also Mössbauer spectroscopy
Spin coupling, 74
Spodoptera
   littoralis, 188—189, 192—194
   littura, 189, 194
      antifeedant activity of organotins in, 208
      body protein in, 209
      organotin bioactivity in, 202—204, 207
Spore germination, inhibition of, 70
Stannoxide, 62
Stannylation, 61—64
Stannylene, 64, 66
Steel production emissions, 7
Sterilization methods, 180—186
Steroid hormone catabolism, 149
Steroids, organotin, 47—51, 54—57
Stream tin, 4
Stream waters, 6
Subcapsular thymic cortex, 140
Subcellular fraction, 118—123
Sucrose, 69, 70
Sucrose phthalate, 69, 71
Sugars, 62, 69—72, see also Carbohydrates; Sucrose
Sulfinates, 225
Sulfur-imidazole separations, 111
Suppressor T cells, 143, 145, 146
Surface antigens, 141—142
Synapsin, 120, 122
Synaptosome fraction, 119

T

Target cells, 146
TBTO effects, 126—135
TCA cycle, 121
T-cell precursors, 141, 144
T-cell progenitors, 141
T cells, 98
   developmental pathways of, 143
   differentiation of, 140, 143—144
      immunocompetence of thymocyte subclasses in, 142—143
      thymocyte origins of, 141
      thymocyte surface antigens and, 142
   effector, 147—148

maturation of, 144
production of, 143
radiation and, 150
regulatory, 148—149
thymic hormones and, 145—146
in thymus, 141
TCHH, see Tricyclohexyltin hydroxide
T conformation, 112, 114
T-derived lymphocytes, 147—149
TdT, see Terminal deoxynucleotide transferase
Tejo River, 6
Tenebrio molitor, 188
Tepa, 182
Terminal deoxynucleotide transferase (TdT), 142, 145
Testosterone, 157
Tetraheterotin compounds, 224
Tetranychid mites, 190—191
Tetranychus urticae, 190
Tetraorganotin compounds, 224
Thermostabilizers, 7
THF, see Thymic humoral factor
Thiolate derivatives, 68—69
Thiol groups, 108—111
Thiotepa, 182
Thy-1, 142
Thylakoid membrane, 13
Thymectomy, 3, 149, 156
Thymic growth factors, 147
Thymic hormones, 141, 143—147, see also Homeostatic thymus hormone (HTH)
Thymic humoral factor (THF), 145—146
Thymic leukemia, 142
Thymic lymphopoiesis, 140
Thymic lymphosaracoma cells, 87—88
Thymic serum factor (FTS), 146
Thymocytes, 85, 86, 94, 139
  cortison-resistant, 98
  mature, 143
  mitogen-stimulated, 94—95, 99
  nonstimulated, 97—99
  organotin cytotoxic effects on, 88—92
  short-lived, 141
  stimulation of, 96
  subclasses, immunocompetence of, 143
  surface antigens of, 142
  as T cell precursors, 141
Thymopoietin, 145, 146, 165, 167
Thymosins, 145, 165
Thymulin, 145—146
Thymus-adrenal interaction, 157
Thymus capsule, 139
Thymus gland, 2—3, see also Thymic hormones
  anatomy of, 139—141
  anticancer hormone of, 57
  atrophy of, 84
  central cell types of, 139
  cortex of, 139—140
  in embryogenesis, 144
  function of, 138
  involution of, 149—150

medulla of, 140—141
microenvironment of, 143—144
phylogeny of, 138
profound atrophy of, 151
radiation and, 150, 158
size of, 139, 149
T-cell differentiation and, 141—143
T-derived lymphocyte function and, 147—149
tin in, 2—3, 15, 151, 152
toxic chemical effects on, 150—151
vascular and lymphatic connections in, 141
xenobiotic tin accumulation in, 54
Thymus- interactions, 157
Thyroid-thymus interactions, 157
Thyroxine, 157
TI (tumor-inducing) principle, 172—173
Tin, see also Tin compounds; Tin steroids
  alloys, 7
  amino acids, 225
  in animal tissue, 13—15
  antitumor activity of, 3, 41
  artifacts, 3
  atmospheric, 7
  in biosphere, 9—11
  circulation of in lymphatic system, 54
  deprivation of, 3
  dietary deficiency of, 2
  environmental, 2, 7—9, 15, 18—19
  in geosphere, 3—6
  in human body, 15—18
  in hydrosphere, 6—7
  immunocompetence and, 151
  immunosuppressive effects of, 152
  inorganic, 6—7, 12—13, 18—19
  mining of, 3—6, 10
  ores, 4—5
  organic, 7, 126—135
  for plant growth, 12—13
  sources of, 4—5
  in thymus, 2—3, 15, 151, 152
  as vital nutrient, 2—3
Tin (II) chloride, 13
Tin(IV) crown-ether materials, 33
Tin-119m Mössbauer spectrum, 108
Tin and Malignant Cell Growth, First International Conference on, 47
Tin-bonded compounds, 225
Tin cans, 3
Tin-carbon bonds, 67—68
Tin-chloride atom bridging, 33
Tin-cholesterol derivatives, 54
Tin-cholesterol linkage, 57
Tin compounds
  4-coordinated structure, 213—224
  5-coordinated structure, 224
  6-coordinated structure, 224
  biochemical, 19
  types of, 213—225
Tin-DNA complex, 40
Tin oxide, 13
Tin-protein complexes, 12

Tin salts, 12
Tin steroids, 3, 54—57
Tin sulfinates, 225
Tin-thymus-anticancer axis, 3
Tin-thymus linkage, 2—3
TL antigens, 146
p-Toluenesulfonyl, 67
Tosyloxy group, 67
TPTA, see Triphenyltin acetate
T quaternary form, 112, 114
Trace metals, 2, 4, 10, 18—19
Trehalose, 70
Tretamine, 182
Trialkyltin/hemoglobin complex, 108
Trialkyltins, 60—64, 129, 185, see also Triethyltin; Trimethyltin
Tribolium confusum, 188
Tricyclohexyltin hydroxide (TCHH), 126—133
Tricyclohexyltins, 126—133, 182
Triethylenemelamine, 182
Triethyltin
  binding of, 115
    donor amino acid residues in, 108—111
    effects of, 111—114
    nature of, 108
    sites of, 108—111
  effect of on hemoglobin, 112
Triethyltin bromide, 118—123
Trimethyltin, 79, 108
Trimethyltin cholate, 202—203
Tri-*n*-butylstannylation, 64
Tri-*n*-butyltin acetate, 191
Tri-*n*-butyltin acetylacetonate, 64
Tri-*n*-butyltin compounds, 68, 70
Tri-*n*-butyltin deoxycholate, 202—203
Tri-*n*-butyltin hydride, 68
Tri-*n*-butyltin sucrose phthalate, 71
Tri-*n*-propyltin, 191
Triorganotin (IV) derivatives, 33
Triorganotins, 47, 151, 224
6,1´,6´-Tri-*O*-tritylsucrose derivatives, 67
Triphenylbenzotriazolatotin(IV), 175
Triphenyl compounds, 47
Triphenylstannyl derivatives, 67
Triphenylstannyl moiety, 67
Triphenyltin(IV) chloride, 174
Triphenyltin acetate (TPTA), 3, 126—129
Triphenyltin cholate, 47
Triphenyltins, 68, 182

Tripropyltin chloride, 13
Trypetid flies, 186
Tumors
  in antiquity, 29—31
  benign, 29
  Crown-Gall, 172—176
  definition of, 29
  growth of, 54
  induction of, 172—173
  inhibition of, 175—176
  in mummified tissues, 29
  occupational, 29
  thymus gland and, 152
  tin steroids and, 54—57
Tumor xenograft test systems, 225

U

Ubiquitin, 145, 165, 167
Urethane elastomers, 7
Uridine derivatives, 44—45

V

Vicinal diol units, 62, 64
Vital nutrients, 2, 5, 10
Vital trace metals, 10, see also Trace metals
Vitamin C, 40, 43
Volcanic emissions, 7

W

Waste incineration, 7
Water, 6, 33—36, 62, 64
Wet-chemical methods, 4, 8
Wood-burning emissions, 7

X

Xenobiotic tin, 54
Xenogeneic T-cell antigens, 146
X-ray crystal structure determinations, 65—66
X-ray fluorescent techniques, 8

Z

Zig-zag units, 34, 35
Zinc, 151